So you want to be a doctor?

The ultimate guide to getting into medical school

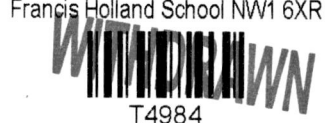

So you want to be a doctor?

The ultimate guide to getting into medical school

Second edition

Harveer Dev
David Metcalfe
Stephan Sanders

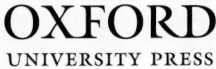
OXFORD
UNIVERSITY PRESS

OXFORD

UNIVERSITY PRESS

Great Clarendon Street, Oxford, OX2 6DP,
United Kingdom

Oxford University Press is a department of the University of Oxford.
It furthers the University's objective of excellence in research, scholarship,
and education by publishing worldwide. Oxford is a registered trade mark of
Oxford University Press in the UK and in certain other countries

First Edition published in 2011
Second Edition published in 2014

Impression: 2

Published in the United States of America by Oxford University Press
198 Madison Avenue, New York, NY 10016, United States of America

British Library Cataloguing in Publication Data

Data available

Library of Congress Control Number: 2013943040

ISBN 978–0–19–968686–5

Printed in Great Britain by
Ashford Colour Press Ltd, Gosport, Hampshire

Dedication

To Sarinder, for her unwavering support and encouragement (HD)

To Mina, my beautiful wife (DM)

To Imogen and Xanthe, for making life marvellous (SS)

Foreword

There has never been a more exciting time to be a doctor. Advances in medical science are allowing doctors to understand human biology, diagnose disease and ultimately treat patients in ways that would have been unimaginable a few years ago.

There are many reasons why medicine continues to attract the most talented university applicants. The profession offers the respect and trust of the public, a team-based work environment, intellectually challenging cases and great job security. However, the best reward remains using your abilities to alleviate the suffering of those in the greatest need and witnessing the results.

Winning a place at medical school is the first step to joining this fascinating profession. The selection process is long, complicated and intensely competitive, so that only the most capable become doctors and care for patients.

Earning *your* place at medical school requires a lot more than just passing exams; at each stage you need to prove that you have the qualities and aptitude required to be a good doctor. This book will take you through the application process and show you how to reach your full potential every step of the way. It will show you how to choose the medical schools that suit your personality and send them a clear message that you are the right applicant for their course.

If you work hard and use this book as a guide, you could be strolling the wards wearing your new stethoscope before you know it! Best of luck!

Professor the Lord Darzi of Denham KBE
Hon FREng, FMedSci, FRCS

Preface

Who has the potential to be an excellent doctor?

Medical schools across the UK wrestle with this question as they confront the thousands of applicants every year. A student's life, skills and personality are reduced to a handful of grades and a single page of writing that will determine their fate. When sorting through these applications, medical schools use fixed criteria to discern 'strong' from 'weak' applications. While this ensures the process is 'fair', these criteria can miss excellent applicants who simply don't know how the system works.

In writing this book, we hope to level the playing field. Regardless of your background or familiarity with the medical profession, this book will help you put together the best possible application.

This book represents the distilled wisdom of over 100 medical students, admissions specialists and faculty members covering every medical school in the UK. It will guide you through every stage of the application process from getting work experience to writing your UCAS form and coping with the first term at medical school. It will also help you choose the medical schools that best suit your personality, meaning you have the best possible chance of being accepted.

Getting into medical school is difficult; we hope this guide helps you show that you have the potential to be an excellent doctor.

Good luck!

Harveer Dev (Cambridge Medical School)
David Metcalfe (Warwick Medical School)
Stephan Sanders (Nottingham Medical School)

Acknowledgements

It would not have been possible to produce this book without the help of many kind individuals and institutions who gave their time and energy for our benefit. In particular:

All the contributors (listed on page ix by medical school) for their informative and insightful descriptions of life at each medical school.

The members of medical school faculty and admissions teams (named on each medical school profile, p. 107) that submitted the text for the Insider's Views.

The members of admissions teams that have collected the data on admissions statistics that we have quoted on each of the medical school profiles.

The superb information provided by the GMC, UKCAT, and BMAT, which made researching this book substantially easier.

Professor Ara Darzi for contributing the foreword.

Kaplan Test Prep and Admissions (*www.kaptest.co.uk*) for the material they contributed for the exams chapter (p. 69) and sample questions (p. 304).

All the contributors of the first edition of *So you want to be a doctor?*

Imogen Hart, Mina Aletrari, and Sarinder Dev for their constant support, exceptional proof-reading skills, and wonderful company.

Our excellent editorial team at Oxford University Press, in particular Geraldine Jeffers, Fiona Richardson, Hannah Lloyd, Abigail Stanley, and Claire Steele. Thank you for your continued support throughout.

Contributors

England

Birmingham
Joseph Higginbotham-Jones

Brighton and Sussex
Tamara Mulenga

Bristol
Rebecca Dwyer
Kayleigh Else

Cambridge
Stephanie Smith
Elizabeth Wheater

Dundee
Craig Maclean

Durham
Joe Selwyn-Gotha

East Anglia
Caroline Anderson

Exeter
The authors

Hull York
Chloe Gelder

Keele
Daisy Clark

Lancaster
Hannah Barlow

Leeds
Jonathan Batty

Leicester
Stefan George

Liverpool
YinYee Susan Ho
Michelle Cheung

London—Barts
Bhavna Gilani
Sanjay Shroff

London—GKT
Vishal Kumar
Thomas Pepper

London—Imperial College
Alexandra Ho
Matthew Murden

London—St George's
Bernard Ho
John Boardman

London—UCL
Alex Nesbitt

Manchester
Rohan Shotton

Newcastle
Matthew Gibson
Josh Patch

Nottingham
Saad Fyyaz
Rebecca Bennett

Oxford
Elizabeth Mumford
Jonathan Dickerson

Plymouth
Emily Adams

Sheffield
Will Sapwell

Southampton
Rachel Colville
Roxana Lachowicz

Warwick
Matthew Bowden

Northern Ireland

Queen's, Belfast
Alan David McCrorie

Scotland

Aberdeen
Mark McInerney

Dundee
Craig Maclean

Edinburgh
John Ferns

Glasgow
Rebekah Wilson

St Andrews
Joanna Aithie

Wales

Cardiff
Maimoona Ali

Swansea
Leifa Jennings

Overseas

Charles, Prague
Nabeel Siddiqui

Contents

Becoming a doctor

There are few careers that offer as vast an array of human experience as that of a doctor. It includes the privilege of being present at the birth of a child, relieving pain, taking actions that save the lives of others, and comforting patients and families in times of distress. It is a noble and exciting profession that attracts the most intelligent and caring individuals of each generation.

Getting into medical school

This book is written to help you face the biggest hurdle on the route to becoming a doctor: getting into medical school. Drawing on the experience of over 100 medical students and doctors, it will guide you through every stage of the process, helping you make the best possible decisions for the perfect application.

Medical school applications are amongst the most competitive of any at university. Having top grades is essential but this is not enough. Medical schools are looking for well-rounded individuals who will make good doctors and who know what the job entails. To ensure that you are the right type of person they expect to see a range of extracurricular activities (p. 41), medical work experience (p. 49) and high marks on your admission tests (p. 69).

Timeline

A successful application to medical school requires almost three years of planning from deciding which A-levels or Highers to study to starting medical school, (see Figure 0.1). The busiest time is year 12 (England, Wales, and Northern Ireland) or S6 (Scotland), during which you must obtain suitable work experience and engage in extracurricular activities, choose

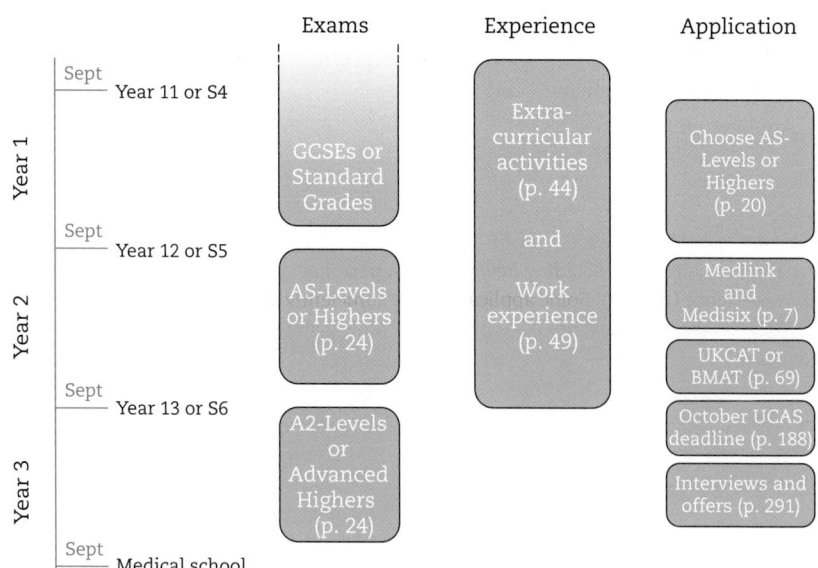

Figure 0.1 Timeline for applying to medical school

which universities to apply to, sit admission tests, and complete the UCAS application whilst studying full-time.

The stages of getting into medical school

To help plan your application the process has been broken down into five stages:

Figure 0.2 The application process

Deciding

The first step on the road to being a doctor is deciding that you want to be one. Chapter 1 discusses some vital factors including what being a doctor is like and how much medical school will cost (p. 15). It is also important to consider which A-levels or Scottish Highers to take, as this influences which medical schools you can apply to (p. 20). Finally you must decide if you want to apply for deferred entry and take a gap year (p. 31).

Preparing

Once you have chosen to apply to medical school you need to start gathering experience for your application. Extracurricular activities such as volunteer work, sport, and music are an essential part of this process and Chapter 4 describes how to make the most of these opportunities (p. 41). Many students find getting the necessary medical work experience to be one of the hardest parts of the application process. Chapter 5 discusses how to arrange this experience and what to expect (p. 49). The final step of preparation is taking the necessary medical school application exams (e.g. UKCAT, BMAT, and GAMSAT), which are discussed in Chapter 6 (p. 69), including which are necessary for each medical school.

Choosing a medical school

Chapter 7 covers how to decide which medical schools to apply to, with an overview describing the different types of medical school (p. 85). This chapter is followed by a detailed description of every UK medical course written by medical students currently studying there (p. 107). There is also a separate description of each graduate entry medical school (p. 229).

Applications and interviews

Once you know where you want to apply, you can start the UCAS form. This process is described in Chapter 9, including how to write a personal statement that makes the most of your experience (p. 192). Some applications are sufficiently different that they are described separately. These are applying to Oxbridge (p. 203), applying as a graduate to standard courses and graduate entry courses (p. 229), and non-traditional routes including access and foundation courses (p. 255). Finally interview technique is discussed in Chapter 14 (p. 263).

Outcome

Hopefully after all this work you will gain a medical school offer and achieve the necessary grades. If not, Chapter 15 describes what options are available to you (p. 281). If you are successful then Chapter 16 outlines what to expect when starting medical school and how to make the most of the experience (p. 289).

Making the decision

Chapter 1
Making the decision

Do you want to be a doctor?

Applying to medical school is like asking someone to marry you. This might seem like an exaggeration; however, over your life you will spend more hours working than you will spend awake with your life partner. Like marriage, being a doctor will change who you are, influence where you live, and affect what you can do with your life. For the right person this can be a wonderful, life-affirming experience. Otherwise, divorce from a medical career can be messy, painful, and upsetting.

Would you make a good doctor?

Medicine includes a huge number of specialities (p. 13), which attract many different personalities. A few qualities are common to all good doctors:

- **Academic ability** While you don't need to be a rocket scientist, you need to be clever to get into medical school and learn medicine.
- **Communication skills** These are the core of medicine; without them you will be unable to diagnose or reassure patients.
- **Caring** This is essential; it is what keeps doctors going when they are busy, tired, hungry, and stressed.
- **Common sense** A lot of medicine involves discerning the key facts and making sensible, rational decisions based on them.

A student's experience ...

I had wanted to be a doctor from an early age and, the older I got, the more determined I became. After the competitive application process I was delighted to get in and the first two years were everything I had dreamed of: fascinating science lectures, great friends, and a stellar social life. However, as the clinical phase began the magic seemed to fade. I found the work unrewarding and disliked the imprecision and unanswered questions of medical life. I stuck at it (I don't do failure well) and graduated with good marks to start the Foundation Programme, which only intensified my dissatisfaction.

Two years later, aged 25, I took the decision to leave clinical medicine and spent a year travelling with the money I'd saved. On my return I was surprised by the number of interesting job options available to 'ex-doctors' and settled on a pharmaceutical company. While I don't regret doing medicine I wish I'd thought about it more at the time. I guess I got lost in the challenge of applying to medical school without thinking about what being a doctor was really like.

Why do you want to be a doctor?

This is a question that will keep coming up throughout the application process, particularly when writing the Universities and Colleges Admissions Service (UCAS) personal statement (p. 192) and at interviews (p. 263). It is important to have thought about the answer very carefully if you want to really convince the reader or interviewer (p. 4, p. 214, and p. 296).

There is one other person you need to convince: yourself. It is vital that you are honest with yourself about your true motives; not just the positive and noble ones that you'll tell other people, but the less honourable and selfish ones too. There is nothing wrong with liking the fact that doctors are quite well paid or being excited about being called 'Dr'.

By admitting these reasons to yourself, you can then decide whether medicine is the best way of fulfilling your ambitions or whether it does not fit your aspirations as well as an alternative career might.

I want to help people...

This is a phrase that many applicants volunteer when asked why they want to be doctors. However, if this is the *only* reason you have for wanting to be a doctor, then medicine may not be the best career. This might seem surprising, since the entire point of doctors is to help people, but consider:

- If your only desire is to help people there are better ways of achieving this goal. Bringing clean water to people in developing countries will save far more lives than being a doctor. Even in the UK the biggest life-saving effects have been policy changes (e.g. seat-belts, sanitation, and widespread vaccination).
- Doctors try to help people in the long term, which often leads to short-term suffering, including medication side effects, painful needles, telling them not to do the things they enjoy (e.g. smoking, drinking), or giving bad news.

While all doctors should want to help people there need to be other motives that keep them going when patients don't get better or the job is difficult.

The importance of being selfish

It is your life. What will make you happy? There is no point becoming a doctor to please parents, impress friends, or satisfy teachers' expectations. Lots of people apply to medical school, so patients will have doctors even if you do not apply. The only sensible reason to become a doctor is because in your heart (and mind) you know that medicine is the career most likely to provide a happy and fulfilling life.

A student's experience...

I was unsure if I was the right sort of person to train as a doctor so my parents suggested that I try work experience at a local hospital. It was difficult to arrange and it took a lot of attempts, but eventually I managed to get three days on a respiratory ward. I was surprised by how old most of the patients were and at the amount of time the doctors spent writing and filling in forms (very different from TV!), but overall I loved it. One of the younger doctors tried to explain what was going on with each patient and how they were treating them, which was fascinating. She also told me about some of the exams and job applications that she was doing. I'd never considered that there would be more exams after medical school—it made me realize how much doctors have to learn.

I thought long and hard about whether I would enjoy being a doctor and eventually decided it looked better than any other career I had seen. I'm pleased to say that I got into medical school and am now working as a junior doctor, which, despite the anti-social hours, hard work, and responsibility, I am thoroughly enjoying.

Deciding to be a doctor

This is not a decision that comes to you in a flash of inspiration; it is one that you make carefully over several months or years, having considered alternatives and researched what a medical career entails.

How to make the decision

The more you know about the lifestyle of being a doctor, the more likely you are to make the right decision about going to medical school. To help learn about this:

- Consider going on a medical school preparatory course.
- Read 'Being a doctor' on p. 10, which includes a description of the average day for doctors at different stages in their careers.
- Do work experience (p. 49) with as many doctors in as many settings as possible. If you do not find your work experience fascinating this is a bad sign.
- Talk to anyone with healthcare experience about what it is like to be a doctor.

Medicine on TV

The practice of medicine includes emergencies, ethical dilemmas, life and death decisions, bodily fluids, and rare diseases—a great recipe for dramatic TV. While many TV shows work hard to create realistic scenarios, the vast majority do not reflect the day-to-day life of a doctor very well. Many aspects of a real doctor's job are far less exciting: partially conscious patients unable to communicate; ordering investigations over the phone; taking blood from people with poor veins; and writing a summary of your examination in the notes. While the rare moments of drama can be exciting you need to be sure that the day-to-day work will satisfy you.

Medical school preparatory courses

There are numerous preparatory courses that can help you to decide if you want to be a doctor and give you advice on getting into medical school. The majority of successful applicants attend at least one such course. There are numerous benefits:

- **Meet other applicants** The value of this cannot be overstated. It allows you to share ideas, get a feel for the quality and enthusiasm of other applicants, and make friends with others going through a similar experience.
- **Learn about medicine** Most courses have doctors sharing details of their job and lifestyle. This is extremely useful for deciding whether medicine is a career that you want to follow and also for getting a feel for how the NHS works (very useful for UCAS applications and interviews).
- **Learn about the application process** Learning from books and websites is no substitute for meeting doctors and admissions experts in the flesh.

Key points Medical school preparatory courses are not essential to getting into medical school and much of the information they impart can be gleaned elsewhere (e.g. websites or meeting doctors through work experience). They do offer a great opportunity to learn the essential facts about medical school applications and what being a doctor is like in a short time with minimal effort.

Examples of medical school preparatory courses

- Medlink (www.medlink-uk.net) This is the most widely attended medical school entry course in the UK with over 5,000 students every year. Two four-day courses take place in mid-December on the Nottingham University Campus and Medical School. Students stay in university halls of residence and attend lectures and practical sessions led by doctors from a range of different medical specialities. The course includes an exhibition day where you can meet representatives of the admissions teams from most medical schools to ask them specific questions about their medical school or university.
- Medisix (www.workshop-uk.net) This takes place around Easter and lasts between two and five days depending on the options you choose. Students stay in halls of residence at Nottingham and attend lectures at Nottingham Medical School. The group size tends to be slightly smaller than for Medlink.
- Medsim (www.workshop-uk.net/medsim) As its name suggests, this course aims to be a 'medical simulator'. Attendees get the chance to perform simulated medical procedures and diagnose simulated patients. Three courses take place in July, each lasting three days. It is much more 'hands-on' than the other courses and gives more of a flavour for clinical medicine.

Key points Many students attend medical preparatory courses. Along with having a great time students usually come away with a much clearer idea about whether they want to be a doctor or not. The courses cost £50–70 a day, which includes accommodation.

Training to be a doctor

Medical school is just the first step in training to be a doctor and getting in is just the first hurdle. Further training after medical school lasts between six and ten years depending on the speciality and includes several rounds of competitive interviews and exams (see Figure 1.1).

Foundation Programme In the last year of medical school students apply for the two-year Foundation Programme (FP) jobs. Applicants are ranked according to their medical school performance, other achievements, and score on an invigilated test of professional judgement. Students are allocated to the jobs they choose in order of the ranking. Although the vast majority of UK graduates are appointed, the recent expansion of medical school numbers and influx of doctors qualified overseas could see this change in future.

Core training and specialist training In the second year of the Foundation Programme, doctors apply for core training jobs in a speciality (e.g. surgery) and region (e.g. East Midlands) of their choice. Jobs are allocated according to each doctor's CV, application form, and performance at interview. There is a similar selection process for specialist training two or three years later. Both stages can be highly competitive depending on the speciality and region selected; applicants may need to have passed part of the professional membership exams (see p. 9).

Final career Doctors who complete their membership exams and specialist training can apply for a job as a consultant (p. 11) or general practitioner (p. 12). These can be very competitive in some regions and specialities. Doctors who do not want this level of responsibility or who have been unsuccessful in their exams or applications become Staff and Associate Specialists doing similar hospital work as consultants but without managerial responsibility and usually for a lower salary.

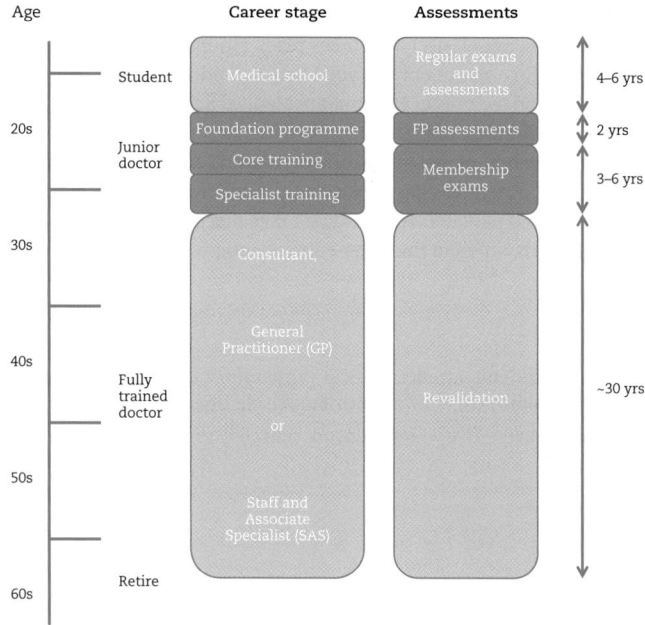

Figure 1.1 Career and assessment timeline

> ⓘ **More information** See *So you want to be a brain surgeon?* by Oxford University Press for details on medical careers, exams, and the different types of medical specialities.

Assessments and exams

Medical school Medical school exams are challenging and stressful, but the majority of students pass. Those who fail usually get a chance to re-sit and, because there are so many exams, a lot of students re-sit at least one during their time at medical school. Failing the re-sits is more serious and a few students have to re-take the year or leave medical school (about 1–5% per year). The details of exams vary widely between medical schools, although they often follow the following pattern:

- **Pre-clinical years** Exams in multiple subjects at the end of each semester (twice a year) with some continuous assessment throughout the year.
- **Clinical years** Exams in specialities recently studied once or twice a year with some continuous assessment throughout. Finals are taken in the last years and encompass a mixture of specialities. The exams are usually multiple choice or true/false but most medical schools also include a practical exam.

Foundation Programme After medical school there is a brief break from exams. Doctors are assessed continually throughout these two years; however, these assessments are rarely failed. For some specialities doctors must take the first part of the relevant membership exam in the second year.

Core and specialist training (membership exams) The exact format and timing of exams varies between specialities, but almost all have to take membership exams during core training. Membership exams are the hardest that a doctor faces in their career. They are designed so that only the best will pass, with 30–60% of doctors passing at each stage. It is common for doctors to re-sit at least one part although each sitting entails two months of intense study alongside a full-time job. They usually follow this format:

- **Part 1 written (science)** A multiple choice exam testing medical science relevant to that speciality (e.g. anatomy, genetics, physiology) and relevant clinical knowledge.
- **Part 2 written (clinical)** A multiple choice exam based on diagnosing and managing clinical scenarios. Some specialities also have a viva section where senior doctors grill the doctor being tested.
- **Part 2 practical (clinical)** An exam testing history and examination skills on real patients.

Some specialities also have an 'exit' exam at the end of the junior doctor training. Throughout their training doctors also need to complete an annual appraisal (e.g. Record of In-Training Assessment, RITA; or Annual Review of Competency Progression, ARCP), although this is rarely an obstacle.

Consultants, GPs, and SAS Once doctors have reached their final career grade they are regularly assessed by the hospital and the re-validation process organized by the General Medical Council (GMC) every five years to ensure that they remain up-to-date. Very few doctors have problems at this stage.

Failing exams

There are two main stages in a medical career where exam performance can have very serious implications. The first is A-levels (or Highers) where missing your offer can prevent you getting into medical school (p. 19). The second is membership exams, which must be passed by certain deadlines. Before each deadline it is simply a case of re-sitting, but after the deadline, doctors may be forced out of the standard career path to work in a Staff and Associate Specialist (SAS) post.

Being a doctor

Unlike most university courses, applying to medicine is a lifelong commitment to one career. It is easy to focus on the choice of medical school (p. 85), affecting the next five years, instead of whether to become a doctor (p. 4), which defines the next 40. Many medical students are surprised to find that the job doctors do is different from their expectations. It is essential to learn as much as possible about being a doctor before you apply through work experience (p. 49) and understand the different roles that a doctor performs.

Foundation Programme

This is the most junior level for doctors and it starts at the end of medical school (it used to be called the Pre-Registration House Officer or PRHO). It is two years long and these doctors are responsible for day-to-day management of patients on the wards. This can include a lot of paperwork and organization alongside reviewing patients' progress and simple procedures. They also perform on-calls where they diagnose and treat patients with new problems.

The Foundation Programme is two years long and is usually composed of six four-month rotations in different hospital specialities or in general practice. A typical job would be:

- Year 1 Medicine (endocrine), Paediatrics, Surgery (vascular)
- Year 2 General Practice, Anaesthetics, Cardiology

A day in the life of a Foundation Year (FY1) doctor...

07:30 Quick shower and breakfast then jump on a bus to the hospital.

08:30 Prepare for ward round by writing summaries of new patients on the ward and checking for any new problems or results overnight.

09:00 Ward round led by a registrar; my job is to present each patient, make sure the results are up-to-date, write the summary of the ward round in the notes, and keep a list of jobs. We cover 14 patients on the main ward and ten 'outliers' on other wards around the hospital. I write requests for investigations (e.g. X-rays) on the way to save time.

12:15 Ward round finishes and I divide up the list of jobs with the specialist trainee; most of the jobs are taking blood, referring patients to other teams, or chasing results. Lunch is a sandwich consumed on the way between jobs. The work is often interrupted by bleeps asking me to review patients, re-write drug cards, and prescribe take-home medications.

16:03 Cardiac arrest call! Elderly patient with no pulse. A specialist trainee leads the team and asks me to take blood from a vein and artery; I manage, but sadly the patient does not survive.

17:15 Frantically write blood request forms for the phlebotomist round tomorrow morning and finish any remaining jobs that must be done today.

17:30 Start on-call for the acute ward where I clerk patients admitted from GPs or A&E. I check my management plans with seniors, but otherwise do all the work myself. I get 30 minutes for dinner, which is just long enough to eat at the canteen.

21:30 Hand over my last patient to the night doctor, head home to watch some TV (Scrubs!) then collapse into bed.

Core training and specialist training

By the end of the Foundation Programme doctors need to have an idea about what type of doctor they want to be (p. 13) because they must apply for core training in that speciality. The format and length of this phase varies between specialities, with general practice being the shortest (four years) and super-specialists being the longest (may include a research period taking the total to over ten years). Core training is often quite general (e.g. mixture of medical specialities) while specialist training is more focused (e.g. renal medicine).

As doctors become more experienced, they gain new responsibilities including leading ward rounds, seeing patients in clinic, and learning new procedures or surgery. The on-calls also involve more responsibility and the management of sicker patients.

A day in the life of a Specialist Trainee (ST3) doctor...

08:00 Drive into work hoping I'll be able to find a parking space easily.

08:30 Check in with the night registrar about new patients and problems.

09:00 Lead the ward round, checking the progress of each patient and making any changes to medications, nursing instructions, or investigations necessary; there is a consultant-led round the next day so we need to try to get all results ready.

12:00 Leave juniors to handle the ward jobs and check on two patients who have been referred to our team.

12:45 Meet consultant in clinic and discuss the ward patients and reviews over a quick lunch and coffee. Thirty-two patients in clinic that we divide between us; many of them are reviews of known patients, but the handful of new cases can take time.

17:15 Check in with junior staff on the ward and discuss latest developments, then review another patient referred from a different team.

17:30 Handed the on-call bleep; on-call entails discussing referrals from A&E and GPs, supervising the management plans of junior staff, and reviewing the most unwell patients on both the acute ward and the other hospital wards.

21:30 Hand over to the night registrar with a summary of new patients or worryingly ill patients. Drive home to finish an audit presentation.

Consultants

At the end of specialist training doctors can apply for consultant jobs. Consultants have ultimate responsibility for all the patients on their ward as well as those seen in clinic. While much of the day-to-day work is performed by junior staff, consultants regularly lead ward rounds to supervise the management of patients. This can be a weekly event or happen several times a day depending on the speciality. Much of their working time is spent in clinic or performing procedures/surgery assisted by the more experienced junior doctors.

Consultants also have a managerial role including supervising the training of their junior doctors, ensuring the smooth operation of their ward, and meeting with hospital management to plan new services and improvements. In teaching hospitals they will also be expected to teach medical students.

The on-call burden varies greatly between specialities, from offering advice from home to being called into the hospital a couple of nights a week.

General Practitioners (GPs)

Fifty per cent of doctors leave the hospital environment to work in the community. As the name suggests, they see a wide range of medical issues across the complete spectrum of patients (in terms of age, socio-economic background, etc.). Alongside the medical side of their job, GPs have to run their practice, which operates as a small business; for some this is an exciting opportunity, for others a major hassle.

The GP role generally offers more control and flexibility than medicine in the hospital environment. The training is shorter (two years of Foundation Programme and four years of specialist training) and the pay is similar. The job can be busy and stressful since the average appointment lasts less than ten minutes, which is not a lot of time to distinguish a cold from early meningitis.

Types of doctor

The role and lifestyle of a doctor varies greatly according to the speciality they choose. This page covers some of the most common jobs.

Anaesthetics/intensive care

- Patients The sickest in the hospital and those undergoing surgery.
- Work Almost entirely based in the intensive care unit or operating theatre.
- Lifestyle Work is intense, both day and night, but predictable hours.

Surgery

- Patients Variable, but average patient younger than other specialities.
- Work A mixture of ward-rounds, clinics, and time in the operating theatre.
- Lifestyle Early starts and late finishes; can be unpredictable.

Medicine

- Patients Often elderly with multiple problems; can be admitted for months.
- Work Mostly ward-rounds and clinics; some specialities do procedures (e.g. endoscopy, bronchoscopy).
- Lifestyle Usually a bit more relaxed than surgery but not always.

Paediatrics (children)

- Patients From premature babies to teenagers, though usually under five years.
- Work Mostly ward-rounds and clinics.
- Lifestyle Hours are usually better than those in medicine and surgery.

Psychiatry (mental illness)

- Patients Wide range of ages; patients often admitted for long periods.
- Work Mostly clinic-based, but some ward-based medicine.
- Lifestyle More predictable 9–5 hours than many other specialities.

Obstetrics and gynaecology (pregnancy and women)

- Patients Women! Young in obstetrics, often older in gynaecology.
- Work Mixture of ward-rounds, clinics, and time in the operating theatre or birth-unit.
- Lifestyle Childbirth is unpredictable. Busy on-calls.

Pathology (laboratory-based diagnosis)

- Patients Mostly looking at samples from patients, but some see patients in the flesh too.
- Work Laboratory-based techniques, e.g. microscopes, chemical tests.
- Lifestyle Predictable 9–5 hours and light on-calls (if any).

Radiology (imaging)

- **Patients** Complete age range of patients.
- **Work** Mixture of performing procedures and looking at images.
- **Lifestyle** Relatively predictable hours, though on-calls can be busy.

Emergency medicine (A&E)

- **Patients** Complete mixture of patients and problems.
- **Work** Ranges from twisted ankles to heart attacks.
- **Lifestyle** Predictable hours (as shift pattern), but intense and busy whilst at work.

The cost of medical school

The average medical student graduating in 2011 was £24,049 in debt (£25,120 for those qualifying in London). However, tuition fees have increased substantially since this cohort graduated and debt will be correspondingly higher for a student starting medical school now (e.g. ~£75,000). Many students are worried by these costs although it is important to understand them fully before letting them affect your decision making.

Where the money goes

The cost of medical school varies depending on type of accommodation, year of study, and location (the pages on each medical school (p. 107) give an estimate of this cost). The cost also varies widely between frugal and extravagant students. Tables 1.1 and 1.2 give an estimate of the costs of a year at medical school.

Table 1.1 Typical first year UK medical student (30-week term-time)

Costs	per week of term	per month of term	per year
Tuition fees*	£300	£1,200	£9,000
Campus accommodation	£78–£175	£312–£700	£2,340–£5,250
Living costs	£80–£140	£320–£560	£2,400–£4,200
Expenditure	**£158–£315**	**£632–£1,260**	**£4,740–£9,450**
Total (including deferred fees)	**£458–£615**	**£1,832–£2,460**	**£13,740–£18,450**

*Paid through salary after qualification

Table 1.2 Typical clinical year UK medical student (48-week term-time)

Costs	per week of term	per month of term	per year
Tuition fees*	£188	£750	£9,000
Rent	£70–£150	£280–£600	£3,360–£7,200
Living costs	£100–£180	£400–£720	£4,800–£8,640
Expenditure	**£170–£330**	**£680–£1,320**	**£8,160–£15,840**
Total (including deferred fees)	**£358–£518**	**£1,430–£2,070**	**£17,160–£24,840**

*Paid through salary after qualification

Tuition fees These are fees charged by the university towards the cost of teaching. The fees are typically ~£9,000/year for all UK students except: students from Scotland studying in Scotland (~£1,820/year); students from Wales studying anywhere (~£3,465/year); and students from Northern Ireland studying in Northern Ireland (~£3,465/year).

Accommodation Most medical students spend the first year in university accommodation then move to private accommodation from the second year. Sixteen per cent live at home

(27% in London). Mean monthly expenditure on accommodation is ~£400 (~£530 in London).

Transport About 50% of medical students have a car (only 18% in London) which is almost essential at some medical schools during the clinical years. Car ownership costs about £1,000/year, though it can result in unexpected large bills when things go wrong. Medical students report spending ~£500/year on travel to clinical placements.

Where the money comes from

There are several sources of funds to support medical students, although the system is complex, which makes it difficult to calculate what to expect. It helps to know the main organizations/schemes involved:

- **Student Loans Company** A non-profit organization that administers student loans and grants on behalf of the government.
- **NHS Bursary Scheme** Offered to students on graduate courses (GEM, p. 229) or undergraduate courses from the fifth year onwards.
- **SAAS** (Students Award Agency for Scotland) pays most of the tuition fee for Scottish students studying in Scotland. The equivalent agencies elsewhere in the UK are Student Finance England, Student Finance Wales, and Student Finance Northern Ireland.

Student Loans Company

All UK undergraduates starting university for the first time should be eligible for a student loan to cover tuition fees and contribute towards other costs. Check out the student loan calculator under 'education and learning' on the www.gov.uk website.

Loans These need to be repaid over several years once you start earning over £21,000/year and are usually claimed directly from your salary like tax and national insurance. The loan has a low rate of interest calculated from inflation, which has varied from 3.8% to 0%/year. Tuition fee loans are always set at the level charged by your institution and are paid directly to the medical school. Maintenance loans are partially means tested and paid directly to you for living expenses.

Maintenance grant These do not have to be repaid but note that entitlement to a large grant will mean receiving a smaller maintenance loan. Maintenance grants are means tested which means the amount you are allowed depends on the income of your parents, partner, or spouse. For example, if they earn <£25,000 you could be entitled to ~£3,354 but you might receive no maintenance grant if they earn >£42,611.

NHS Bursary Scheme

Final year students on undergraduate medical degrees or second, third, and fourth year students on graduate entry courses receive an NHS Bursary instead of the usual student loan. This pays the tuition fees, includes a reduced maintenance loan (administered by the Student Loans Company), and offers a non-repayable bursary (see Table 1.3). The latter is composed of £1,000 for all eligible students and an additional means-tested bursary award. It may also reimburse mileage and parking expenses incurred travelling to clinical placements. Experiment with the bursary calculator at www.nhsbsa.nhs.uk.

Table 1.3 NHS Bursary Scheme (only available in specific years, see p. 16)

Type		Rest of UK	London
*Tuition fees paid**		*Up to £9,000*	*Up to £9,000*
Maintenance loan (not income assessed)		About £3,263	About £3,450
NHS bursary (income assessed)	Pre-clinical (30 wks)	Up to £3,591	Up to £4,128
	Clinical (48 wks)	Up to £5,395	Up to £6,460
Income		**£6,854–£8,658**	**£7,578–£9,910**
Total assistance (including tuition bursary)		**£15,854–£17,658**	**£16,578–£18,910**

*Paid directly to medical school

The shortfall…

Any shortfall between income and expenditure is made up through parental contributions (66% of students), part-time jobs (25% of students), and professional trainee loans up to £25,000 (20% of students). More than a quarter of students work part-time during term and 43% work during vacations, earning an average of just over £2,000/year. Over 50% believe paid employment has a detrimental effect on their academic performance. There are also scholarships, hardship funds, and other bursaries available. See www.money4medstudents.org.

Stay up to date Undergraduate student finance will remain a controversial issue for years to come. Medical student finance is even more complicated and most applicants will need to carefully review the situation for their particular year of entry. Places to look for up-to-date information include:

- BMA Medical Student Finance Guide http://bma.org.uk/developing-your-career/studying-medicine/guide-to-medical-student-finance
- Royal Medical Benevolent Fund www.money4medstudents.org
- UK Government www.gov.uk

Succeeding at A-level

Chapter 2

Succeeding
at A-level

Choosing subjects

Medical careers are plagued by exams. School exams are just a first step that will determine whether you win a place at medical school. Most applicants sit a combination of AS and A-levels, although the International Baccalaureate and Scottish Highers are acceptable alternatives.

A-levels

The transition from GCSE to AS and A-levels is a significant one. Whilst the number of subjects you study is much reduced, your knowledge of each must be far greater. It is this trade-off, from breadth to depth, that requires students to get to grips with the core material in a way quite unlike anything they have done before. This demands time and commitment independent of classroom teaching, so it is essential that you enjoy the subjects you choose.

Which subjects? Admission requirements differ hugely between medical schools; for a full list see p. 107. Almost all require A-level chemistry and most like to see another science subject at A-level as well. Some courses require a third science, at least to AS-level. Others prefer breadth and reward candidates taking a non-science subject, such as history. As a general rule, traditional medical schools prefer a spread of science subjects (see p. 85). For many applicants this means chemistry, biology, physics, and maths. Chemistry and biology are particularly helpful to save learning these disciplines from scratch at medical school. However, the 'all sciences' option is by no means the only route to obtain a place for studying medicine.

There are two ways to choose your A-level subjects. If you have particular medical schools in mind then check their profiles (p. 107) and double-check on their websites to find their subject requirements and preferences.

Most admissions tutors will tell you to use the second method, which is simply to choose subjects you enjoy. This is not just to satisfy a cliché. Subject requirements (e.g. chemistry) aside, grades are many times more important than subject options. They are so important that you should be confident of achieving an 'A' in every subject you choose. As you probably found at GCSE, you are far more likely to score highly in subjects you enjoy.

Choosing AS and A-levels: A safe bet

If you follow this strategy you should be able to apply to almost any medical school:

- Only choose subjects in which you can realistically achieve at least an 'A'.
- Use the medical school profiles (p. 107) to check admissions requirements.
- Take chemistry and biology unless you have a particular reason not to.
- Choose two out of physics, maths, and a 'rigorous' non-science (see p. 21).
- Continue chemistry, biology, and one other to A2.

How many? Studying extra A-levels can show breadth of interest and impressive academic ability. However, this strategy requires more work and risks a lower set of grades overall. Almost all medical school offers require at least three A2-level grades; some require a minimum grade in a fourth subject at AS-level too. It is extremely uncommon for medical schools to require four A2-level grades.

Many students choose to take four subjects all the way to A2. There are potential benefits to this strategy:

- If you drop a grade in one of the subjects, one of the other ones may allow you to still make your medical school offer.
- Some of the 'academic' medical schools may be slightly more impressed by four A2 subjects than three A2 and one AS.
- If you apply after year 13, once you have received your grades, it may make your application slightly stronger.
- It provides a challenge and fulfils personal interest.

There are also risks to taking additional subjects. 'AABC' looks far worse on a UCAS form than 'AAB'. If you decide to take additional subjects, you must be prepared to drop one if your overall workload is too high and your results begin to suffer. Nothing should threaten your three core subjects. On balance it is safer to concentrate on a manageable number of A-levels instead of hedging your bets with extra subjects.

What grades? Applicants successful at interview are made an 'offer'. For most candidates this offer is conditional on meeting certain grades. In many cases applicants are offered 'AAB', perhaps with additional conditions, e.g. one 'A' must be in chemistry. A few medical schools (such as Oxbridge) usually make an offer of A*AA. Others may offer ABB, perhaps following a strong interview performance, but they are unlikely to go lower. See p. 107 for specific course requirements.

If you are applying before your final A-level results, your application is based on predicted grades. These are determined by your school and will be influenced by your performance at AS-level. Since there are so many highly qualified applicants applying to medical school, your predicted grades should be at least straight 'A's. This is not an absolute requirement (the minimum required to win an interview at some medical schools is 'ABB'), but the competition is fierce and predictions really do matter. This means working as hard as you can: firstly to convince teachers to predict good results and secondly to make the grade.

'Good' and 'bad' A-levels

Medical schools want to see evidence that you can complete at least three academically rigorous subjects in two years. Some A-levels are not considered sufficiently rigorous, in particular:

- General Studies
- Critical Thinking

There are also combinations that are 'too easy' when taken together, including:

- Combinations of maths, further maths, and statistics.
- Combinations of biology, human biology, and sports science.

Succeeding throughout the year

Unlike GCSEs, A-levels are modular. First year modules lead to an AS-level, which, combined with second year modules, becomes an A-level (also called A2-level). Together with coursework and assessments, this system means you have to stay committed throughout the year.

Formulate a plan Whatever you read in the press, achieving 'A' grades is not easy. Few people rely on talent alone to earn and achieve medical school 'AAB' offers. Instead you must treat A-levels like a military campaign—and every campaign begins with a plan. First, visit the website of the exam board (e.g. AQA, Edexcel) used for your course. Find your specific course (beware of similarly named courses; biology and human biology are not the same!) and download its syllabus. Sometimes the syllabus is called a 'course specification'. While you are there, download past papers, mark schemes, and examiners' reports as well.

The syllabus is a list of topics covered by each module. It is what examiners will have in front of them when they write your exam questions. Use this document to guide your studying. If a topic is not in the syllabus, you do not need to know about it. If it is there, you really do.

Coursework Assessed coursework can count for up to 50% of your final A-level grade. You cannot afford to be complacent for any piece of assessed work. Even if a piece of coursework is only worth 10%, a 'D' grade (50%) can significantly damage your chances of scoring an 'A' overall. In fact it would mean needing to average 84% in your exams instead of the normal 80%. To lose a medical school offer for the sake of a few extra hours on a piece of coursework would be heartbreaking.

Begin coursework as soon as it is assigned. If there is a practical component, go the extra mile to get a reliable set of results. Work hard and re-do experiments if they do not run smoothly at the first attempt. Your teacher may be assessing your practical work and, at the very least, will gather an impression of how seriously you are taking the assignment.

Write clearly and ask someone more experienced (e.g. a parent) to proofread everything you produce. Aim to write formally but do not get carried away using a thesaurus. Avoid writing in the first person (e.g. using 'I' and 'we') and use course textbooks to see the kind of style you are aiming for. Be sure to follow any instructions you are given; mark schemes rarely award credit for originality.

Very few A-level students will use academic references to support their work so, to distinguish yourself, use the internet to find research papers relevant to your assignment (e.g. www.pubmed.gov) and never reference Wikipedia as a source.

Don't be afraid to ask your teachers for help and pay careful attention to any advice they offer. They may assess and grade your completed work. If not, they at least have a clear idea of how the mark schemes work. If you finish work early, some teachers will provide comments before you hand it in. It certainly never hurts to ask politely.

Key points Do not, under any circumstances, copy from textbooks, websites, or other students. This is easily spotted. Not only will you lose marks and may score zero on the piece of work, but also medical schools are very unlikely to accept someone caught plagiarizing at school.

Making the most of your time

- **Be consistent** Throughout your A-levels you should be aiming to be at the top of your class. This includes presentations, coursework, and exams. Build an impression of an 'A' grade student and you're half way there.
- **Set achievable goals** Be ambitious but the aim is to achieve goals, not set yourself up to fail them.
- **Work hard and work effectively** Hard work is certainly rewarded but don't waste effort that could be invested elsewhere. Use the course syllabus and past exam papers to maximum effect.
- **Revision guides** Invest in revision guides early on. It's difficult to make good notes throughout the year and even the best students miss things out. A good revision guide based on the correct syllabus fills gaps in your teaching, understanding, and notes.
- **Find a study partner** This doesn't work for everyone but if working alone isn't your thing, find someone to study with. Other potential medical applicants studying similar subjects make ideal study partners.
- **Network with teachers** Always be polite and enthusiastic around teachers. Not only are they a great resource, but also they write your references, make your A-level predictions, mark your practical work, and assess your coursework. Your career aspirations will be easier to achieve with others helping you.

Preparing for exams

Exam success follows successful revision. Central to this formula are endurance and efficiency. A-level revision requires more independence and commitment than GCSEs. You will need to begin reviewing your work early on and develop an effective strategy to maximize the time you spend revising. During this time you should clarify your understanding of material covered in class and identify knowledge gaps. Your goal is to reach a point where you can answer past paper questions confidently under exam conditions.

There are no fixed rules for revision; to succeed you must be flexible. But this should not stop you from producing a timetable to organize your revision.

Planning revision Create a timetable, ideally a few months before your exams begin. The more time you have to revise the better. Include key events such as exams and non-academic obligations. Be sure to leave a week or two before the exams to review important topics and practise past papers. Distribute topics evenly, beginning with those you are least confident about. Remember to be realistic about how much you can achieve in a single day.

Revising
- Once you have a schedule, stick to it. Wake at a set time so the morning doesn't just pass you by.
- Experiment with different environments to find where you learn most effectively. You could try working in your bedroom, at the dining table, or in the library, staying in one place or changing location throughout the day.
- Remember to find somewhere away from distractions: the internet, mobile phone, and talkative friends should be saved for scheduled revision breaks.
- Work hard but be careful not to compromise your normal lifestyle. Sleeping, eating, and regular exercise are particularly important. Exercise breaks up the day, keeps the mind alert, reduces stress, and improves quality of sleep.
- Try to ensure revision isn't the last thing you do before sleeping. Reading a novel or talking to your parents will help you think about something other than revision.

A student's experience...

I spent hours 'studying' in my room and everyone seemed very impressed. It wasn't until the exams that I realized how little I knew from all the 'work' I had done. Looking back, 90% of my time was spent on the internet. Most of the other 10% was spent rearranging stationery and re-writing my revision timetable. Thirty minutes of studying a day is not enough—even if it is spread across the whole day.

Key points Don't get too carried away with one topic. The law of diminishing returns states that, beyond a certain level of success, continued effort becomes increasingly wasteful. Learn a topic adequately and then move on.

Making notes There are many different ways of revising and you will need to find the revision strategy that suits you best. The most successful methods require active engagement with your course material.

Making notes helps to reduce masses of information and makes you think as you express it in your own words. Keep re-writing your notes to condense them even further. The aim is to be left with only a few pages of prompts to review shortly before each exam. Numbered lists and coloured diagrams can also be great to stick around the house. Why shouldn't your family learn about the Kreb's cycle too? But don't forget that you need to learn, not just create a great set of revision notes. There is only one way to check you have not slipped into the trap of passively copying out words. You have to stop, put your notes away, and challenge yourself. Choose a subject at random and write down everything you know. Then go back and see how well you did. Be ruthless. This is the only way to guarantee you are learning. The exam is not the place to find out!

If you use textbooks, avoid becoming carried away with unnecessary detail. Instead, use textbooks to fill crucial knowledge gaps. Make revision notes from work in class or, even better, invest in a revision guide. This should cover what the course syllabus requires you to know in just the right amount of detail.

Memorizing notes

Three things help with memorizing information: concentration, repetition, and emotional response. Ideally revision should encourage all of these; for example, copying things out forces repetition and concentration; getting a question wrong (and to a lesser extent right) results in an emotional response. The hippocampus (your memory store) receives strong inputs from the emotion-sensing 'limbic system' of the brain. For this reason, imagining something funny/sad/surprising alongside your notes can help you to remember them.

Past papers You wouldn't take a driving test without practising in a car and you should never sit an A-level exam without making the most of any available past papers. Past papers are undoubtedly the most effective way to assess your knowledge of the subject matter. A-level exams are consistent in terms of difficulty from year to year so past papers are an opportunity to find out how you will score in the real exam. Clearly it is important to assess this while you still have revision time left!

At regular intervals in your revision, complete a past paper under exam conditions: timed, in a quiet room away from your notes. Mark it fairly afterwards. Do not award extra marks because you know what you meant: examiners are not that forgiving. Try to find the examiners' report for that particular past paper. These offer a great insight into what the examiners were looking for and what they got. When you have marked the exam, honestly appraise your strengths and weaknesses. If you scored an 'A' (usually over 80%) then keep up the hard work. If you didn't quite make the grade then assess which areas are your weakest and go back to your revision with a vengeance.

Private tuition

Most school teachers are fantastic but they will face obstacles when teaching an A-level curriculum. In particular, they have to teach large groups of students, each of whom has a different set of learning needs. Not every student needs straight 'A's across difficult subjects. This is where private tuition can help. Although it can be expensive, it may be worth it to avoid dropping a grade and missing your hard-earned medical school offers.

Do you need a tutor? In many cases the answer is 'probably not'. A bright student supported by good teachers and motivated to work hard for two years has a very good chance of achieving 'A' grades. Before hiring a tutor, think hard about whether you are actually using your school resources to maximum effect. Do you concentrate throughout every lesson? Do you look things up if you do not understand them? Do you approach a teacher if you are still stuck? If you already use everything your school has to offer, but still feel you could achieve more, private tuition is certainly an option worth considering.

What does it involve? A private tutor is usually a teacher, retired teacher, or graduate providing one-to-one lessons outside of school hours for a fee. They can be self-employed or work for an agency. Fees vary depending on your locality, the tutor's qualifications, and where the lessons take place. Most A-level tutors charge between £25 and £35 per hour, including travel expenses.

Who to choose Finding the right private tutor can be difficult. There are no league tables and, although many are highly qualified, this says little about their ability to teach. For this reason, the most reliable way to choose a tutor is by personal recommendation. If you don't know anyone who was tutored, use the internet or a local newspaper to make a list of potential tutors. There are several major online directories of tutors whom you can search for based on subject and your geographical area.

It's not unusual for a tutor to offer tuition in several different subjects but be aware of multi-specialists. At A-level, it is difficult to keep abreast of so many modules, let alone different exam boards. Medical applicants are already strong candidates and may have more challenging needs than other students. Your tutor needs to help push 'B' grades to 'A', not simply guarantee reasonable A-level grades. Avoid those who have recently finished their own A-levels. Undergraduates are unlikely to have the breadth of knowledge and teaching experience needed to keep you on track. If possible, try to find someone currently teaching your subject at A-level in a school. They will implicitly understand the level of detail you require as well as the importance of working to a course syllabus. With any luck they will be A-level examiners as well!

A student's experience...

After speaking to a few of my friends, I realized I wasn't alone in wanting a little extra help in one of my subjects. To save on costs, we decided to receive private tuition as a group. The tutor charged extra for teaching more than one student, but it still worked out a lot cheaper than one-to-one lessons. Just make sure that the other students are not included to the detriment of your own work.

Arranging your first lesson Try to speak with potential tutors by telephone before hiring them. It is likely that your parents, if they are picking up the fee, will want to speak with them as well. A telephone call is important to make sure your tutor is familiar with your subject, exam board, and particular needs. It can also provide a preliminary assessment of their suitability.

If it is not already clear, use this time to agree the lesson fee and any travel expenses. If travel expenses raise the fee, consider finding someone closer to home, or perhaps meeting your tutor elsewhere. Many tutors will agree to a free introductory meeting, which is worth taking advantage of. This allows you to get to know each other and discuss how future sessions should be organized. Give your tutor an example question or topic that you would like to go through in the first session; this way you can ascertain how much preparation they have done. Try not to agree on a fixed number of lessons at any stage. This number should depend upon how well you are progressing and the productivity of each session.

Getting the most from your tutor
- Remember these private sessions are an expensive asset: if you feel you would benefit from approaching the sessions in another way, let your tutor know as soon as possible.
- Make a list of topics you need help with. Be as specific as possible and keep a list of questions that crop up when you are studying.
- Most tutors will happily answer questions by email or telephone. But remember they may have a number of students and a full-time job as well.
- Make sure your tutor sticks to the course syllabus as far as possible. They may want to teach outside of the syllabus and, while no education is wasted, this is less likely to boost your exam performance.
- Most students opt for 60–90 minutes of tuition a week. Don't arrange lessons if there is not something in particular that you want to work through.
- To make the most of private tuition, use it sparingly. Ninety-five per cent of your work should take place before the lesson. Always prepare adequately by reading the relevant section in your revision guide and then re-reading it after the lesson.
- Never be afraid to hire a different tutor. This might be awkward but private tuition is too expensive a luxury to be wasted. Speak to whoever pays the bill if you think you could achieve more with a different tutor.

Key points Of course many students cannot afford the luxury of private tuition. This is rarely a problem. Many of the advantages brought by a private tutor can be obtained in school. Very few teachers will refuse to see a motivated student at break or lunchtime to discuss a particular learning need.

Exams

Nobody likes exams but you will meet them again and again while training to be a doctor. In fact, many doctors are still sitting exams at the age of 40 and beyond. Exams are not only a test of knowledge, they also test technique. After revising hard, avoid making simple mistakes in exam week.

The night before

Make sure you have everything ready for exams the following day. You do not want to rush around in the morning or, worse, forget something. Make sure you have an exam timetable, identification if required, appropriate stationery, and a calculator. Aim to take three good writing pens just in case.

A student's experience...

I'd stayed up late revising for a biology module. Even though I had covered most of it already, there were still some gaps and I wanted the opportunity to cover everything again. I couldn't believe my luck when I reached the last question—an essay worth 15 marks. It was the subject I had covered just before going to bed and I could still remember every word on that page of my revision guide. If I didn't get every one of those 15 points I shall be disappointed.

Staying up vs. sleeping This is a delicate balance and, to some extent, the answer depends on your body and what you are used to. As a general rule you are more likely to do well if you feel refreshed: an alert brain will read the questions more accurately, make better decisions, and allow better recall of memories.

Despite this, many students choose to slave away, 'cramming' facts until the early hours of the morning. For some students this can work surprisingly well; the stress allows them to absorb large numbers of facts into their short-term memory (technically medium-term...) and they experience only a mild reduction in alertness. For others the revision is time wasted and they risk sleeping through the exam, missing questions, or putting in an awful performance. It can be extremely difficult to be aware of the effects of tiredness on your own brain; however, if you are finding it hard to make decisions then that is a bad sign.

Critical A-level exams are not the time to experiment with new revision strategies; go with what you know works for you.

A student's experience...

A friend spent ages locked away revising in his room and seemed to think he could keep going while everyone else was sleeping. His valiant efforts came to an end about half way through one of our maths exams. I looked up to see him fast asleep on the desk. Fortunately an invigilator saw him at the same time and woke him up. But he had lost almost 30 minutes. Needless to say he stayed awake for the rest of the exam!

During the exam

- **Check the paper** Check you have the correct exam paper (mistakes do happen!) and confirm the number of questions you should answer (including the back page).
- **Time per question** Divide your time according to the weighting of each question and write down the finish time for each one.
- **Reading ahead for short answer questions** If there are multiple parts to a short answer question have a quick glance over all of the parts before you begin. This can sometimes give you a clue as to where the examiners want you to go with your answers.
- **Reading ahead for long answer questions** It is worth starting long answer/essay papers by reading all of the questions that you will have to answer first. This allows your brain to work subconsciously on the later questions whilst you're answering the earlier ones.
- **Understand the question** Be sure you understand the question before attempting an answer. This is more applicable to longer essay-based questions, but it can still be applied to the short-answer type. If necessary, define specialist terms in your question before attempting a response.
- **Anticipate the mark scheme** There are often marks for obvious statements, so write these down before showing off your detailed knowledge.
- **Keep moving** If you find yourself unable to answer a question then simply move on. If you keep a fast pace throughout the exam there will be time at the end to return to difficult questions. It is best to get full marks for answers you do know rather than waste time getting partial marks for those you don't.
- **Concise essays** Essay questions, particularly in science modules, often have set facts that must be written down to score each mark. You are not publishing a literary masterpiece so write what you know as clearly and concisely as you can without repetition.
- **Use diagrams** Science answers can often benefit from appropriate use of correctly labelled diagrams, which are faster to produce than text. You do not score double marks for repeating everything in the diagram in text as well.
- **Don't panic!** If you've revised everything the answer is in there somewhere: re-read the question and write your best answer if you are still unsure. You may find the answer is obvious when you come back to the question later on.

After the exam

Having wrangled for hours with an exam paper, it is often tempting to conduct a post-mortem. Most students discuss the exam with friends. Others use notes to answer questions they struggled with in the exam room. If you do this, bear in mind that it will create a false impression of your performance. Because memory is so influenced by emotion, you will forget questions you answered with ease and focus on those you were less sure about. For this reason you should put aside each exam once you've left it, at least until the last one is finished. Students rarely estimate their exam performance accurately and there are always surprises on results day. You won't know how you did until then!

Taking a gap year

Chapter 3

Taking a gap year

Should you take a gap year?

This might be the last time you can *ever* spend 12 months doing whatever you want. As many as 250,000 young people choose to take 12 months away from full-time work and education every year. You could seize this opportunity to backpack around the world, help a deprived community, or follow your sporting dreams. If you want to try something else before a lifetime of lectures and early morning ward rounds, this chapter will help.

There are good and bad reasons for taking a gap year. The decision could have a massive impact on your life and, like any big decision, needs to be thought through carefully. The list below provides some common reasons for taking a gap year.

- **Life experience** Medicine is a structured career and time out later on is sometimes difficult to arrange. The time between school and university is your own and a great opportunity to pursue your dreams.
- **Maturity** Most medical schools emphasize the importance of early exposure to patients. This means students have to adopt a professional image from their first weeks at medical school. Lots of applicants (and some new doctors!) feel they are not yet ready for this responsibility and would benefit from some personal development time.
- **Skills development** Maturity doesn't come from 12 months of watching daytime television—it's the result of experience. Gap years are an opportunity to develop transferable skills (e.g. professionalism, communication) and practical skills (e.g. a new language).
- **Money** Medical school is an expensive undertaking (p. 15) and some applicants take a gap year to boost their finances. An applicant living at home in a £15,000/year job could go some way to funding their tuition before approaching the Student Loans Company. However, don't forget that a year of lost earnings over your career could cost £100,000. See Table 3.1 before taking a gap year for financial reasons.
- **Work experience** A year away from education means 12 months to collect work experience. This could be long-term employment in the NHS, exotic healthcare placements abroad, or a mixture of UCAS-friendly experiences. However, don't forget that the best experience for being a doctor is a year *working* as a doctor. If clinical experience is your reason, remember that those 12 months could be spent as a doctor if you went to medical school straight away.
- **Four medical school rejections** Whether you planned to take a gap year or not, many good applicants find themselves filling time before the next round of UCAS applications. See p. 34 for how to make the most of this time.

Table 3.1 The true 'savings' of working during your gap year

Gap year spent working		Not taking a gap year	
Money earned over year	£15,000	Extra year working as a senior doctor	£100,000
		Extra year of pension contributions	£20,000
Total	**£15,000**	**Total**	**£120,000**

Why not take a gap year? Gap years are increasingly common but most students start higher education straight after school. There are reasons why you should think twice about taking a year out.

- **Time** It's all in the name: a gap year means 12 months out of education. If you include the summer after school ends, it's closer to 15 months. Some people are keen to get started on their career; this might be particularly important to mature applicants (p. 228) and anyone hoping to be a consultant (p. 11) by their early 30s.
- **Money** Gap years are an opportunity to boost or break your finances. You can earn a lot of money working (p. 62) but a whole year travelling costs between £5,000 and £8,000 even if you're frugal.
- **Lack of ideas** Many candidates never think about a gap year. It is always worth considering (if only for a few minutes), so keep reading.

How do medical schools view gap years? Medical schools are broadly in favour of gap years. Admissions tutors understand that they are an opportunity for applicants to develop skills and reflect on their decision to study medicine. However, they will expect a good idea of what you intend to *do* and *gain* from your time off. This doesn't mean that all gap years have to be spent building villages and saving orphans in remote locations. It simply means you have to think hard about your gap year plans and be clear about what you stand to gain from them.

Deferring offers to study medicine There are two routes to taking a gap year. The first is to apply at the 'normal' time, a year before finishing school, indicating your wish to defer by checking a box on the UCAS form. This will give you the peace of mind of a guaranteed medical school place if you are successful or a second opportunity to apply if you are not. The UCAS reports that between 13,000 and 30,000 higher education applicants (2–7%) choose this option every year.

Although some medical schools (e.g. Cardiff, Sheffield) explicitly welcome deferred applications from those who can justify their gap year plans, others (e.g. Warwick) are unwilling to defer offers without good reason. They may tightly match offers to places and cannot cope with successful candidates disappearing around the world each year. Others only permit a limited number of deferrals each year. If in doubt, ask your preferred institutions about their policy towards deferred applications.

Key points Twelve months invested wisely can be a huge asset to your application and career. But, like any valuable resource, time should be spent with a clear strategy for achieving a return on your 'investment'.

Applying a year later The alternative is to apply after A-levels for admission the following year so that you already know your A-level grades at the time of applying. The obvious disadvantage is that, if your application is unsuccessful, you might be forced into a second year off or into another contingency plan (p. 281). You also need to consider if being available for interviews will interfere with travel plans.

Of course there is no rule against doing both. You *could* apply the year before finishing school to see whether or not your deferred application is successful. If so, you could choose to accept or decline the offer. In the event of being rejected, you could start the gap year you were hoping for and submit a better application the following year. This means a year to improve your UCAS application and, potentially, interview experience to learn from.

Where to go

Once you've decided to take a year out the next stage is to decide where to go. Gap years in the UK are very different from those abroad and this decision is fundamental to your gap year plans.

Staying at home

There are advantages to staying in the UK, not least because you're guaranteed three meals a day, flushing toilets, and a hot shower.

- **Money** If your gap year is designed to save money, it's not best spent gallivanting around the world. Round-the-world tickets (four stops) start at £850 before factoring in accommodation, food, visa, and activity costs. Staying at home minimizes expense while permitting work in stable employment. However, if your reasons are purely financial, remember that a year out will cost (at least) £100,000 in lost earnings over the course of your career (p. 32).
- **Work experience** You can arrange healthcare work in any country (p. 35) but NHS experience is limited to the UK. For this reason, experience at home could provide a better insight into work as a NHS doctor. If you are available for a long period of time (e.g. a year), you could become an experienced healthcare assistant or phlebotomist (p. 63). But remember (as on p. 32), the best experience for *being a doctor* is being a doctor. Don't spend a year as a phlebotomist in the NHS at the expense of a year working in medicine later on.

The only 'bad' reason for staying at home is fear of new experiences. As a medical student you will be exposed to a huge range of human experience, from helping to assess an acutely psychotic patient to performing chest compressions at a cardiac arrest. If you want to be a doctor you will have to learn how to thrive outside of your comfort zone. A gap year is a good place to begin.

> **Key points** Try to get away from home for at least part of your gap year. Although you don't have to spend 12 months overseas, making the most of your time means acquiring a broad range of experience. These experiences can be in the UK or abroad; however, a decision to take a year out to stay at home will take some explaining to admissions staff.

Going abroad

Most gap year students go abroad, at least for part of their time. There are many reasons to go overseas:

- **Opportunity to travel** If you are the typical British medical school applicant, you will have lived in the UK all your life. Experience of the wider world will be limited to television, the internet, and family holidays abroad. A year out is an opportunity to experience just a few of the other 195 countries in the world. Although medical students can travel on their elective (p. 107), few manage to visit more than one country. After graduation, employment impedes travel opportunities for all but the most adventurous doctors.
- **New experiences** Although experience overseas will undoubtedly be different from the UK, it will depend on *what* (p. 36) you do.
- **Interview ammunition** New and varied experiences mean lots of things to talk about at interview. An interesting gap year will help you stand out and relate questions to your

own experiences abroad. Other candidates will be using examples (e.g. grade 8 flute and the Duke of Edinburgh Award) that the interviewers will have heard many times before. However, deferring applicants might be interviewed before their gap year begins to bear fruit.

- **Making a difference** Many communities in the developing world are resource-poor and benefit from gap year volunteers. Volunteering opportunities could include working in a hospital, building a school, teaching English, or disseminating health information to local people. Unfortunately, many small projects are without financial support and rely on volunteers to fund them in return for the opportunity to help.

Where to go abroad Every country is different but there are similarities (cultural and geographical) within regions. If you want to stay in the English-speaking developed world, where things are broadly similar to the UK, the USA, Canada, Australia, and New Zealand are all possibilities. Travelling through Europe is simple (travel is more or less unrestricted between European Union member states) and flights are cheap. Budget airlines fly from London to key European cities for ~£10, less than a train ticket between most British towns. Although flights are cheap, other expenses (e.g. food and accommodation) are less so and European travel can end up becoming expensive. A further disadvantage is that many people in continental Europe will not speak fluent English. This is of course an opportunity to resurrect your rapidly dissipating memories of GCSE French.

The developing world (much of Africa, South and Central America, and Asia) promises amazing cultural experiences. After visiting these regions, you will be telling stories of your travels (whether or not others want to hear them) for years to come. Backpacking in the developing world is cheap and money lasts a long time—especially if kept safe in a money belt. The disadvantages are largely practical (e.g. booking transport) and related to comfort. If you're willing to forgo flushing toilets for the experience of a lifetime, consider visiting these types of countries.

Other regions promise culture without a need to sacrifice home comforts. These include developed parts of Asia (e.g. Singapore, Japan) and stable countries in the Middle East (e.g. Oman, Jordan, and the United Arab Emirates). Gap year students rarely visit these destinations and you would be breaking new ground!

Should you stay or should you go? A gap year is probably your longest period of 'freedom' before retirement. With very few limitations, you can choose to do whatever or go wherever you want. For most students the ideal gap year includes working to earn money then going away to do something interesting. If you *can* afford (and choose) to spend the whole year travelling, you're unlikely to regret the experience. If you're not keen on heading out by yourself, consider taking a friend or don't travel *too* far out of your comfort zone, just a little to push your own personal boundaries.

If you don't choose a gap year If you remain unconvinced by the value of a gap year, you can still go abroad. There are three months before A-level results day and the start of medical school. This is an ideal opportunity to work, relax, travel, or try all three. Think carefully about how to make the most of this time—it might be the last study-free period you have for the next 40 years.

Key points The potential of your gap year is only limited by your imagination. You can do (or try) almost anything in 12 months. Make the most of your time and you will shine at interview as well as earning memories that will remain with you for life.

What to do

What to do is at least as important as where to go. These pages set out the benefits, disadvantages, and skills associated with popular gap year activities.

Working

There are many different ways to work during a year out, either at home or overseas. Most students work for some of their gap year. While health or social care employment is ideal, don't worry if the work you find is less immediately relevant to medicine. Some of the skills you can gain from work include:

- **Teamwork and communication** Most jobs require work with colleagues and/or customers. Some people are not instantly likeable and human interaction always requires communication skills. Your medical work experience should illustrate how important communication is within the NHS.
- **Working under pressure** Do you become stressed and ineffective when deadlines (or even food orders) are stacking up? If so, gap year work is an opportunity to learn to work under pressure.
- **Problem solving** Almost everyone is employed to solve problems and initiative will be important at every level of your medical career.

The disadvantage of finding employment is that you have a lifetime of work ahead of you. The trick is to look for a job with added value: either one you really enjoy or one that challenges you to develop new skills. By limiting the time you spend working, you can squeeze other experiences out of your gap year too.

Volunteering

There are many projects needing international volunteers. Many expect a financial contribution to support the project before you start work. You should be wary of projects that resemble commercial tourist activities. If you're travelling to Malawi to build a school, ask yourself why local people (even local builders) can't construct a school themselves. They probably could if they had the necessary resources. Your donation of £1,000 pays for bricks and mortar but, in return, you buy the 'privilege' of building the school yourself. There is nothing wrong with such projects as long as you realize how they work. Projects might include:

- **Health promotion** This could include speaking to local people or visiting schools to disseminate health information (e.g. malaria or HIV prevention).
- **Basic hospital work** Undertaking tasks similar to a healthcare assistant (p. 63) in the UK. Responsibilities could include basic patient hygiene and monitoring blood pressure, pulse, temperature, and respiratory rate. Do your research before working in countries with high prevalence of infectious diseases (e.g. HIV). You should always wear some form of protective equipment (e.g. gloves) when exposed to bodily fluids.

Key points Be very careful if volunteering abroad that you avoid working beyond your competence. Knowing your limitations is vitally important to working as a doctor. Medical school interviewers will not be impressed to hear how you were taught—then practised—limb amputations in a hospital overseas. As a general rule, if you feel uncomfortable taking on a task then you should politely decline.

As well as seeing the rewards of your labours, volunteering is a way to integrate with a community, as you are not simply there as a tourist. It can also be a good way to gain work experience (p. 49). Don't forget that most medical schools provide volunteering projects overseas during university vacations.

A student's experience...

A friend and I headed 'down under' to Australia and New Zealand. We had a great time staying in backpacker hostels and making our way slowly through Australasia. We organized work permits and were able to find temporary jobs to fund our most extravagant activities. And we gained our PADI diving qualification!

Backpacking

Backpacking is a good way to see the world without remortgaging your parents' house. It essentially means travelling with nothing more than a backpack of gear. Backpackers often use local hostels (travel guides are a good place to start, p. 38) as a base in each new location. As there are thousands of young people backpacking at any one time, you'll almost certainly meet others and end up travelling for a while together. As well as collecting stories for your new (and envious) friends at medical school, think about the kinds of skills you will gain from backpacking.

- **Surviving in a new environment** Junior doctors move jobs every few months to work in a new speciality, team, or hospital. Coping with change will be an important part of your postgraduate training.
- **Meeting new people** You cannot fail to meet new people backpacking. This will mean lots of practice establishing rapport and building relationships with those around you. It won't be long before you notice an improvement in your response to other people, even if you weren't doing badly before. Your ability to 'get along' with new people will be fundamental to your career.
- **Problem solving** You are unlikely to travel without encountering challenges. Cancelled trains, dwindling funds, crime, and disorganization are all possibilities. Meeting these challenges head on is not unlike the work of a doctor, whose role is almost always to solve problems.
- **Perspective** It might be difficult to articulate, but backpacking is great for developing perspective. You will see for yourself how priorities, attitudes, and behaviours differ around the world and this can lead to a more sophisticated, mature outlook. It has to be an improvement on life spent learning about the world from television and teachers.

How to decide

Although few students regret their gap year activities, careful planning will stop you from missing valuable opportunities. There are 15 months between finishing school and starting university; more than enough time for a combination of working at home, volunteering, and travelling overseas.

A student's experience...

I bought a 'round-the-world' ticket that included five stops. One took me to South Africa and I went to a lion-breeding programme in nearby Zimbabwe. I spent eight weeks feeding and exercising young lions and working in other areas of conservation.

How to find out more

These pages will point you towards informative and reliable sources of information to help in planning your gap year.

The internet The most obvious place to look for gap year information is online. There are many different online resources, including official websites (e.g. the Foreign and Commonwealth Office), charities, commercial gap year organizations, forums, and travellers' blogs. Before embarking on a project (and certainly before parting with money), find out as much information as possible. If an organization seems well organized, provides lots of information, and is commended by online travel journals, you should be on to a winner. If information is sketchy, think twice, and certainly don't shy away from asking questions. Most reputable companies and charities will put you in contact with previous customers or volunteers for a semi-independent perspective.

Useful websites include:

- **Foreign and Commonwealth Office** Up-to-date travel advice by country. Find out in advance whether your intended destination is considered 'safe' by people in the know: www.gov.uk/fco
- **TrailFinders** Links to all types of travel experience: www.trailfinders.com
- **Madventurer** Useful search engine for healthcare, sports, and educational projects seeking volunteers worldwide: www.madventurer.com
- **Gapwork.com** Connects gap year travellers to temporary work in jobs around the world. Also lists volunteering and adventure activities: www.gapwork.com
- **Responsibletravel.com** Travel 'holidays' from basic to luxurious, including visits to the Arctic and Antarctica for students not short of cash: www.responsibletravel.com

Books If you're someone who likes to see information on the printed page, there are some great travel guides available. Backpacking favourites include:

- **The Lonely Planet** A series of travel guides covering almost every country you could ever hope to visit. These books are beloved and bemoaned by experienced travellers in equal proportions, but if you're going anywhere unusual, add the relevant Lonely Planet guide to your kit list.
- **On a Shoestring** Another popular travel series, although also published by The Lonely Planet. These guides differ as they're written with the budget traveller (i.e. gap year student) firmly in mind. They're also titled by region (e.g. Africa) so you get less detail for your money but don't have to buy a separate guide for every country you visit.
- **Rough Guides** These are the major competition for The Lonely Planet. Rough Guides tend to include more information but at the expense of glossy pictures. They are often larger than Lonely Planet guides. Take some time in a bookshop or library before committing to one guide or another.

Advice from real people It's a small world and more people travel now than ever before. Perhaps those in the year ahead at school are away on gap years now. Teachers and other students might know how to contact them; email and social networking sites are a good place to start. Those currently travelling will have the best idea of the pros and cons of each individual project or trip.

If you don't know people who are travelling, or even if you do, consider speaking to an experienced travel provider as well. STA Travel has branches around the world (including 47 in the UK) and years of experience negotiating affordable flights for students and other young people. Staff in STA branches often have travel experience themselves and might have an 'insider's view' of your chosen destinations. However, you can often find cheaper arrangements yourself online. Remember to ask whether you can change ticket details later on and, if so, whether this costs extra.

A student's experience...

After a gruelling selection process I was invited to accept an Army gap year commission. I spent three weeks ironing, running, and trying to avoid my drill instructors' tirades at the Royal Military Academy Sandhurst before joining my new regiment as an officer. At 18 I was responsible for the discipline, administration, and welfare of 40 soldiers. In my year with the Army, I was paid £15,000 for the privilege of gaining a driving licence, learning to ski, and following my unit around the world from Belize to Bosnia.

Things to consider

- **Budget** Travel can be cheap but it can also be very expensive. Flights from London to New York cost as little as £420 return whereas a 15-day voyage to the North Pole doesn't leave change from £20,000. It's often much cheaper to book accommodation, internal flights, etc. from within a country rather than booking through agents in the UK.
- **Medical school application** If you don't yet have an offer, make a note of the UCAS deadline and potential interview dates.
- **Parents** Parents may be alarmed by your newfound independence. Try to involve them in your planning and negotiate sensitively!
- **Visas** Many countries require visas organized in advance of travel (e.g. from the Embassy or High Commission). Others allow travellers to buy visas when they arrive. Find out so you're not caught out.
- **Vaccinations and disease prevention** Organize vaccinations in good time as some require multiple doses over a period of months. A yellow fever vaccination certificate is required for entry to some countries. Remember that, as a potential medical student, you must take special care to avoid blood-borne viruses that could negatively impact on your career (p. 261). These include HIV and hepatitis viruses B and C. Identify potential health risks (e.g. from a reliable travel guide) and take care to avoid them.
- **Travel insurance** Insurance might be an unwelcome expense but it is a necessity. Cancelled gap year plans (e.g. due to bereavement or airline failure) can be financially disruptive as well as disappointing. The average cost of medical repatriation from the USA currently stands at £30,000 without paying for hospital care in that country. Tropical disease and injury are real possibilities for any traveller. Serious injury with multiple operations, a prolonged intensive care stay, and medical repatriation would be sufficient to bankrupt most parents without adequate insurance coverage.

Key points Do plenty of research when organizing your gap year, particularly if you intend to travel. This is the best way to stay safe *and* to make the most of your time away.

Getting a life

Chapter 4

Getting a life

Why do extracurricular activities?

Medicine is about science and patients; why does it matter if you play rugby or the violin? An easy answer is that it is one way that medical schools can choose between straight 'A' students, but that's not a complete explanation. Medical schools need candidates who can relate to patients and resist being overwhelmed by the demands of their profession. Having interests outside of medicine is essential to maintaining your mental health and showing you are a well-rounded individual. This chapter will help you think about activities that could help demonstrate these qualities to course selectors.

Discriminating between candidates Extracurricular interests *are* necessary to win a place at medical school. But don't just see them as a 'box to tick'. They are an opportunity to distinguish yourself from other applicants, almost all of whom will boast straight 'A's. In short, you want to stand out. Admissions staff understandably want to select interesting candidates and one way to be interest*ing* is to have interests. These are best found outside the classroom.

An insider's view...

One of the ironies of medical school selection is that we pick students with lots of hobbies for a time-intensive course where such activities are difficult to sustain. We know that it's not enough just to accept academically successful applicants. The grades are a minimum requirement. We really want rounded students who will go on to become resilient, insightful, and reflective doctors.

Transferable skills Transferable skills are those that are learned in one environment but can be applied elsewhere. For example, working with people of different ages and from different backgrounds on a charity project could help you as a doctor working in a multi-disciplinary team. You are not expected to have everything you need to be a doctor before getting into medical school. However, admissions tutors expect to see that you have started to develop the qualities necessary for work as a doctor. For this reason it is important to write about them in your personal statement (p. 192). It is worth taking a few minutes to consider which qualities are helpful for a doctor. There is no correct answer but your list could include leadership, effective communication, teamworking, and time management, among many others (p. 192). With a range of appropriate interests you should be on your way to developing and demonstrating these skills.

An insider's view...

It can be tedious shortlisting candidates for medical school interviews. Almost all are predicted 'AAA', play a sport to a high level, finished the Duke of Edinburgh Award, and play a musical instrument to grade eight. These things are all very important and many will succeed, but it's the candidate who did something *different* who catches my eye and whom I really want to meet at interview.

Broadening your personality One of the most important transferable skills you can develop is your personality. This is shaped, at least in part, by life experiences and will continue to develop throughout your life. There is no 'right' personality to have as a doctor—good doctors can be shy, scholarly, contemplative, confident, outgoing, or boisterous. However, you can broaden your personality by making the most of extracurricular opportunities.

Adaptability is a vital aspect of any doctor's personality and an important transferable skill. For doctors, no patient, colleague, or working day is ever exactly the same as the last. This is one of the great advantages of a career in medicine—boredom is a rarity—but it can be stressful for people who don't thrive on new experiences. Fortunately there is a solution. Trying new things will make you more adaptable, achieving will make you more confident, and meeting new people will stretch your communication skills. Almost all experiences will have a positive impact on your personality and, even if you don't realize it at the time, give you a better chance of shining at your interview and beyond.

Relaxation Of course, extracurricular interests should also be fun. Most students work hard to achieve the grades required to win a place at medical school. It is easy to become preoccupied with this aim at the expense of everything else. This can lead to stress and anxiety, which negatively impact on grades, as well as causing health problems. Unfortunately, this is an easy trap to fall into after winning a place at medical school as well. This is one reason why there are such high levels of divorce, addiction, and suicide among doctors. However, stress can be relieved by maintaining a good social circle and a range of hobbies. An hour spent exercising or reading a novel before work can increase your productivity far more than hitting the books straight away.

Key points Medical schools understandably avoid taking on candidates who cannot strike a balance between work and play. These students might not complete the course or struggle to cope with life as a doctor. This is a key reason why admissions tutors look for evidence of extracurricular interests.

A warning

Extracurricular interests must be considered as part of your overall strategy. They are different from activities that everyone does to relax such as chatting to friends, watching soaps, or going to the cinema. These alone are unlikely to impress course selectors. Instead, you need to consider more 'interesting' activities. This chapter provides some suggestions but don't forget that extracurricular interests, however important to your application, are also supposed to be fun.

Key points Extracurricular *achievements* are even better than extracurricular *interests*. This is because most applicants can think up a string of unconvincing hobbies to include on their UCAS application. Examples commonly used include walking, reading, and swimming. If you're going to rely on an example later on you might want to distinguish yourself from the casual swimmer. Strong candidates achieve in their extracurricular life as well as in their academic work.

What can you do?

Choosing extracurricular interests is a personal choice that should be made as early as possible. Of course, your interests should be interesting to *you*. However, a couple of strategic choices can make a difference to the outcome of your application. Applicants often make the mistake of choosing several hobbies that demonstrate similar skill sets (e.g. hiking, climbing, and orienteering). Another trap is to accumulate a long list of activities without ever really committing to any of them. The key is to be *selective* in your choice of activities. If you have achieved something amazing—perhaps you are an Olympic athlete or West End actor—one activity may be enough. But most applicants find they need three or four to impress the admissions team.

There is no single list of extracurricular activities that must appear on every successful application. Although some course selectors award points for playing sport to county level, a musical instrument to grade eight, or the Duke of Edinburgh Award, such an inflexible approach is unusual. The trick is to choose activities you can engage with and gain from. For this reason, it is helpful to pick activities you enjoy. Here are a few ideas to get you on your way.

- Sports and music A large number of applicants play a musical instrument or team sport to a reasonable level. These can certainly help show that you are a rounded individual with interests outside of school. However, it is worth noting that *achievement* says more than simply listing an interest. Admissions tutors know 'I enjoy football' could simply mean you once played in PE class. Being captain of the school team is far more impressive than simply enjoying the game. Although sport and music are great additions to an application, they are by no means required. Musical success often depends on taking lessons at a young age and no-one expects your medical school strategy to have begun at age seven. Although it doesn't hurt to step out of your comfort zone and pick up a new sport, or even an instrument, there are many other ways to demonstrate a rounded personality.
- Uniformed youth groups There are many uniformed youth groups, usually led by volunteers and separated by age range. They are typically well organized and operate at a local level across the country. Groups usually meet on the same evening each week, but may require additional time commitments as well.

  'Cadets' are associated with different professions (e.g. Police, Army, Navy, Ambulance Service). Although most cadets do not pursue these careers, they learn a lot about themselves and develop lots of transferable skills (p. 192). These include an appreciation of hierarchy, command, teamwork, and professionalism. Whilst each group has its own unique qualities (insignia, drills, ceremonies, etc.), these serve as a foundation for community involvement and developing good citizenship.

Key points Uniformed youth groups include St John Ambulance, Scouts, Boys/Girls Brigade, Police Cadets, and military cadet forces (e.g. Army, RAF, Navy).

- **School activities** Although extracurricular activities are about non-academic achievements, this should not stop you utilizing opportunities at school. Your school is likely to have resources and contacts that are difficult to find elsewhere. A number of schools also permit access to national programmes such as the Duke of Edinburgh Award. Many of these activities occur during or immediately after school, which can reduce travelling time. On the other hand, make sure any hobbies taken up at school do not impact negatively on your lessons.

  Most schools provide opportunities for student representation. A position as head boy/girl or school president can be taken very seriously by admissions tutors. You will be communicating with senior adults in your school and will have to balance deference with assertiveness. This would undoubtedly improve your confidence and adaptability.

Key points Don't worry too much if the 'top job' eludes you. Many other committee positions offer the chance to demonstrate these qualities. Examples include joining the school council/committee, working as a prefect, mentoring junior students, and/or helping to organize school clubs.

- **Community involvement** Wherever you live there will be opportunities to help out in the community. This can be distinct from work experience (p. 49), which is more about finding out what it's like to work in healthcare. Examples of community work include working in an animal shelter, charity fundraising, and volunteering (e.g. in a homeless shelter). Community work can provide opportunities for working with people outside your peer group. It can also provide a great insight into 'real life' as it affects those in your community.

Key points If you don't remember what your school has to offer, your teachers will know. Check notice boards regularly and ask around to ensure you're not missing out!

Hobbies

Never forget that hobbies will be interpreted as an outward reflection of your personality. For this reason you should think twice about developing or describing an interest that could have negative connotations. However, this can sometimes work to your advantage and finding an 'unusual' interest shows sincerity and ingenuity. It can also serve to make your application more memorable, but do be prepared for probing questions at interview.

How many?

This depends on the activities and how much time you can squeeze out of your schedule. Your first priority is achieving strong A-level grades. However, most good personal statements mention three or four activities, which is enough to demonstrate a range of skills. If you only manage one activity it will need to be exceptional and should speak for itself as to why it is the key focus of your spare time.

A few examples

Applying to medical school is not simply a competition to showcase the most creative hobby. However, it is a distinct advantage to stand out (for the right reasons) from other applicants. The following examples give an idea of what other strong applicants have done in the past and what they believe they gained from their experiences.

World Challenge

I had never travelled further than France on family holidays so became really excited when someone told me about World Challenge. I raised enough money through working and sponsorship and went on a four-week expedition to Uganda, trekking through the jungle and savannah. I also helped build a classroom for a local primary school. The best thing about travelling through Africa is that I matured and gained a great sense of perspective from seeing how some communities survive with few resources.

Air Cadets

I joined my local Air Cadets when I was 15. As well as learning drill, I made lots of new friends and experienced camping, shooting, abseiling, water sports, flying, and parachuting in just three years. The Air Cadet Organisation helped me through the Duke of Edinburgh Award as well. Having led other cadets on cold and wet weekends away, I was able to provide lots of examples of having worked as part of a team under pressure.

School visit to Russia

To further my interest in Russian literature, some friends and I organized a visit to a school in St Petersburg with the help of our literature teacher. We stayed with some of the local students, which kept the costs very low, and raised money from sponsored activities to pay for the flights. Along with having a fascinating trip, I learned about a different culture and developed lots of organizational skills.

Bagpipes

Although I have no Scottish ancestry, I decided at the start of my GCSEs to learn the bagpipes. I wrote about this on my UCAS form and my interviewers seemed to think it was really amusing. In fact they spent most of the time talking about how it's possible to blow into the pipes whilst inhaling at the same time, though they were disappointed to hear that is not how bagpipes work. This really wasn't a topic I'd prepared for!

School photography club

I was very interested in photography and, with two like-minded friends, I set up a photography club. Our school was very supportive and one of the teachers, also a keen photographer, offered to help. In our first year I helped to run a photography competition across the school, which generated lots of interest in photography and earned us quite a few new members as well.

Homeless shelter

During a shadowing placement at a local shelter I met a homeless man who explained some of the difficulties he faced. I spoke to a general practitioner about the problems that homeless people have accessing healthcare and he helped me write a leaflet on this subject that the council has agreed to publish. While working on this I learned about the impact of social circumstances on health and the structure of community healthcare.

Genealogy

I started tracing my family tree and became really interested in population migrations. In fact I became involved with a group of local historians and even co-wrote a chapter for a book that was published about my town. It might sound like a geeky hobby but the admissions tutors seemed impressed that I had an 'academic' interest outside of what was required by the A-level curriculum.

Form prefect

As a prefect I was responsible for mentoring younger students. In this role I helped with project ideas, assisted with a class drama production, and tutored students who were struggling. A year eight student approached me on one occasion to say he was finding maths difficult and felt the teacher picked on him. I arranged a lunchtime meeting at which the teacher explained he believed the student to be very bright but under-motivated. Their relationship improved after this meeting. This taught me that many different problems can be resolved by clear and honest communication.

Work experience

Chapter 5

Work experience

Work experience

Medical school is not just about a university degree; you are choosing a career. Both you and the medical schools you apply to need to know that you understand what it means to be a doctor. This is why work experience is essential.

It is becoming increasingly difficult for school students to find medical work experience. Hospitals and GPs need to protect the personal medical details of their patients from the general public, a principle called patient confidentiality. This can include potential medical students. Although it is difficult, you are unlikely to win a place at medical school without work experience. This chapter will help by suggesting ways to find work experience (p. 52), make the most of your time (p. 58), volunteer (p. 60), find healthcare employment (p. 62), and experience research (p. 64), as well as what to do if all else fails (p. 66).

How much is enough? The short answer is that you can never have too much. The practical reality is that you have to balance work experience with your work and social life during the school terms and vacations. Although there are no hard and fast rules, the best applicants spend two or three weeks shadowing and several months volunteering or working part-time in a role connected with the caring professions. Many positions only require a few hours a week of commitment but you will have to begin early to maximize your chance of winning a place at medical school.

It is important to remember why work experience is so valuable. This will help you distinguish between good and better (there are no 'bad') experiences. Your goal should be to find work experience that helps you to make an informed decision about a career in medicine.

Timeframe

The earlier you begin collecting work experience, the stronger your application will be. Applicants often organize their shadowing placements up to a year before submitting their UCAS form. However, it can take a long time to arrange work experience and last minute panic is best avoided by good planning. Long-term volunteering (e.g. at a hospice or nursing home) shows great commitment to medicine but obviously takes even more time to accrue.

Why work experience is important to medical schools

- Medical schools are choosing doctors not just students; applicants must show a good understanding of what doctors do.
- Between two and ten applicants apply for each place at medical school. Work experience is a way for course selectors to determine which applicants are genuinely committed to medicine.
- Work experience provides material to discuss with applicants at interview.

Why work experience is important to students

- It provides an insight into what it really means to be a doctor, although bear in mind that doing the job is very different from watching someone else do it.
- It provides an opportunity to talk with doctors about their experiences and lifestyle.
- Students can gain a realistic understanding of the pros and cons of a medical career.
- Students can learn about how hospital and community medical services work.
- It provides plenty of positive (and perhaps negative) experiences to discuss with medical school interviewers.

Problems with work experience

- It can be very difficult to arrange. The next few pages should help.
- Work experience can leave applicants with false or misleading impressions of life as a doctor.
- Medicine is a hugely varied profession. It is impossible to experience every speciality so it is inevitable that applicants go into medicine without properly appreciating the range of roles available (p. 13).

A student's experience...

I remember my work experience like it was yesterday...

'We're losing him, doctor.'

'PADDLES????!'

'Charging 360...CLEAR!'

'Sorry to interrupt your break, doctor, but Mr Wilson in bed four has just been sick again and he's insisting that you look at it.' We grudgingly switched off the TV. It was a great episode...the sick, on the other hand, was less great. I followed the junior doctor for another four hours, getting in the way and insisting that every patient I saw was having a heart attack (after seeing one earlier that morning).

Of course being a doctor is not quite as it looks on television. There are considerably fewer crash calls and lots more paperwork! But this was as useful an insight as any; I learned that if it's hourly crash calls I am after, then perhaps I should have applied to drama school.

Arranging work experience

Finding contacts First, compile a list of everyone you know who works in healthcare. Think laterally. Perhaps a family friend, teacher, or distant relative knows a GP. Maybe a neighbour is a practice nurse or GP receptionist. Any personal connection, however tenuous, could provide a lead. Ideally, try to find contacts working in different healthcare settings (e.g. General Practice and hospital). Be thorough and keep returning to the list; at the very least almost everyone has a GP. Ask older relatives if they are, or have recently been, under the care of a hospital specialist.

Using contacts Once you've found a contact, ask for advice. Try to find out which doctors are approachable and likely to help. Ask if your contact would mention you to the health professional before you get in touch. It might seem odd seeking an introduction at this stage but it can reduce the risk of your efforts being 'filed' in the recycle bin. Try to find an email or postal address so you can follow up in person with the doctor (or their secretary). If you are confident, telephoning can be more effective. It is certainly harder to say 'no' to someone in person. Practise what you are going to say before calling and don't be shy about using your contact's name if you have permission to do so.

If contacts don't help If you cannot find a personal contact, drop in to your own GP practice. Ask the receptionist how you could approach the doctors about work experience. They may have a pre-planned scheme for arranging placements. Your own GP might feel a responsibility to help but may worry about confidentiality. If they cannot help, you need to look further afield.

You could have more luck writing to GPs in neighbouring towns where you are less likely to know the patients. You could start by asking each doctor simply to talk with you about medicine. It will be hard for doctors to turn down this humble request. Talking to doctors will be useful in itself but may lead to work shadowing later on. If you have written a letter or email, you should always expect a reply. Many hospitals and GP practices will be unable to help but it is only polite to say so if you have written to them. You may have to write a second time or follow up with a phone call. Lots of people ask for work experience so you need to be persistent (but not annoying) to be 'heard'. Whenever anyone says 'no', don't forget to ask if they can suggest a colleague who can help.

Should your efforts fail, book a normal appointment with your GP. Apologize for taking up their busy schedule and ask if you can discuss their experiences of medicine. Find out whether they could help arrange work experience for you or at least offer advice about who else you could contact.

Key points Don't give up. However you approach them, some people will say 'no'. It's not your fault; don't be upset, simply move on and find someone else to ask. It doesn't matter how many 'no' answers you collect as long as you have one 'yes'.

Special interests If you have a particular interest in a speciality (e.g. elderly medicine), phone nearby hospitals to ask for the names of consultants who work in that department. Alternatively, most hospital websites list consultant names and email addresses. Once you have a list, telephone the hospital switchboard and ask to speak with the secretary for each consultant. Secretaries will probably pass on your message and call you back to say whether their consultant can help. Call the secretary a second time if you have not heard within a few days. If you have an email address, you could contact the doctor directly. However, it is worth remembering that many senior doctors are not confident with technology. They are also not renowned for strong organizational skills and your message does risk getting lost. This is less of a problem if you have found a good secretary to help you.

Most students try to organize placements in specialities such as cardiology, paediatrics, and A&E. Don't neglect less well-known specialities such as pathology, microbiology, anaesthetics, or ophthalmology.

> **Key points** If a doctor can't help, ask them to suggest a colleague who may be willing. You will not get anything if you don't ask and asking (politely) will rarely leave you at a disadvantage.

Be creative If you cannot find a contact in healthcare, become one yourself. Lots of healthcare jobs are part-time and require few qualifications. You could volunteer (or find paid work) typing up patient notes in a GP practice, portering in a hospital, or serving tea in a hospice. Many successful applicants find work as a healthcare assistant. Consider working in any job related to healthcare. Ask doctors, nurses, and other healthcare staff about their jobs, the health service and, of course, about shadowing!

No luck? Don't forget to contact the Royal Colleges or medical schools themselves if you are having trouble arranging work experience. They might also have advice (or contacts) for medical school applicants. You should also remember that shadowing is just one type of work experience. Although it is a very useful thing to organize and to have on your application, it is possible to find out about and show commitment to medicine in other ways. These include volunteering (p. 60), healthcare work (p. 62), and research (p. 64). If after all this you're still short of ideas, see p. 66.

A student's experience...

I was having difficulties shadowing my doctor because many patients didn't want a student present. One day the hospital porters offered to look after me for an afternoon and this was the turning point in my work experience. I found out one of the porters was leaving and I was taken on straight away until a replacement could be found. As a hospital porter I was moving patients around the hospital, preparing surgical kits in theatre, and sitting with patients as they recovered from anaesthetics. I even carried a cardiac arrest bleep! This was great work experience and I got paid to be there; it's definitely worth grasping opportunities in hospital as you never know what might come of them.

Preparing for work experience

Before starting your placement, it is useful to have an understanding of how the NHS works (see p. 10 as well).

General Practice When a person feels unwell or is worried about their health, they often seek help from their general practitioner (GP). In many cases, the GP is able to give advice or treatment (e.g. a prescription for a medication). If the problem requires specialist skill or knowledge then the GP refers the patient to another health professional (e.g. hospital consultant, physiotherapist). For this reason, GPs are often described as the 'gatekeepers to the NHS'. GPs have an important role in preventing illness, managing acute health problems, and caring for patients with long-term (chronic) illnesses.

Emergency Department If a patient needs urgent medical attention they can go directly to the Emergency Department or ED (which used to be called accident and emergency or A&E). Most patients are treated directly; however, if further care is required they can be admitted to a Medical or Surgical Admissions Unit (MAU or SAU). GPs can also refer patients directly to the ED, MAU, or SAU. Patients usually stay on an MAU/SAU for less than 24 hours before being discharged or admitted to a specialist ward in the hospital.

Specialists Most specialist doctors (consultants) work in hospitals where they look after patients who have been admitted for treatment (e.g. surgery, antibiotics). Specialists also see patients from outside the hospital in clinic; these are either patients who were admitted and are now being followed-up or patients referred by other doctors such as GPs or other specialists.

A student's experience...

One of the patients I spoke to had called his GP to say he felt a crushing pain in his chest. His GP thought he might be having a heart attack and called 999. An ambulance went to the man's house and the paramedics brought him straight to A&E. They found out *en route* that he was indeed having a heart attack and so the A&E doctors were waiting and ready to treat him as soon as the ambulance arrived. He was then moved to the Coronary Care Unit. When he left hospital, he returned for consultations with a cardiologist and later had an operation to improve his heart function. His GP is now managing his blood pressure to prevent a second heart attack. This showed me how every department is vital to patient health. A failure at any step could have been fatal.

Who's who?

- **Foundation doctor** Also known as Foundation Year 1 or 2 (FY1/FY2) doctors. They are involved in the day-to-day care of patients while still learning the skills of medicine. They also ensure that tasks are completed on the wards, such as form filling, taking blood samples, and chasing chest X-rays. See p. 10.
- **Specialist Training (ST)** After the FY2 year, doctors specialize in a hospital department or general practice. These doctors are training to become either consultants or GPs. See p. 11.
- **General Practitioner** These doctors have overall responsibility for a large number of people in their area. They are usually the first contact for patients and may refer for specialist advice to secondary or tertiary care. See p. 12.

- **Consultant** Consultants are the most senior hospital doctors with ultimate responsibility for patients. Having trained for over a decade they are very knowledgeable and experienced. Most teach students, research, hold clinics, and lead ward rounds. Some also work privately in their own time. See p. 11.
- **Allied healthcare professionals** Doctors work as part of a multi-disciplinary team with nurses, physiotherapists, occupational therapists, speech and language therapists, social workers, midwives, and many others.

How the NHS is structured

The National Health Service (NHS) is the main UK healthcare system; it was launched 60 years ago, is funded by taxes, and aims to be 'free at the point of use'. It costs the UK taxpayers about £100 billion every year to pay for staff, buildings, equipment, and medications. The NHS is a very complicated organization (1.7 million employees make it the fifth largest employer in the world) but its structure is something you should learn about during the application process. To complicate matters, the way the NHS is run underwent a complete revamp in April 2013 following implementation of the new Health and Social Care Act. See Figure 5.1 for a diagram explaining the structure of the NHS from April 2013.

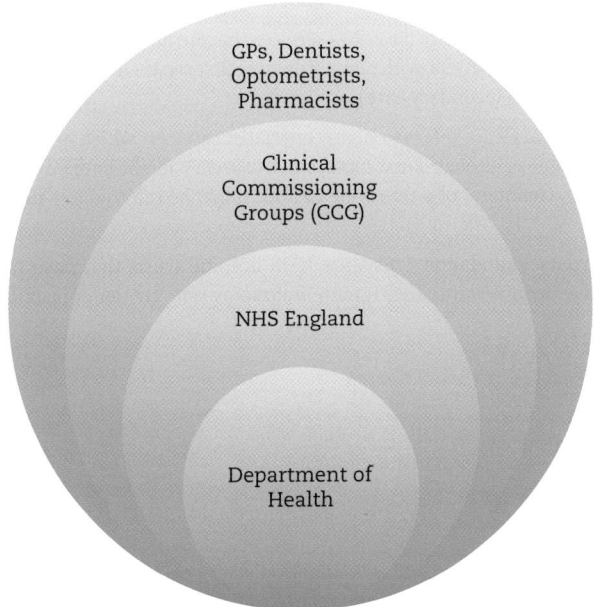

GPs, Dentists,
Optometrists,
Pharmacists

Clinical
Commissioning
Groups (CCG)

NHS England

Department of
Health

Figure 5.1 **Structure of the NHS**

The Department of Health (DH) The DH has overall responsibility for the NHS and is led by the Secretary of State for Health who is accountable to Parliament and therefore the voting public. However, since April 2013, the DH has delegated day-to-day running of the NHS to a new organization, NHS England.

NHS England (formerly The NHS Commissioning Board) This organization oversees and allocates resources to around 200 local Clinical Commissioning Groups nationwide.

Preparing for work experience cont...

Clinical Commissioning Groups (CCGs) These are groups (largely led by GPs) with responsibility for around 60% of the health budget. The role of CCGs is to determine which services to 'buy' on behalf of local patients and from which service provider. For example, a CCG might decide to buy all knee replacement services from one local hospital (which is cheapest or has the 'best' outcomes). Or they are might decide not to fund a specific treatment altogether, perhaps because it is too expensive or there is little evidence for its effectiveness. The reason for letting CCGs determine regional treatment priorities is that they thought to be better placed to know what local people want. However, the new structure is controversial (not least because private companies can bid to supply services against existing NHS organizations) and could well come up as a discussion point at interview. Work experience is an opportunity to canvass opinion from NHS employees or to appreciate how few really understand the reforms.

Primary care Primary care describes the 'frontline' services that are the first point of contact for most people, e.g. GPs, dentists, pharmacists, and optometrists.

Secondary care Secondary care describes services that are accessed through a primary care provider. For example, a patient with chest pain may first see their GP (primary care) before meeting a cardiologist (secondary care).

Tertiary care Tertiary care refers to highly specialist services, which are provided in large centres. For example, although knee replacement surgery might happen in most hospitals (secondary care), treatment of a rare bone tumour might be referred to a highly specialized unit in London.

Foundation Trusts Foundation Trusts are NHS hospital trusts that have met specific set criteria and have been rewarded with more autonomy and greater control over their own budget.

Making the most of shadowing

Many students mistakenly try to learn medicine during their placements. This is not what you are there for, as there will be plenty of time for studying later. Instead, try to gain an insight into your future career. Pay attention to what doctors do and how this impacts on the doctor, patient, and other members of the healthcare team. For example, if you witness a complicated patient case, use it to appreciate the uncertainty of medicine rather than learning about the disease processes at work. Interviewers expect a realistic understanding of medicine, not someone ready to work as a doctor.

Who to shadow Doctors are not the only people you will come across in hospital. The truth is that, without a team of healthcare professionals to support them, doctors are not a lot of good to their patients. In fact, if you spend all your time with doctors you may never even meet other members of the healthcare team. So branch out; shadow a physiotherapist, speak to a Macmillan nurse, arrange a lunch date with the hospital chaplain. You could even ask to see the laboratories. Gain as broad a perspective as possible and try to appreciate where doctors fit into the wider team.

Reflect To make the most of shadowing, take some time to organize your thoughts. This will help you understand what you are witnessing and learn from the experience. Consider keeping a diary during each placement as this will help organize your thoughts and provide a space to reflect on experiences that made you think. It might also be a useful revision aid on the train to your medical school interview.

- Before starting, ask yourself what you expect and see if your expectations change throughout the placement.
- What do you hope to get out of shadowing? Obviously there is a metaphorical 'box to tick' on your UCAS application, but there is much more besides.
- What did you learn? Did anything surprise, please, or disappoint you? Perhaps you saw a distressed relative, an elderly patient being restrained, or a very ill child. You might see a rude or abusive relative or dislike how a healthcare professional talks to a patient. Make a note of these events and consider how they could have been avoided. If appropriate, talk to the person you are shadowing, who might have a different perspective on the experience.
- Think particularly hard about any ethical dilemmas you come across. Should the GP have given contraception to a 14 year old? Is it right to sedate an elderly patient with Alzheimer's who shouts on the ward? These questions may well come up at interview and it will be an advantage if you have already thought about them.
- Don't forget the bright side as well; think about how doctors are placed to improve patients' lives. It doesn't always require a crack diagnosis; sometimes a clear explanation or a kind word is all it takes.

The perfect application

Try to shadow each of the following:

- GP
- Hospital specialist (e.g. consultant or registrar)
- Junior doctor
- Another health professional (e.g. nurse, occupational therapist, dietician).

Make sure you also volunteer or work part-time in a hospital (e.g. as a porter, a nursing auxiliary, or in a nursing home). Prepare for interviews by writing down anything that made you *think*.

Ask questions To really engage with work shadowing you need to ask questions. It is much easier to teach a student who is enthusiastic than one who follows silently behind. Remember to be polite when talking to patients and introduce yourself as a medical school applicant so nobody mistakes you for a doctor.

- Talk to patients—they are important to your future career! Ask what ideas, concerns, and expectations they have about their illness. Don't be afraid to ask questions. 'Does it hurt?' and 'How do you cope at home?' are perfectly valid when asked at appropriate times.
- What do they think makes a good doctor? Most patients will have had a lifetime of good and bad experiences. You will be asked at interview what qualities are important for a doctor and now is a good time to find out.
- Use every opportunity to talk with all types of healthcare professional. Talk to doctors about their work patterns, the NHS, and whether they would choose medicine again. What problems do they face?
- Ask other healthcare workers about their role, the challenges they face, and how they interact with doctors.
- Ask doctors about their lifestyle. What do they like and dislike about their job?
- Perhaps most importantly, could you imagine yourself in this job for the rest of your career?

Be proactive You're not just there to ask questions. Offer a pair of helping hands at every appropriate opportunity. This could be as simple as opening the door for patients coming to clinic. You could offer to take wheelchair-bound patients back to the ward to save them waiting for a porter. At the very least you will make a practical contribution to the hospital. At best, the staff will see you are keen and will go out of their way to help you make the most of your time.

A student's experience...

I spent two afternoons with the nursing staff; the charge nurse was so impressed by my willingness to help that he organized for me to work part-time as a health-care assistant. This gave me the chance to record patients' blood pressure, complete fluid charts, and distribute meals. It was also an opportunity to meet more doctors and nurses around the hospital.

Volunteering

There is more to work experience than simply shadowing doctors. It is for this reason that medical schools look for students who have undertaken voluntary work, which can demonstrate:

- Understanding of challenges such as working with ill and/or dying patients.
- Long-term commitment to health or social care.
- A genuine interest in people. This is often more valuable than showing you have simply 'ticked the box'. To some extent, this can also be achieved through voluntary work in a non-medical setting (p. 45).

Where to volunteer

This depends on what is available locally. The ideal volunteer position will involve contact with people, possibly in a healthcare setting. Remember that long-term commitment to volunteering is much more valuable than a shorter time. For this reason, try to choose something you might enjoy and can reach without too much difficulty. Good places to volunteer include:

- **Hospitals** Volunteering opportunities could include work in the hospital shop or reading to elderly patients on the wards.
- **Residential homes** Elderly people living in residential accommodation can often benefit from help with shopping, tidying, or just someone to talk to.
- **Nursing homes** Individuals in nursing homes often require a lot of care, which can sometimes involve volunteers. Other roles can include befriending and/or taking residents out for a change of scenery.
- **Hospices** These institutions help support people with life-limiting diseases. They are often run by charities and require lots of help from volunteers. There are many lessons to learn in this environment for any potential medical school applicant.
- **Support groups** These groups exist for people with a range of different conditions. They usually hold regular meetings, where you could assist by helping set up and welcoming people to the meeting.
- **Campaigns** Many charities benefit from volunteer fundraisers helping run charity events or appeals. Although you might not be directly exposed to patients, you could still demonstrate an interest and will meet lots of different people in the process.

A student's experience...

I spent a year working every Saturday afternoon in a nursing home. My work involved feeding patients during meal times, helping the carers clean immobile patients, and chatting to the residents and their families. I soon found that, most of all, I wanted a career where I could work with so many different people. I'm confident this came across at interview.

How to organize voluntary work

Compared with work shadowing, volunteering is much easier to organize. This is because many organizations rely on support from volunteers. Nevertheless, as with all your work experience, you should organize opportunities as early as possible. Some organizations require interviews, training, and/or Criminal Records Bureau (CRB) checks before you can begin working. This can take a lot of time.

Don't forget that telephoning or personally visiting an organization will provoke a quicker response than a letter or email. If you do write first, you may have to call afterwards to encourage a response. The local phonebook, newspapers, and the internet are useful sources for finding contact details. Wherever possible try to find the name of an individual to write to. This will make a response more likely and provide someone you can call if an answer is not forthcoming.

There are plenty of voluntary opportunities around so don't give up at the first hurdle. If you're having trouble, think laterally. Maybe you have an elderly next-door neighbour who needs help gardening or a family friend requiring a babysitter. There are opportunities all around you and very few experiences will be wasted. Remember that your ultimate aim is to learn more about a healthcare role and to be able to demonstrate that you have learned this on a UCAS form or at interview.

Key points www.do-it.org.uk is an excellent resource for finding local volunteering opportunities. You can search projects based on the group you want to work with (e.g. the homeless, young people) or what you want to do (e.g. build, mentor, counsel). The WRVS also offers a range of volunteering roles in the hospital and community: www.wrvs.org.uk.

Making the most of voluntary work

The same principles of productivity and reflection apply to volunteering as to other types of work experience. You should certainly not dismiss opportunities because there are no doctors present. Great opportunities and insights often arise from a 'less interesting' post, so commit yourself to whatever you sign up for. You never know where it might lead.

Don't forget to ask yourself and others questions about everything around you. What do elderly people who live alone worry about? How did women in a breast cancer support group receive their diagnosis; could their experiences have been improved? You may come across some sensitive issues concerning fairly vulnerable people. If it is appropriate to approach these topics you should do so with care and sensitivity. You will learn far more by thinking about your volunteering experiences as much as possible than by simply going through the motions each day.

Needless to say, if you come across a doctor (or other health professional), ask if you can shadow them!

Employment

Many applicants find it hard to set aside time for work experience alongside studies, hobbies, and part-time work. Fortunately it is possible to combine work experience with employment, essentially getting paid for improving your medical school application.

Advantages

There are many reasons why you might combine employment and work experience:

- **Responsibility** You can often feel as if you are in the way when you do work experience; this is not the case for a paid employee who is an integral part of the team. Doing a job forces you to concentrate more than watching other people at work.
- **Duration** While work experience might only last a few days, employment will usually continue over a period of months or years. It takes time to become familiar with any new experience and the longer duration will help you feel comfortable in a healthcare setting and around patients. It also demonstrates commitment and interest in working with sick or disadvantaged people.
- **Contacts** Any job in healthcare will be alongside healthcare professionals. These people may respect your initiative and offer further opportunities such as shadowing (p52)—don't be afraid to ask, but expect any shadowing opportunities to be outside of your working hours.
- **Pay** Employers must pay at least the minimum wage to all employees. There are different rates available for those aged <18, 18–20, and ≥21. If there is any doubt, check the minimum wage (http://www.gov.uk/national-minimum-wage-rates) and contact the Citizens Advice Bureau to clarify if you are unsure.

A student's experience...

I worked at a GP practice helping summarize paper notes onto a computer system. I was paid £7.50 an hour, more than my friends working in other jobs, and felt I was making a real contribution to the practice. The GPs were keen to talk to me about a career in medicine and sometimes let me spend a few hours with them seeing patients.

Obstacles

As with all work experience, there are obstacles to watch out for:

- **Age** Many healthcare providers require employees to be above a minimum age, e.g. 16 or 18 years old.
- **Administration** CRB checks often take four weeks to process. It may also be necessary to have immunizations and an occupational health check-up, so apply early.
- **Timing** Residential homes and hospitals may need evening workers but other employers, such as GP practices, might only open during the day. Summer holidays are ideal for working.

Types of work

There are thousands of jobs in healthcare but most require specialist qualifications. Work experience applicants often find certain jobs more accessible than others:

- **Healthcare assistant** Healthcare assistants (HCAs) work alongside nurses and help with washing and dressing patients, bed-making, and monitoring vital signs (e.g. pulse and temperature). This is an ideal way to experience 'hands on' care.
- **Clinical support worker** This is a similar role to that of an HCA although clinical support workers usually assist a therapist (e.g. physiotherapist, audiologist) rather than nursing staff.
- **Carer** Many agencies employ carers to visit elderly or disabled patients in their own homes. Carers will often have a similar role to HCAs, although many posts require a means of transport to visit clients.
- **Phlebotomist** These healthcare workers take blood from patients and ensure it is transported safely to the appropriate laboratory. It is a useful experience as you will meet lots of patients, learn a vital skill, and develop methods of helping patients deal with painful procedures.
- **Hospital porter** Porters move patients and equipment around the hospital. They work everywhere from wards to operating theatres and get to see a wide range of departments, patients, and practices.
- **Domestic services** This includes cleaners, catering, stores, and laundry workers. These roles are easiest to organize and some allow patient contact.

A student's experience...

As a cleaner on a cardiology ward I got to know many different patients. They often confided in me so I learned all about their worries, home lives, and thoughts on the hospital staff. In particular, I learned there is more to each patient than a disease.

How to find employment in healthcare

First choose the organization you want to work for (e.g. hospital, GP practice, residential home). Use the internet or local paper to identify any jobs being advertised.

Small organizations (e.g. GP practices) should be approached directly, whereas hospitals may have their own Human Resources (HR) department. There is no reason why you should not visit HR departments in person to ask what type of work they have available. You are more likely to be offered employment if you are available for an extended period of time (e.g. the summer vacation) rather than evenings and weekends.

Large hospitals will often have a website complete with an up-to-date list of vacancies. Many hospitals (and residential homes) take on staff through an employment agency. If you cannot find which agencies place healthcare staff, ask the organization you want to work for which one they use. Most jobs will require you to complete an application form and attend an interview. This will probably be followed by a period of training.

Key points www.jobs.nhs.uk lists all the NHS jobs available in your area. For non-NHS jobs, use Google to find agencies supplying staff to local care homes.

Research experience

Although it is not a common form of work experience, some applicants organize time in a laboratory helping with research. There is a growing commitment in the NHS to 'evidence-based medicine' (EBM), which means finding out which treatments actually *work* rather than using them just because they have been used for a long time. Millions of pounds are spent every year on this process. Research is not a substitute for spending time with patients, although it can add a further angle to your application.

Advantages The main advantage of research experience is that you will see another side of modern medicine. Although not all doctors are researchers, many undertake a research project at some point in their career. It would be great if you could show an understanding of this early on. More importantly, seeing research might help you understand the importance of evidence-based medicine and how doctors and scientists learn about disease.

Disadvantages There are three things to consider for any applicant thinking about research work. The first is that it can be very difficult to organize. Laboratories have lots of expensive and potentially dangerous equipment; electron microscopes cost £1 million each. Laboratories also contain sensitive research work. It is not unusual for a PhD student to work for three years developing a cell line, which could easily be destroyed by an inexperienced work experience student. However, this will depend on the laboratory and most could accommodate showing a student around for an afternoon.

The second point to consider is that you are unlikely to achieve very much with only a short period of time available. This is because it takes a long time to learn laboratory techniques before they can be used to 'discover' anything. It may also be tedious simply watching researchers go about their work. However, going along for a day could be useful in helping to inform your career decisions.

Finally, it may be difficult to explain to interviewers why you chose to find out about research. They will prefer experience with patients and may need convincing that research is a useful addition to your work experience portfolio. This will depend on where you apply and who the interviewers are. But have an explanation ready in case this unusual part of your application is picked up. Talking intelligently about evidence-based medicine could work very well at this point.

A student's experience...

I spent a summer working in a laboratory with my neighbour, who is Professor of Physiology at a nearby university. Some of the techniques were hard but I think I was useful to the team in the end. I was given a long time to talk about my project at interview and the interviewers were particularly impressed that I was named on a research paper! I am now a medical student and will be returning to the lab to continue my project as a paid research assistant in my first summer holiday.

Should you try to find research experience? Research is never a substitute for experience with patients. Admissions tutors want to see evidence of your interest in people above everything else. There are, however, a number of reasons why you might consider looking for research experience:

- You want to learn the importance of research to medicine through first-hand experience. Selling this idea appropriately at interview could show maturity and insight far beyond what the interviewers are expecting.
- You already have a lot of shadowing and volunteering experience. If you are looking to add breadth to your application, research is a possibility.
- You are applying to a medical school with a strong emphasis on basic sciences. These include Oxford (p. 152), Cambridge (p. 118), and Imperial College London (p. 138).
- You are applying to biomedical science through UCAS in addition to medicine (p. 189). Research could fulfil the same role for biomedical science as hospital work does for medicine. Unlike medicine, very few applicants to these courses will have relevant work experience and your chances of acceptance will increase dramatically.
- You are interested in research after graduating as a doctor. Experience now could help confirm this interest or put you off altogether.

Finding research There are many different types of research. It is unlikely you would be involved in the type of research that goes on in hospitals as this involves patients and may take years to finish. You may, however, hear doctors talk about research projects and/or see patients who are part of clinical trials. Don't forget to ask questions if you do!

You are more likely to find work experience in a laboratory. Although there are research laboratories in some hospitals, most are found in universities. You could try contacting a nearby medical school or Department of Biological Sciences for advice. Most will have websites that list their researchers and current projects. Choose a researcher or project that is relevant to medicine. If you are already interested in a particular field, write to a researcher with similar interests for permission to visit his/her laboratory. Alternatively, don't be shy about exploiting personal contacts. If you or your family know anyone in research, a PhD student, technician, or professor, consider asking them. They may know someone you could approach to supervise you.

The most important thing to remember is that research experience is not a vital part of your medical school application. Very few applicants will have any. If the opportunity arises then seize it; however, it is unlikely to affect your application if you cannot, or do not want to, experience medical research.

Key points Research experience is not a substitute for work with patients. It should probably only be considered by a small number of applicants such as those applying to very academic courses, those who already have an existing interest in research, and/or those who have already undertaken a wide range of different work experience placements.

If all else fails...

Successful applicants often have a long record of experiences such as shadowing, volunteering, and part-time employment. These are important and often necessary, but an additional tactic is to find something that makes you stand out from the other applicants. Have a look at some of the examples below for ideas but don't feel limited by them!

Hospitals abroad

On holiday with my parents, I visited a small clinic in a remote area of Malawi. I had finished two hospital attachments in the UK but was interested to see how things worked abroad. Fortunately, the medical assistant in charge understood my interest and spoke good English. He showed me around his clinic and I was amazed to see how much could be achieved without expensive equipment. This taught me that many conditions can be diagnosed simply by talking and examining patients. These are vital skills anywhere that medicine is practised.

Occupational therapists

Occupational therapists help people who have restricted activity as a result of their illness. During a shadowing placement I spent a couple of days with the occupational therapy team. I watched them conduct assessments, provide vital equipment, and even visit patients in their own homes. If I am honest, I hadn't really thought about healthcare taking place outside hospitals and GP practices. I was able to see first-hand how much important work goes on in the community and how it is not just doctors and nurses who treat patients.

Pathologist

During a summer vacation, I worked as a lab assistant in the histopathology department of a hospital. Although I didn't think this would be useful for medical school, as I didn't see many live patients, I was wrong. At interview I talked about the importance of hospital support services, which often go undervalued because they are hidden away from patients. This seemed to please the pathologist on my interview panel!

I was also invited by one of the consultants to see deceased patients being prepared for post-mortem. This was fascinating, although I was apprehensive at first, and writing about it on my UCAS form led to a discussion at another interview about when and why post-mortems should be carried out. Fortunately I had asked the consultant very similar questions so found myself in a great position to answer them.

Mountain rescue

As a keen climber, I read an article in a climbing magazine about mountain rescue teams. This seemed like an ideal opportunity to combine work experience with something I already enjoyed. Although I wasn't able to join one of the teams because of my age, I met with the team doctor who gave me a tutorial on the effects of low temperature on the body. This helped me see how basic science, anatomy, physiology, and biochemistry all fit into clinical medicine. It also gave me some ideas about what I might like to do when I finish medical school.

Army doctors

During my time as an Army cadet, I listened to a talk by an Army doctor. He described his journey through medical school and working in NHS hospitals, before touring conflict zones such as Afghanistan. This helped me identify another reason for studying medicine: the skills learned as a doctor can be applied in thousands of different situations. Wherever there are people in need of help, there is an important role for doctors.

A brief warning Finding work experience abroad can be a great way to have fun and set your application apart from the competition. This is much easier to organize during a gap year after school (p. 36). Always remember to put patient safety and dignity before your own need to gain experience. Do not put yourself in a position (e.g. by doing things you are unqualified to do) whereby patients are put at risk. Any suggestion of this could result in a premature end to your application.

If things still aren't working out Work experience is difficult to arrange. However, successful applicants will almost always have managed to organize something; if you think laterally enough there will always be opportunities available. You could contact local pharmacists, hospital laboratories, travel clinics, hospices, or baby weighing clinics, all of whom might be able to help.

An insider's view . . .

Students often want to know what experience they need to win a place at medical school. There is no simple answer. We want to know that applicants have learned something about being a doctor and are enthusiastic about medicine. At the very least, applicants should have read about healthcare. They should have spoken to doctors (at least their own GP) and patients about the qualities needed to be a good doctor. Students struggling to find work experience should remember that there are many ways to learn about medicine. Even simple things can help persuade interviewers that you want to be a doctor.

Preparing for admission tests

Chapter 6

Preparing for admission tests

The use of admission tests

Most medical schools require an admission test to help identify the best candidates. You only get one chance to take each test each year but with careful preparation it is possible to maximize your score.

The tests are very different from A-levels and appreciating this difference is the key to doing well. They do not test what you know; rather they test how well you can think under considerable time pressure. To succeed you must focus on answering lots of questions well rather than a few questions perfectly. The test designers claim that preparation does not help since the questions are based on intellect and not knowledge. However, in practice, being familiar with the tests and refining your technique can make all the difference.

The following chapter describes the format of these tests, how the scores are used by medical schools (p. 71), strategies to get the best marks (p. 74), and an overview of the UKCAT (p. 78) and BMAT (p. 82). The GAMSAT, a test usually reserved for graduate entry courses (p. 228), is described on p. 221. To help explain the format of the different question types we have included sample questions in the appendix (p. 304); these were contributed by Kaplan (www.kaptest.co.uk) who run preparation courses for these tests.

The admission tests

There are two main tests used by medical schools in the UK: the UK Clinical Aptitude Test (UKCAT) and the Biomedical Admissions Test (BMAT). They are used by all medical schools except:

- The graduate courses at Exeter, Nottingham, Peninsula, St George's (London), and Swansea, which use the Graduate Medical School Admissions Test (GAMSAT), see p. 221.
- Birmingham, Bristol, Lancaster, and Liverpool, which do not use an admission test.

The UKCAT has five sections: Verbal Reasoning, Quantitative Reasoning, Abstract Reasoning, Decision Analysis, and Non-Cognitive Analysis (p. 78). The BMAT consists of three sections: Aptitude and Skills, Scientific Knowledge and Applications, and the Writing Task (p. 82).

The purpose of admission tests

Tests have become a necessary part of the admissions process due to the high number of students applying to study medicine. They offer:

- A way to distinguish between candidates Nearly all medical school applicants are predicted straight 'A's (or at least 'AAB'). The admission tests offer universities a way to distinguish between them.
- A fair comparison The admission tests allow the medical schools to compare all applicants using a fair and consistent standard. Unlike A-levels, where students taking the same subject sit exams set by different exam boards, every candidate answers the same standard of questions.

- Identical mark schemes The marking is done to the same standard; in fact the UKCAT is marked by computer and the BMAT is multiple choice except for the occasional short answer question and the essay, which has a consistent mark scheme (p. 333).
- Teaching independence Since the tests require limited background knowledge the benefits or disadvantages of different schools and teachers are minimized.

Key points The admission tests are very different from other exams. You need to be willing to skip questions, make quick guesses, and prioritize which questions to go back to. Practising the tests under time pressure will make a big difference to your technique (p. 72).

How are the tests used by medical schools?

This is not an easy question because the use of admission test scores differs between medical schools. Furthermore, many institutions do not describe their selection methods. As a general principle the tests are used to filter out the 'best' applicants:

- Is there a cut-off score? Anecdotally, it appears that most medical schools set a 'cut-off' score: those above the specific score get invited to interview while those below do not. Other medical schools derive a total score by assessing GCSEs and UCAS forms alongside admission tests and set a cut-off for this value instead.
- Are the cut-off scores available? Medical schools generally keep quiet about their cut-off scores and many do not acknowledge using them. Accordingly, information is hard to come by, although thorough internet searching and recent applicants can provide estimates.
- What is the estimated cut-off score? A UKCAT score of 2,400 out of 3,600 (i.e. an average of 600 out of 900 in each of the first four sections) appears to be a common cut-off score. There is less information about the BMAT cut-off, but it is generally thought to be 13 out of 23 (5 out of 9 in each of the first two sections and 3C out of 5 on the essay—see p. 333).
- Is it difficult to reach this estimate? Not for above-average applicants: in 2012 the average scores for the UKCAT were 580, 656, 633, and 646 for sections 1–4 respectively. For the BMAT the median scores were 4.7, 4.6, and 3.5A for sections 1–3 respectively. The cut-off scores are not unreachable but you need to do better than average.
- Test scores in context Admission tests are an important component of your medical school application; however, they are considered alongside GCSEs, AS-level results, predicted A-level grades, and the personal statement (p. 192). For some medical schools, a bad admission test score means no interview; at others it means that the rest of your application must be outstanding.

Preparing and taking the tests

There are several resources that you may call upon to help you prepare for admission tests:

- **This chapter** These pages should be used to gain tips about how to answer admission test questions. By reading about the format of the UKCAT (p. 78) and BMAT (p. 82), you will learn more about what is involved in each section. You can then practise the sample questions in the appendix (p. 304).
- **Specimen questions** The UKCAT and BMAT websites offer sample question papers for each section. These have the advantage of being identical in format and style to the questions you will receive on the day. However, there are limited numbers and you risk them becoming over-familiar if you practise too often. This can lead to a false sense of security.
- **Practice books** These usually consist of a bank of questions similar to those in the UKCAT and BMAT. Make sure that the book has explanations along with answers so you can learn what to do more easily. Such books have two limitations: lack of individual feedback and inability to assess BMAT essay performance (p. 83). You could try asking your teachers to look at your practice essays, together with a copy of the mark scheme (p. 333).
- **Websites** Alongside practice books, a number of websites have practice questions for UKCAT and BMAT. They range in quality and cost; up-to-date lists and reviews can be found on medical student forums (p. 338).
- **Preparatory courses** These offer the opportunity to practise test questions under timed conditions with experts who can provide tailored feedback and explain the answers to questions you don't understand. Practice courses are also invaluable for going through answers to BMAT essays. Kaplan, who provided the test material (on p. 304), offer preparatory courses in the UK and in real-time online.
- **Further reading** There are various books available on thinking skills, logic, and critical reasoning that may be used to better understand these areas. These skills are particularly useful for sections 1–3 of the UKCAT and section 1 of the BMAT. It may also be worth investing in some GCSE physics, chemistry, biology, and mathematics revision books for section 2 of the BMAT.

Preparatory courses and websites

Almost all students prepare for their UKCAT or BMAT using a combination of the resources above. The questions in the appendix (p. 304) were provided by Kaplan Test Prep and Admissions who offer class-room courses that teach methods and strategies for the test and also provide website resources (www.kaptest.co.uk).

UKCAT practicalities

Taking the UKCAT The UKCAT is taken before completing the UCAS form and choosing the medical schools to which you will apply. The test can only be taken once a year, before the beginning of October (see www.ukcat.ac.uk for exact dates) and you need to book a test date, often four to six weeks in advance. It is a computer-based test performed at one of the official Pearson VUE test centres. There are many centres across the UK and internationally; an exemption list of countries without a test centre in which students do not need to take the test is available on the UKCAT website. An extended version of the test is available for candidates with special needs (UKCATSEN). In both versions you can mark questions for 'review' and go back to them at the end.

Practical hints Aim to sit the UKCAT as soon as possible, allowing you to focus your efforts towards your UCAS application form and preparing for interview. This also allows you to re-schedule if you are feeling unwell or unprepared in the days leading up to your test date. Make sure you have been given your pen and laminated booklet to make notes on before the test begins. Ear plugs might be available, but take your own to ensure your comfort while helping to prevent distractions.

UKCAT results Your test answers are marked by computer and the result is available immediately after the test. The test centre then sends your result to UCAS, which will pass it on to universities to which you send an application.

If your results aren't quite what you expected, don't panic! UKCAT results are usually considered alongside other factors such as exam results and your personal statement (p. 192). If it is obvious that you scored very low, you should consider applying to medical schools that are not strict about cut-offs (although identifying these medical schools can be tricky— p. 107) or institutions that do not use the UKCAT at all (pp. 70 and 72).

Key points The UKCAT costs around £65 for EU students, provided they take the test before 31 August. It costs EU students £80 after this date and non-EU students pay £100. For further details, including information on bursaries, see www.ukcat.ac.uk.

BMAT practicalities

Taking the BMAT This test is taken after choosing medical schools and submitting your UCAS form. Applicants must register with the Cambridge Assessment Group before 15 October (the same closing date as UCAS applications); however, there are late booking fees so it is best to register earlier. The BMAT is a written test that must be taken at an official test centre. The majority of candidates will sit the BMAT at their own school or college, around the beginning of November. A soft pencil should be used for sections 1 and 2 (take an eraser as well) and a black ink pen for section 3.

BMAT results Most people leave the BMAT test feeling that it did not go well. Nevertheless, you should avoid trying to anticipate your results until they arrive, as the BMAT is not the type of test that you leave feeling you've nailed! It's designed so that you feel you could have done better with more time. The BMAT results are usually released online at the end of November.

Key points The full BMAT specification and additional specimen questions can be found on the Cambridge Assessment Group website. This is also where you will need to register to sit the BMAT as well as find further details regarding reimbursement: www.admissionstests.cambridgeassessment.org.uk. The BMAT costs around £40 for EU students and around £70 for late registrations after 31 August. The non-EU standard entry fee is around £70, while the late entry fee is around £100.

Admission test strategy

There are three ways to improve your performance in the admission tests: practise, practise, and practise! You are very unlikely to learn a question that will come up. But you will learn to manage your time, concentrate on questions you can answer, and become familiar with the format so that you don't waste valuable seconds on instructions on the day.

The admission test strategy

- 'Revising' will not help Your strategy for the admission tests needs to be different from your A-levels. 'Cramming' before the test won't help you since outside knowledge is irrelevant to the UKCAT and is only required to a limited degree in the BMAT.
- Learn the format Instead, you need to focus your efforts on learning the format of the questions so no time is wasted trying to understand the task (p. 78).
- Learn about the mark scheme You should be familiar with what the sections are examining (p. 82) and, in particular, those taking the BMAT should be aware of what examiners are looking for when marking the essay question (p. 83).
- Maximizing your marks In the multiple choice sections you can maximize your marks by answering as many questions as you can in the time allowed. On the BMAT essay marks are maximized by an essay that directly answers the questions and meets or exceeds the requirements of the marking criteria (p. 333).
- Do not be afraid to skip questions It is not a realistic aim to answer all of the questions correctly. In order to succeed you must be prepared to leave questions and return later on if there is time.
- Guess Because there are no negative marks, if you do not know the answer, guess (p. 76).
- Practise You need to practise mock tests under timed conditions in order to maximize your mark on the test day.

> Key points By practising your pacing you can learn to triage questions, rather than waste time answering long or complicated ones. You can guess strategically and move on to quicker marks later in the section. Knowing this, and practising for it properly, can make all the difference in qualifying for interview.

Practise your pacing

Many students have their first experience of sitting the UKCAT or BMAT under properly timed conditions on the test day. For many this experience is stressful and ultimately disappointing since they find there are far more questions than they can answer in the time available. These test-takers tend to score below average in one or more sections, which means that they miss the cut-off score and fail to qualify for interview. It's a hard lesson to learn and an unpleasant way to learn it. This can of course be avoided by adequate preparation.

There are a few things you can do as part of this practice to get yourself in the test day mindset:

- Average time per question   Work out the average timing per question for each section of the test. For example, the Quantitative Reasoning section of the UKCAT requires you to answer 36 questions in 23 minutes. Be careful here, as the minute to read directions cannot be used to answer questions; so instead of having 23 minutes, there are only 22. With only 22 minutes to answer 36 maths questions, you must answer each question in about 36 seconds and that's without allowing extra time to look over the charts and tables that accompany the questions. See pp. 78–83 for timing calculations.
- Triaging the 'stinkers'   'This highlights the importance of triage (p. 76). You may find that with a bit of timed practice you have no trouble answering most maths questions in 30 seconds. Unfortunately the test designers have thought of this, so they mix in questions that are more complicated. These could be complex because there is more information to read or because the maths required is significantly more elaborate. Instead of taking about 30 seconds, these questions might take three or four minutes. Working even one of these out completely could cost you five or more marks on later, quicker questions. In the UKCAT you can guess an answer, mark the question for review, and come back to it. In the BMAT, guess an answer then place a star in the margin.
- Timed practice   You've probably never had a test that required answering so many maths questions so quickly. The good news is that, with timed practice, you can improve your speed and accuracy. But this practice must be timed and it must include questions that are similar in terms of their format, structure, and range of difficulty.

An insider's view . . .

Every year we have many students on our admission test prep courses who sat the UKCAT or BMAT in the previous year and failed to qualify for interview. They simply didn't score highly enough, despite having mostly 'A's at A-levels. Although these students are incredibly bright, they made the mistake of assuming that the UKCAT and BMAT are similar to school exams. They had never encountered a test that is designed to be difficult for a bright student to finish. In fact, most of them had never left questions on an exam unanswered until they sat the UKCAT or the BMAT. Unfortunately, they had this experience of leaving questions unanswered on the test day, which destroyed their hopes of getting a place to study medicine that year. These students always say the same thing: they wish someone had told them about the benefits of practising beforehand, because they would have invested time preparing for the test then and earned the score required the first time around.

Brian Holmes—Head Writer at Kaplan for UKCAT and BMAT
Kaplan Test Prep and Admissions (www.kaptest.co.uk)

Admission test strategy cont ...

The following tips apply specifically to the multiple choice-type questions you will face in the UKCAT and/or BMAT.

Triage

Triage is a French word meaning *to separate, sort, or select*. Imagine that you are the only medic in the A&E ward of a rural hospital on a quiet night. Following a car crash, five patients come in at once. Assessing them quickly, you find that one is unconscious, not breathing, and has no pulse while the other four are bleeding profusely but are conscious. By ignoring the unconscious patient initially you can save four lives by quickly stopping them from bleeding (elevate and compress). Once the bleeders have been stabilized you can see if there is anything you can do for the last patient.

- Why triage? When resources are limited, triage is essential. It allows you to achieve the most benefit with the time, equipment, and experience that are available.
- Triage in admission tests To maximize your marks on the UKCAT and BMAT you must triage each question as it appears. If a question appears to be time consuming, you do not have time for it. This includes questions with unusually long sections of text or pages of information with them. There are more marks, and quicker marks, in the questions you have yet to encounter.
- Returning to the rest If you have time left over after a first pass through the questions in the section, you can come back to the ones you've skipped. This approach may be unfamiliar, but these tests have been designed to give you a hard time finishing if you answer all the questions in order. Triage is the surest way to success.

This strategy works because virtually all the questions on the UKCAT and BMAT are multiple choice; this means there's another strategy you can use as well...

Strategic guessing

- No negative marking An essential fact: there is no penalty for incorrect answers on the UKCAT or BMAT so there is no penalty for guessing. Thus, it's essential that you put down an answer for every question. Leaving questions blank means giving up on marks that could have been yours.
- Strategic guessing Guessing strategically means doing a quick assessment of a question to eliminate one or more answers before guessing from the remainder. Since a multiple choice question can only have one correct answer, there must be a reason why all the other answers are wrong. You can either work out the correct answer through straightforward reasoning/maths, or you can work out the correct answer by eliminating all of the wrong answers. Guessing strategically is a variation on this latter option: when you don't have time to eliminate all of the wrong answers, simply eliminate the obvious ones and make your best guess from the answers that remain.

Consider the odds of guessing correctly when guessing blindly, as compared to guessing strategically, shown in Table 6.1.

Table 6.1 The odds of strategic guessing

Number of answer choices	Odds of correctly guessing blindly	Odds of correctly guessing strategically after eliminating:	
		1 answer	2 answers
3	33%	67%	100%
4	25%	33%	50%
5	20%	25%	33%

When you can eliminate one or more answer choices, guessing strategically gives you a much stronger chance of answering correctly and picking up the mark.

- Blind guessing The odds of guessing blindly are not bad, particularly when there are only three answer choices. Still, you should only guess blindly if you are running out of time and at risk of leaving questions unanswered. In that situation guessing blindly gives you some chance of picking up the mark. If you leave a question unanswered, the odds of picking up the mark are nil.
- BMAT exceptions Note that the BMAT sometimes includes a few questions in section 1 or section 2 that have write-in answers, e.g. a number or a phrase. These questions are relatively uncommon and not susceptible to strategic guessing. As you triage the BMAT, it's usually best to leave the write-in questions for later, unless, of course, you find they are quick work and easy marks.

Key points You must be prepared to guess strategically and maximize your marks with questions you don't have time to work out properly.

The UKCAT

The UK Clinical Aptitude Test (UKCAT) is currently employed by:

- England Brighton and Sussex, Durham, Exeter, Hull York, Keele, Leeds, Leicester, London—Bart's, London—Imperial (graduate entry only), London—King's, London—St George's, Manchester, Newcastle, Nottingham, Peninsula (undergraduate only), Sheffield, Southampton, University of East Anglia, Warwick (graduate entry only).
- Northern Ireland Queen's (Belfast).
- Scotland Aberdeen, Dundee, Edinburgh, Glasgow, St Andrews.
- Wales Cardiff.

The UKCAT is produced by the UKCAT consortium to assess a wide range of 'mental abilities and behavioural attributes' that medical schools have identified as being important. The entire test takes two hours and each of the five sections of multiple choice questions are timed separately.

Section 1: Verbal reasoning

44 questions—11 reading passages, 4 questions per passage

21 minutes—less than 2 minutes per passage

Section 1: Verbal reasoning

The first section assesses your ability to think logically about written information presented in a passage of text and reach a reasoned conclusion. For each passage you are given there are four corresponding questions. Your answer must be based *only* on the information you have been given in the passage, not on any personal prior knowledge. For some of these statements you will be asked to choose: 'True', 'False', or 'Can't tell'. Other questions will require you to select the most suitable response to a question or incomplete statement. For this section there are four sample questions based on a single passage of text on p. 306, which you should aim to complete within two minutes. The answers are on p. 318.

Section 2: Quantitative reasoning

36 questions—9 sets of graphs/charts/tables, 4 questions each

22 minutes—approximately 2½ minutes per graph/chart/table

Each question has five options, one of which is correct

Section 2: Quantitative reasoning

After the verbal reasoning section comes an assessment of your ability to solve numerical problems. You will need to be able to quickly extract relevant information from graphs, charts, and tables. Although good mathematical ability helps, it is less a test of numerical competency and more to do with problem solving, such as manipulating simple ratios, fractions, percentages, and averages. For this section there are four sample questions based on one set of charts on p. 308, which you should aim to complete within two minutes. The answers can be found on p. 319.

Section 3: Abstract reasoning

65 questions—13 pairs of sets, 5 test shapes to assign to one of each pair

15 minutes—approximately 1 minute per pair of sets

Section 3: Abstract reasoning

This section assesses your ability to infer relationships from information by convergent and divergent thinking. You are presented with two *sets* of shapes, labelled 'set A' and 'set B'. All the shapes in each set are similar to each other, but set A is not related to set B. You have to determine whether the test shape belongs to set A, set B, or neither set. The items include irrelevant material, so it is important that you remain focused in identifying a rule that relates each item of a set to all the others. Once you are sure you have identified the rule for each set, it should be easy to get all five marks. For this section there are five test shapes based on one pair of sets on p. 312, which you should aim to complete within one minute. The answers can be found on p. 320.

Section 4: Decision analysis

26 questions

31 minutes—approximately 2 minutes' reading time to familiarize yourself with the codes and any additional instructions and approximately 1 minute per question

Section 4: Decision analysis

The penultimate section investigates your ability to deal with various forms of information, infer relationships, make informed judgements, and decide on an appropriate response in situations of complexity and ambiguity. Deciphering each code will require a skilful combination of logic and judgement to reach an answer. There are four or five options for each question and in some questions more than one option may be correct. For this section there are five sample questions based on one code on p. 314, which you should aim to complete within seven minutes. The answers can be found on p. 320.

Section 5: Situational Judgement Test

13 scenarios each consisting of between 4 and 6 potential response options to rate

26 minutes

Section 5: Situational Judgement Test

The final section is being piloted from 2012, in order to evaluate its usefulness in the future. Currently, the UKCAT consortium has decided not to include this component in your final UKCAT score, nor will they communicate your score for section 5 to your chosen medical school, although make sure you keep up to date with information on the UKCAT website, as this is continuously changing (www.ukcat.ac.uk).

The UKCAT cont...

The Situational Judgement Test assesses your judgement in healthcare-related scenarios, by assessing for the interpersonal skills, self-awareness, professionalism, and ethical values necessary for successful medical practice. After reading a hypothetical clinical scenario you will be asked to make judgements about a series of options relating to the scenario, by selecting their appropriateness or importance. Each response option must be considered irrespective of the timeframe (i.e. short-term options may be more or less important/appropriate than long-term options) and independently; therefore you may choose the same option multiple times for any given scenario. The list of options is not meant to be exhaustive, and you are asked to make a judgement only about the options presented to you.

For this section there are eight sample questions based on one scenario on p. 316, which you should aim to complete within three minutes. The commentary to this section can be found on p. 322.

> **Key points** If you wish to see more examples of Situational Judgement Test-type questions, you could try some (harder!) questions intended for the Situational Judgement Test sat by final year medical students—*Oxford Assess and Progress: Situational Judgement Test*.

The BMAT

Cambridge, Imperial, Oxford, and UCL require applicants to have completed the Biomedical Admissions Test (BMAT). The BMAT is produced by the Cambridge Assessment Group and consists of three sections. The following pages describe the structure and format of each section, the qualities they are testing for, and the approach you should take when answering them.

Section 1: Aptitude and skills

35 questions—multiple choice or short answer questions

60 minutes—1 minute 40 seconds per question

Section 1: Aptitude and skills

According to the specification, this section of the BMAT aims to test generic skills that will be used as an undergraduate medical student. These are:

- Problem solving This refers to encoding and processing numerical information into simple numerical and algebraic operations in order to solve problems. Around 13 marks are available for your ability to select relevant information, recognize analogous cases, and apply appropriate procedures.
- Understanding argument A series of logical arguments are presented that require the candidate to reason, make assumptions, and form appropriate conclusions. There are ten marks available for these questions.
- Data analysis and inference You will need to interpret and reach appropriate conclusions from verbal, statistical, and graphical information. There are 12 marks available for these questions.

Drawing diagrams can help you to answer these questions and often single letters can be used to represent different names/groups. You must also be able to manipulate integers and fractions easily. You are unlikely to be able to solve all the questions in your head and a single question often needs extensive jottings on scrap paper. There are four sample questions on p. 324 for this section, which you should aim to complete within seven minutes. The answers can be found on p. 329.

Section 2: Scientific knowledge and applications

27 questions—multiple choice or short answer questions

30 minutes split between biology (6–8 questions), chemistry (6–8 questions), physics (6–8 questions), and maths (5–7 questions)—just over 1 minute per question

Section 2: Scientific knowledge and applications

The designers of the BMAT have created this section to test whether candidates have the core biomedical sciences knowledge necessary for studying medicine, as well as the capacity to apply their understanding. The material is restricted to that normally included in non-specialist school science and mathematics courses, i.e. equivalent to (dual award) science and mathematics at GCSE.

Many students become obsessed with revising GCSE material for section 2 of the BMAT. While the questions are based on GCSE science and maths, the GCSE content is used as a basis for multiple choice questions that test the *application* of knowledge and quick thinking. You only have a minute for each question in section 2 so it is important to remember that you will face time pressure.

Drawing diagrams, especially when faced with dense descriptive passages, will often help you towards the correct answer. There are four sample questions on p. 326 for this section, which you should aim to complete within four minutes. The answers can be found on p. 332.

Section 3: Writing task

Answer 1 question out of 4—answer to be handwritten on a single page of A4

30 minutes—including any planning time

No dictionaries or reference books allowed

Section 3: Writing task

For this section you have half an hour to answer one from a choice of four questions. The questions will be based on topics of general, medical, or scientific interest. They are often preceded by a short proposition, such as a famous quote or theoretical hypothesis. You will then be asked to consider the argument that has been proposed, as well as its implications, propose your own counter-argument, and/or resolve the conflict raised by the proposition.

You are limited to a single side of A4; therefore selection and organization of your ideas is critical. You should spend at least five minutes planning your essay (up to 20% of marks are given for organization and structure of the essay). That will leave you with 22 minutes to translate this plan into a concise and accurate piece of written work, leaving three minutes spare to read it through and correct any mistakes.

Outside knowledge is necessary to complete the BMAT essay since you will need to provide examples from real life to illustrate the points you make, i.e. historical or current events. It is difficult to prepare, other than by writing practice essays in the proper format (i.e. limiting yourself to 30 minutes and one side of A4, handwritten). You could also try learning a few common ethical dilemmas (see also p. 274) and the merits and pitfalls of science, law, and the arts. BMAT essay titles almost always require examples from science and/or medicine, so preparation for your medical school application should be sufficient for this essay.

There are three sample questions on p. 328 for this section; you should aim to answer one on a single side of A4 within 30 minutes. Advice can be found on p. 333.

Choosing a medical school

Chapter 7

Choosing a medical school

The medical school

Once you have decided to become a doctor, the next big decision you have to make is where to study. The years spent at medical school will be some of the most important of your life as you acquire the necessary skills and knowledge and develop professionally to be a doctor. The choice of medical school also greatly affects your chances of getting an offer to study medicine. You need to select medical schools that match your individual academic and non-academic skills.

This chapter will take you through what you need to consider about the medical school, including course type (p. 88), university type (p. 89), how difficult each medical school is to get into (p. 91), your own personality (p. 92), teaching styles (p. 94), medical school league tables (p. 98), and where to find further information (p. 104). The next chapter shows details of every undergraduate medical school in the UK (p. 107).

Factors to consider about the medical school

If you want to become a doctor, the medical school you choose is unlikely to affect your career path. Your focus should be on finding a medical school that will accept you. Start by making a shortlist based on the following:

- **Basic eligibility criteria** You need to check basic admissions criteria for the university and course for which you are applying. This includes age, nationality, GCSE grades, AS/A-level subjects, and health and criminal record checks. If you are in any doubt about whether you meet their criteria, check with the admissions office before applying. See p. 108.
- **Competition** It is hard to know how you compare with the other medical school applicants; however, it is worth considering how competitive the different courses are so that you always include a 'safe bet'. See p. 91 for competitiveness.
- **Types of course** These can be divided into problem-based learning (PBL), integrated, and traditional (Table 7.1). It is worth bearing in mind that elements of PBL are increasingly being incorporated into all types of course. Similarly, don't expect to avoid scientific theory in PBL courses—you will need a minimum amount to become a safe and competent doctor. See p. 94.
- **University** The geography of the university/medical school will either be campus, city-based, or collegiate. See Table 7.2.
- **Intercalated degree** Consider the chance to obtain an additional degree during your medical studies—see p. 87.
- **Reputation** This is difficult to define and less important for most medical careers than for other careers (although see p. 103). Generally universities with medical schools have strong reputations; furthermore they all receive a stamp of approval from the GMC (p. 278), which guarantees high standards of education. For the very small minority of high fliers who may benefit from attending an internationally renowned medical school, the league tables on p. 98 are worth considering. Everyone else should concentrate on finding a medical school that fits them, rather than listening to hearsay.

The intercalated degree

In addition to a medical degree, most undergraduate courses offer the chance to complete an additional degree (often a Bachelor of Science or BSc). These last an additional year and provide an opportunity for you to research another subject that you are interested in. It is worth considering whether you want to pursue an intercalated degree when making your list of possible medical schools.

Advantages The degree is a great chance to explore an area in which you might want to specialize later in your career. It also provides an opportunity to become involved in original research and earn CV points, especially if your project leads to a conference presentation or publication. With increasing numbers of medical students taking intercalated degrees, there is an increasing need to have one if you are applying for the more competitive medical specialities. There are also many transferable skills to be gained, such as learning to critically appraise research literature. It also provides a pleasant break from the dictatorial routine of medicine, providing a more self-directed learning experience.

Disadvantages It is worth remembering that, whatever you spend your time studying, it is unlikely to be relevant to general medical practice. This is because most research projects are very specialized. If you attempt a research project, most students fail to come away with publishable data during their limited laboratory time. A degree will also delay you from paid employment by one additional year (as well as adding an additional year of costs).

Choice Intercalated degrees are offered as an option at all UK medical schools (except for graduate students) but the following universities have a compulsory intercalated degree year: Cambridge (p. 118), Imperial (p. 138), Oxford (p. 152), St Andrews (p. 176), and UCL (p. 144). Nottingham (p. 150) includes a BMedSci qualification within their five-year course and without requiring an additional year of study. Other medical schools only permit students to intercalate based on their academic performance during the core medical degree. See individual medical school profiles (p. 107) for details.

A student's experience...

The year I spent studying for a BSc in pharmacology was divided between lectures and laboratory time. These lectures were different from those in medicine as we were expected to familiarize ourselves with important relevant developments in the scientific literature. In the second half of the year I worked full-time in a lab, using a special type of microscope to assess the structural composition of a protein. The majority of this time was spent on long, repetitive, and often fruitless procedures. However, hours of work were rewarded by publishing in a good biochemistry journal. After passing my exams at the end of the year, I was successfully awarded a BSc.

Key points www.intercalate.co.uk has good up-to-date information on most of the intercalated degrees offered across the UK. It also specifies whether the courses are available for external candidates, should you wish to consider conducting an intercalated BSc at a different university (though this is uncommon).

Types of course

Use Table 7.1 to help you decide which type of course would suit you best.

Table 7.1 Types of course offered by UK medical schools

Course	Problem-based learning (PBL)
Description	Students meet their weekly learning objectives by working in teams to solve a clinical scenario, e.g. management of a 72-year-old male with poorly controlled diabetes in the community. Each student's findings are presented to the facilitator and the rest of the group at the end of the week.
Pros	• Large element of teamwork and encourages problem solving, both of which are required daily by doctors. • Develop lifelong skills of self-directed learning. • Engaging and 100% clinically relevant from day one. • Early clinical exposure to supplement the problems presented.
Cons	• A less established technique subject to the criticisms of some older doctors. • Less standardized teaching and the experience is highly dependent on the quality of the non-medical facilitator. • May have large gaps in scientific understanding.

Course	Integrated
Description	Lectures on systems of the body (their normal function and aberrations in disease) are integrated with clinical attachments.
Pros	• Good relevant scientific understanding delivered at the appropriate stage. • Early clinical exposure.
Cons	• Early clinical exposure may unnerve those who prefer grasping all the theory before facing patients. • Still receiving lectures in the final years of the course. • Lack of depth in theory may frustrate those favouring scientific detail.

Course	Traditional
Description	Pure sciences are taught in the first half (the pre-clinical course), followed by hospital/GP attachments in the clinical half of the course.
Pros	• Best understanding of the theoretical science underpinning medicine. • Clinical exposure only after a substantial knowledge base has been built.
Cons	• Out of touch with *real* medicine during pre-clinical time. • Less clinical exposure in total. • Hours spent learning unnecessary scientific detail that is often quickly forgotten after exams. • Clinically relevant details can be lost in the ocean of facts.

Types of university

Use Table 7.2 to help you decide which type of university appeals to you.

Table 7.2 Different types of university

University	Campus
Description	The students live and work in a fairly self-contained area, separate from the local town/city.
Pros	• Sense of community between students. • Very student-orientated services/facilities; cheap and convenient.
Cons	• Students everywhere! • Quite artificial and distant from the 'real world'.

University	City
Description	The university buildings are dispersed throughout a town/city.
Pros	• The experience of living within a real town/city. • The benefits of the local facilities of a town/city.
Cons	• Can be expensive. • Living arrangements and travel to work can be impractical. • May live far away from other students on your course.

University	Collegiate
Description	Independent colleges that are dispersed throughout a town/city providing catering, accommodation, social, and welfare services. Members of different colleges are brought together in practical laboratories, lecture theatres, and GP practices/hospitals.
Pros	• Close contact with non-medical students. • Wealthy institutions that can often provide additional financial support (although very variable).
Cons	• Often provide additional regulations, e.g. mandatory minimum attendance for evening dinner; college fees for international students, etc. • Little interaction between colleges—lack of central Students' Union/bar, hence poorer sense of university spirit.

An insider's view...

It's impossible to appreciate the different types of university until you've spent at least a day exploring each one with someone familiar with the area. Open days are ideal for this and you should avoid making any decisions about which medical schools to apply to until you have had a good look around.

Summary of medical schools

Table 7.3 shows the key details of each undergraduate medical school in the UK for quick comparison. The full details of each medical school are shown in the next chapter (p. 107). See also Table 11.2 for graduate entry courses on p. 227.

Table 7.3 Summary of undergraduate medical schools in the UK

Medical school	Type[1]	Grade[2]	BSc	Location	Length (years)
Aberdeen	Stone	AAA	BSc	Campus	5
Barts	Carbon fibre	AAAb	BMedSci, BSc	City/campus	5
Birmingham	Red brick	A*AA–AAA	BMedSci	Campus	5
Brighton and Sussex	Plate glass	AAA–A*AB	BSc	Campus	5
Bristol	Red brick	AAA	BSc, BA	Campus	5
Cambridge	Stone	A*AA	BA[3]	Collegiate	6
Cardiff	Red brick	AAAc	BSc	Campus	5
Charles, Prague	Stone	Exam	Not available	City	6
Dundee	Red brick	AAA	BMSc	Campus	5
Durham	Plate glass	AAA	BA, BSc	Collegiate	5
Edinburgh	Stone	AAAb	BSc, BMedSci	Campus	5
Glasgow	Carbon fibre	AAA	BSc	Campus	5
Exeter	Carbon fibre	A*AA–AAA	BA, BSc	Campus	5
Hull York	Carbon fibre	AAAb	BSc, MSc	Split campus	5
Imperial College	Stone	AAAb–AAAC	BSc[3]	City	6
Keele	Carbon fibre	A*ABb–AAAb	MMedsci	Campus	5
King's College	Red brick	AAAb	BSc	City/campus	5
Lancaster	Carbon fibre	AAA	BSc, MSc	Campus	5
Leeds	Red brick	AAA	BA, BSc	Campus	5
Leicester	Plate glass	AAA	BSc, MA	Campus	5
Liverpool	Carbon fibre	AAAb	BSc, MSc	Campus	5
Manchester	Carbon fibre	AAA	BSc, MSc	Campus	5
Newcastle	Plate glass	AAA	BSc, MRes	City/campus	5
Nottingham	Red brick	AAA	BMedSci[3]	Campus	5
Oxford	Stone	A*AA	BA[3]	Collegiate	6
Plymouth	Carbon fibre	A*AA–AAA	BSc, MSc	Campus	5
Queen's, Belfast	Red brick	AAAa	BSc, MSc, MRes	Campus	5
Sheffield	Red brick	AAA	BMedSci	Campus	5
Southampton	Plate glass	AAA	BSc	Campus	5
St Andrews	Stone	AAA	BSc[3]	City	6
St George's	Plate glass	AAAb–BBCb[4]	BSc	City	5
UCL	Red brick	AAAc	BSc[3]	City	6
University of East Anglia	Carbon fibre	AAAb	BSc, MRes	Campus	5

[1] See p. 94 for descriptions; [2] AS-levels are indicated by a lowercase letter; [3] Compulsory intercalated degree; [4] If you are offering grades higher than BBC with a 'B' in your fourth AS, St George's will consider your application if this achievement is 60% higher than the average performance of your school/college—see website.

Competitiveness of medical schools

It is important to avoid applying only for the most competitive medical schools. The obvious number to consider is applicants per offer; however, this is not a complete picture. Prestige gives an idea of how sought after each place is; a lower score is more prestigious. The final score is subjective, based on considerations of the quality of applicants, required grades, and applicants per place. Table 7.4 ranks each school in the UK by competitiveness. See also Table 11.1 on p. 226 for graduate entry courses.

Table 7.4 Competitiveness of undergraduate medical schools in the UK, 2013

Medical school	Competition (applicants per offer)	Chance of interview (applicants per interview)	Success after interview (offers per interview)	Prestige (offers per place)	Competitiveness score
Oxford	9.5	3.5	2.8	1.0	5
Cambridge	5.6	1.0	5.6	1.0	5
Imperial	5.4	3.8	1.4	1.4	4
Edinburgh	7.6	N/A	N/A	1.5	4
Nottingham	7.2	3.7	2.0	1.5	4
St Andrews	5.8	2.1	2.7	1.5	4
UCL	4.5	3.6	1.3	1.7	4
Plymouth	8.9	3.9	2.3	1.4	3
Glasgow	5.0	3.2	1.6	1.4	3
Cardiff	6.0	3.0	2.0	1.5	3
Bristol	10.0	4.2	2.4	1.7	3
Southampton	8.6	N/A	N/A	1.7	3
Leeds	8.4	7.0	1.2	1.7	3
Manchester	4.0	2.7	1.5	1.7	3
St Georges	4.1	2.6	1.6	1.8	3
King's College London	5.5	3.3	1.7	2.0	3
Brighton and Sussex	10.9	5.6	2.0	1.7	2
East Anglia	5.1	2.5	2.0	1.8	2
Sheffield	2.3	1.7	1.4	1.8	2
Liverpool	5.5	3.0	1.8	1.9	2
Barts and The London	3.9	2.6	1.5	1.9	2
Queen's, Belfast	2.7	N/A	N/A	1.9	2
Aberdeen	6.7	3.9	1.7	2.0	2
Dundee	6.0	3.0	2.0	2.0	2
Newcastle	4.6	2.1	2.2	2.0	2
Keele	6.6	3.7	1.8	2.2	2
Birmingham	3.4	2.6	1.3	2.3	2
Hull York	3.7	2.3	1.6	2.1	1
Durham	2.5	1.8	1.4	2.1	1
Leicester	6.3	2.2	2.8	2.2	1
Lancaster	4.6	3.1	1.5	2.2	1

The applicant

Once you've made your shortlist of possible medical schools (p. 86), it's time to be introspective to identify the courses that suit your own talents, learning style, personality, and circumstances.

Factors to consider about you

Teaching/learning styles Choose a type of course (p. 88) that suits your preferences, skills, and CV. If you have a particular penchant for molecular sciences, a traditional course will probably suit you best. If you cannot wait to have your first exposure to clinical medicine, an integrated course may be what you're looking for. Or if you would prefer self-directed learning, group work, and seminars over lectures, a PBL course might suit you better.

Equally, look at what you can realistically achieve. If interpersonal skills are your strength, you might be more successful on a modern, clinically focused course. If you're a closet scientist or enjoy rote learning, a traditional course might be better suited to your particular talents. There is always a mix of teaching styles so you cannot avoid a particular one in its entirety, but the emphasis does vary between courses. Take the time to find the most suitable mix for you.

Competition Use objective measures (e.g. your grades, practice admission test results) and subjective judgements (e.g. teacher's advice, amount of preparation) to estimate your relative strength as an applicant. Table 7.4 on p. 91 estimates how competitive each medical school is; try to apply to those appropriate to your estimation of your abilities, but remember that it is sensible to choose one of the less competitive schools too.

Assessment methods A variety of assessment strategies are used by most courses, including vivas (oral exams), multiple choice questions, extended matching questions, short answer papers, and essay papers (p. 210). Some courses involve exams at the end of every module while others hold them at the end of each year. Again, play to your strengths. Make sure you ask at the open days which methods are used as this may change from year to year (also see p. 107).

University life Do you enjoy the busy city life or would you prefer a more peaceful suburban environment? If you are moving away from one extreme, think carefully about this. Stay with a friend or relative for a few days—you never know what will make you love or hate a new place until you've experienced it properly. Birdsong at 6am or crowded underground trains might make this decision for you.

An insider's view...

The most successful applicants are usually those who have applied to a medical school that suits them. Anyone who has read a prospectus can describe the layout of first-year accommodation and a quick Google search will bring up a university's international ranking for that year. What is more persuasive in a medical school application is for the applicant to describe what makes them uniquely suited to that particular medical school.

Hobbies and interests If you have a specific interest outside of medicine (e.g. you play a sport competitively) it may be worth looking at what facilities/opportunities the specific university can offer. Use the Students' Union website of each university as a starting point for more information.

Distance from home This is important for many people and you should consider the practicalities of travel. You need to strike a balance between living an independent life and having your family near enough for support (and potentially clothes washing or food packets...). A common approach is to draw two circles around your home town, one for too near and one for too far.

Costs Given standardized tuition fees, the cost of education will not vary between medical schools unless you are a Scottish, Welsh, or international student (see p. 15). Other costs can vary greatly depending on where you choose to live. In general, London is extremely expensive and the further you travel away from London the cheaper the cost of living is. There are some notable exceptions to this rule, including Edinburgh.

The other key variable is your own frugality. It is easy for a student in Newcastle to spend far more than one in London if they are leading a life of relative extravagance. See p. 15 for estimates of living costs and the next chapter (p. 107) for the relative living costs at specific medical schools.

Future career Choosing a medical school for its expertise in a particular speciality requires unrealistic foresight. By the time you have finished medical school it is likely that your career aspirations will have changed dramatically as you discover more about each speciality.

Future life Most qualifying students tend to work close to the medical school at which they qualified. This is especially true for FY1/FY2 (p. 10) so consider whether you would be happy living in the surroundings of the medical school for the next seven years or more. Although there is nothing to stop you moving away upon qualifying, you are likely to stay put whilst you adjust to your new job.

Key points Once you graduate from medical school, you are free to move anywhere in the UK for work. The application process makes a point of ensuring that hospitals cannot pick and choose doctors who qualified locally. However, many graduates choose to stay in the same region for personal reasons—they know the hospitals and consultants and have made friends locally. For example, in 2008, 74% of Peninsula (now split into Exeter p. 122 and Plymouth p. 154) graduates chose to work at hospitals in the South West.

As the job application process is competitive, graduates of universities in popular locations may find themselves forced to move due to competition. These locations vary from year to year but often include London and Oxford.

A guide to decide

Armed with facts about medical schools (p. 86) and secure in the knowledge of your own strengths as a medical school applicant (p. 92), you are ready to narrow down your options. UCAS permits applications to four medical schools each year (p. 186). The following pages will help you identify the medical schools that suit you best and ease your decision-making process.

The choices

Each medical school has its own character and artificially grouping them inevitably leads to generalizations. For example, Liverpool and Manchester are often described as two of the six 'official' red brick universities but both teach a more modern PBL type of course. Durham lacks the traditional course style found at Oxbridge (p. 202) but is nevertheless divided into colleges (p. 208). With this in mind, use the following groupings as a *guide*, to help focus your attention on similar medical schools to the ones you have already shortlisted.

Carbon fibre Ultramodern PBL courses (p. 88). These are the Marmite of medical schools—you either love them or hate them: *Barts, Exeter, Keele, Glasgow, Lancaster, Liverpool, Manchester, Plymouth.*

Plate glass New, sensible, and made for the city, if somewhat commonplace. Campus- or city-based courses with a mixture of PBL and lectures include: *Brighton and Sussex, Durham, Hull York, Leicester, Newcastle, Southampton, St George's, UEA, Warwick.*

Red bricks These tried and tested courses are likely to feature in your application. Lecture-based city courses with early clinical exposure and minimal PBL include: *Birmingham, Bristol, Dundee, King's College London, Leeds, Nottingham, Queen's Belfast, Sheffield, UCL.*

Stone Established but a little stuffy; old academic (occasionally collegiate) courses with an emphasis on science: *Aberdeen, Cambridge, Edinburgh, Imperial, Oxford, Charles University Prague, St Andrews.*

> Key points You need to be cautious if your shortlist contains medical schools at opposite ends of the spectrum. If you are completely stuck, use the algorithm (Figure 7.1) as a starting point to identify the group of medical schools that you should focus your research on.

> Key points Applicants commonly ask: what is the best medical school? The bottom line is that your choice will not make a huge difference to your professional career. Your knowledge, skills, and attitudes will depend much more on the amount of time you invest in the course than the institution you attend. Regardless of your medical school, you will be as free as anyone else to pursue the speciality of your choice. Choose institutions because you would thrive there instead of perceived indicators of quality or status.

An algorithm for picking medical schools

While Figure 7.1 grossly simplifies a complex thought process, it should help to highlight some of the most important factors and the types of courses that embrace them. Medical schools have many subtle distinguishing factors so don't discount them until you have read more (p. 107).

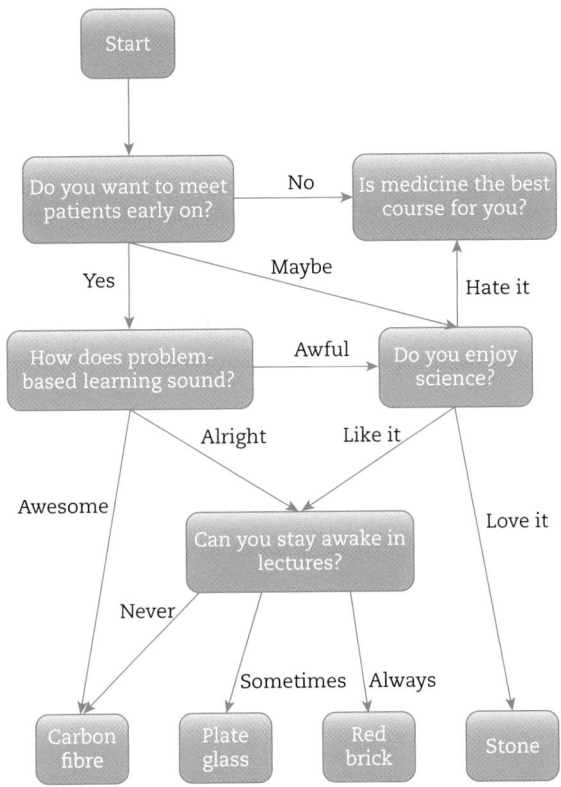

Figure 7.1 An algorithm for choosing a type of medical school.

A guide to decide cont...

Tailoring your application to the shortlist

The preparation doesn't stop once you have chosen four medical schools. You need to work through the appropriate medical school profiles (p. 107) to identify similarities and consider writing your personal statement (p. 192) to fit these specific schools' priorities.

Your four choices should ideally be similar types of course to allow such tailoring of your personal statement. If you've gone for the more traditional science-based teaching, you might want to write about how you've demonstrated an interest in science through learning more about a particular discovery.

Alternatively, if you are applying to PBL-based courses, you could describe an example from your work experience where a doctor discussed a management plan with their colleagues and researched additional options. In this way, you could draw parallels between the self-directed group learning of PBL and everyday clinical practice.

At this stage, it is worth writing some brief notes on the courses to which you are applying for interview purposes. These can be used to refresh your knowledge of the course when it comes to interview day (p. 262). This will help avoid the risk of discussing the prospect of an intercalated humanities degree at a university where this is not an option.

A student's experience...

A large proportion of my Cambridge interview was dedicated to discussing the research project I participated in during my summer holidays. Whilst this appeared successful at Cambridge, my attempt to replicate the conversation a few weeks later at Liverpool was less well received. Eventually we went on to talk about my part-time employment as a Health Care Assistant and the insights I had gained into the challenges of healthcare. This seemed to impress the panel far more! It became quite evident from this experience that different medical schools are not looking for identical qualities and experiences.

An insider's view...

We need to be satisfied that the candidates sitting before us will become safe and competent doctors and this can be achieved by applicants demonstrating a fairly generic set of skills. But we also have to consider the suitability of the candidate to the course that we offer. Assessing whether the medical school and the student are a personality fit is a more subjective decision that is based on our limited exposure to the applicant as they discuss their experiences and answer our questions.

Key points It is possible to write a personal statement (or answer an interview question) that is attractive to all types of medical schools, but having an idea of your target audience is an obvious advantage.

League tables

League tables must be approached with caution. Using medical school and university league tables is often fraught with difficulties because of conflicting results. Even when the popular league tables agree, be cautious in the way you use the information. The following pages discuss this oft-cited but poorly understood topic and include some important tables that you should consider.

How are rankings calculated? League tables use various criteria to reach their final scores. The following criteria are commonly used:

- **UCAS entry score** Average number of student UCAS points.
- **Student satisfaction** Scores based on students' views on teaching.
- **Quality of research** The Research Excellence Framework (REF) score, which rates departments based on academic research.
- **Staff** The expenditure on staff per student or the staff to student ratio.
- **Class of degree** The percentage of 2:1 and 1st class degrees conferred.
- **Employability** The likelihood of securing full-time employment after graduation. This is more applicable to university league tables, which include students studying non-medical degrees.

See p. 99 for a table summarizing the medical school rankings in 2013 from some of the most popular producers of league tables, including: *The Complete University Guide, The Guardian and The Times*. The tables on p. 100 and p. 102 show a detailed breakdown of the scoring for *The Guardian and The Complete University Guide* rankings respectively.

The ranking of universities is discussed more frequently than that of medical schools. University league tables look at all courses offered by a particular university, not just medicine, when assigning scores. The table on p. 99 shows the position of medical schools in both UK and international university rankings.

What really matters? While the rankings of medical schools are unlikely to affect the careers of most doctors, the teaching styles may have an impact. The figure on p. 103 shows the results of an interesting study that assessed performance in a Membership Exam taken after medical school (p. 8), which is required for medical graduates to proceed into a specialist training post. There are many reasons to question the findings, including medical school examination styles giving an unfair advantage, selection bias (i.e. the best applicants choose the more competitive courses), and changes in medical school teaching since the doctors qualified. Nevertheless, this study shows an apparent benefit from studying at Oxford, Cambridge, and Newcastle.

How should rankings be used? Whilst many people (including parents) look at medical schools in this way, you should not rely too heavily on league tables. Ask yourself how important a score for staff research is for assessing the quality of your education. Similarly, the number of 2:1/1st class degrees conferred by a university might not relate to high quality teaching. Whilst weaker applicants may want to avoid higher-ranking universities and stronger applicants may want to consider them, remember that you should use league tables in context, after considering everything else about each medical school.

Medical school rankings, 2013

Table 7.5 shows the rankings of undergraduate medical courses according to four of the most respected league tables—three national and one international.

Table 7.5 Rankings of UK medical schools from four sources

University	League table rankings for medicine			
	The Guardian University Guide 2013[1]	The Complete University Guide 2013[2]	The Times Good University Guide 2013	The QS World rankings, 2012–2013
Cambridge	1	1	2	2
Oxford	2	2	1	5
Edinburgh	3	3	3	21
UCL	4	4	4	26
Newcastle[3]	6	7	7	126
Aberdeen	9	6	5	162
Imperial College, London	11	5	6	6
Dundee	5	9	9	204
Queen Mary's, London	7	8	11	147
Hull York	10	11	10	110
Plymouth	12	13	14	—
Leicester	7	17	17	185
Leeds	14	14	13	94
Sheffield	18	12	12	66
Birmingham	23	10	16	77
King's College, London	16	19	18	26
St Andrews	16	30	8	93
Warwick	13	18	24	58
Nottingham	15	21	20	72
Manchester	19	15	22	32
Southampton	22	23	18	73
Bristol	26	16	25	28
Queen's, Belfast	27	22	23	166
Brighton and Sussex	20	29	26	188
Liverpool	25	24	27	124
East Anglia	21	26	30	236
Glasgow	28	28	21	54
Cardiff	29	20	28	143
Keele	24	27	31	—
St George's, London	30	25	29	—
Lancaster	—	—	—	163

[1] Table 7.6 shows the breakdown from which *The Guardian* ranks were obtained.
[2] Table 7.7 shows the breakdown from which *The Complete University Guide* ranks were obtained.
[3] Note that Durham is not listed separately; use Newcastle figures as a guide.

The Guardian University Guide: league table for medicine, 2013

The medical school rankings are based on objective scores; however, the relative weight of each component (e.g. is student satisfaction more important than research quality?) is open to interpretation. See Table 7.6.

Table 7.6 Breakdown of *The Guardian* 2013 ranking of UK medical schools

University	Guardian score[1] (/100)	Satisfied with course[2] (%)	Satisfied with teaching[3] (%)	Satisfied with feedback[4] (%)	Student:-staff ratio[5]	Spend per student[6] (/10)	Average entry tariff[7]	Value-added score[8]/10	Career after 6 mths[9]
Cambridge	100	94	93	69	5.8	10	630	2	98
Oxford	91.1	99	99	86	7.8		611	2	99
Edinburgh	80.2	92	94	35	5.9	10	577	2	100
UCL	75.9	96	93	57	5.2	7	554	7	99
Dundee	74.8	92	94	52	6.7	10	535		99
Newcastle[1,10]	65.2	94	95	62	7.9	5	528	7	100
Leicester	64.4	95	93	57	6.2	5	505	6	100
Queen Mary	64.4	94	93	66	8.6	6	496	9	100
Aberdeen	64.2	98	95	68	8.4	4	533	5	99
Hull York	63.6	90	92	56	5.6	4	514		99
Imperial College	62.3	93	91	49	7.3	6	556	1	100
Peninsula	60.6	92	92	61	8.3	7	500		99
Warwick	55.1	85	91	44	8.3	8		7	100
Leeds	54.2	96	95	63	8.2	4	494	4	100
Nottingham	53.6	89	92	43	6.7	3	517	8	100
King's College, London	48.9	76	84	27	5.1	7	502	4	100

University	Guardian score/100[1]	% satisfied with course[2]	Teaching quality score[3]	Feedback score[4]	Staff–student ratio[5]	Spend[6]	Average entry tariff[7]	Value-added score/10[8]	Career score[9]
St Andrews	48.9	94	98	53	12	3	536	4	96
Sheffield	45.8	92	92	60	9	3	509	2	100
Manchester	45.4	69	81	39	8.6	8	500	9	100
Brighton and Sussex	43.8	94	95	54	11.4	4	469		99
UEA	42.7	80	89	52	7.8	3	453		100
Southampton	42.6	88	88	51	9	3	469	9	100
Birmingham	41.7	84	87	35	9.2	3	534	5	100
Keele	41.2	87	93	57	9.2	2	464		100
Liverpool	38.1	71	78	33	8.3	6	484	8	100
Bristol	37.3	81	90	38	11.5	5	508	6	100
Queen's, Belfast	34.8	75	86	40	9.9	3	506		100
Glasgow	34.7	64	80	33	8.7	4	517	4	99
Cardiff	34.5	69	81	29	9.6	4	520	7	100
St George's, London	27.2	84	89	49	14.9	5	459	7	99
Lancaster	—	—	—	—	—	—	—	—	—

[1] The *Guardian* score/100 is an exclusive rating of excellence based on a combination of all the other factors. [2] Course satisfaction is the percentage of final-year students satisfied with overall quality, based on the National Student Survey (NSS). [3] The teaching quality score is the percentage of final-year students satisfied with the teaching they received, based on the NSS. [4] The feedback score is the percentage of final-years satisfied with feedback and assessment by lecturers, based on the NSS. [5] Staff–student ratio is the number of students per member of teaching staff. [6] Spend is the amount of money spent on each student, given as a rating out of 10. [7] Average entry tariff means the typical UCAS scores of students currently studying in that department. [8] The value-added score compares students' individual degree results with their entry qualifications, to show how effective the teaching is, given as a rating out of 10. [9] The career score is the percentage of graduates who find graduate-level jobs, or are studying further, within six months of graduation. [10] Note that Durham is not listed separately; use Newcastle figures as a guide.

Copyright Guardian News & Media 2012.

The Complete University Guide rankings for medicine, 2013

The medical school rankings for *The Complete University Guide 2013* are shown in Table 7.7.

Table 7.7 Breakdown of *The Complete University Guide 2013* ranking of medical schools

University	Student satisfaction (/5)	Entry standards (UCAS tariff)	Research assessment (/4)	Graduate prospects (/100)	Overall score (/100)
Cambridge	4.2	630	3.14	100	100
Oxford	4.6	611	3.03	100	99.8
Edinburgh	3.8	577	2.98	100	97.8
UCL	4	554	2.91	100	97.3
Imperial College, London	3.9	556	2.91	100	97.1
Aberdeen	4.2	539	2.86	100	97.1
Newcastle	4.2	528	2.67	100	96.3
Queen Mary	4.2	496	2.93	100	96
Dundee	3.9	535	2.56	100	95.8
Birmingham	3.6	534	2.65	100	95.6
Hull York	3.9	514	2.68	100	95.5
Sheffield	4	509	2.57	100	95.2
Plymouth	4.1	500	2.56	100	95.1
Leeds	4	494	2.63	100	95.1
Manchester	3.5	500	2.81	100	95
Bristol	3.6	508	2.69	100	95
Leicester	4.1	505	2.46	100	95
Warwick[1]	3.7	—	2.53	100	94.9
King"s College, London	3.5	502	2.7	100	94.7
Cardiff	3.5	520	2.51	100	94.6
Nottingham	3.8	517	2.29	100	94.5
Queen's, Belfast	3.6	506	2.47	100	94.5
Southampton	3.9	469	2.7	100	94.4
Liverpool	3.5	484	2.58	100	94
St George's	3.8	459	2.38	100	93.2
East Anglia	3.9	454	2.38	100	93.2
Keele	3.9	464	2.1	100	92.8
Glasgow	3.5	517	2.64	99	92.6
Brighton and Sussex	4	469	2.2	99	91
St Andrews	4.2	536	2.3	98	90.8
Lancaster[2]	—	—	—	—	—

[1]Warwick is a graduate medical school and a UCAS tariff calculated for school-leavers was not included. [2]Lancaster medical school began taking medical students in September 2013, and no data were available for *The Complete University Guide 2013*.

Reproduced with permission from The Complete University Guide 2013.

Performance after medical school

Figure 7.2 shows the performance of graduates by medical school in exams essential for training in a speciality (p. 8). See p. 98 for more details of this study.

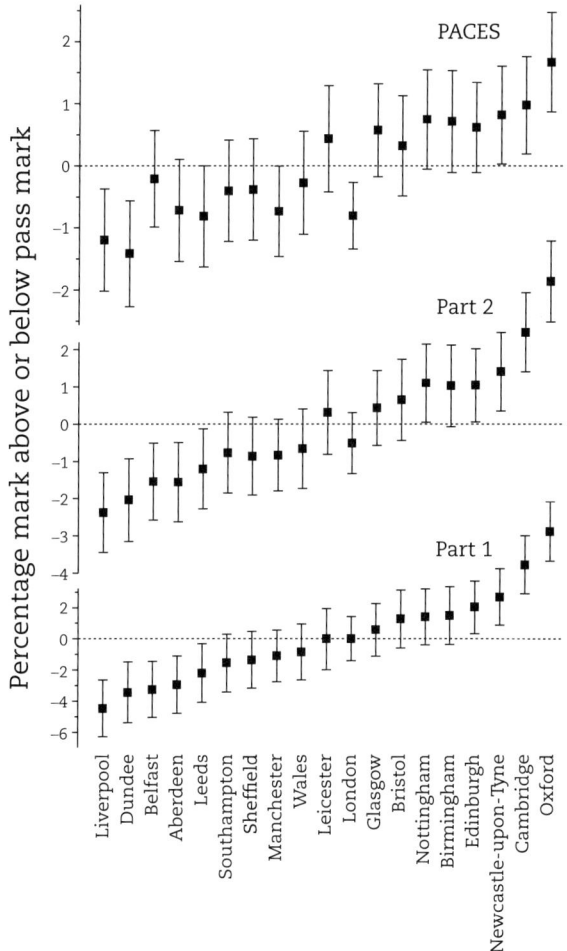

Figure 7.2 Medical schools' effects for Part 1, Part 2, and PACES exams of MRCP(UK). For all three parts of the examination, medical schools are sorted by the size of the effect at Part 1 examination. Error bars indicate ± 1 standard deviation. Note that the absolute values are different for the three examinations

Figure 7.2 is taken from the article by IC McManus, Andrew Elder, Andre de Champlain, Jane Dacre, Jennifer Mollon, and Liliana Chis. Graduates of different UK medical schools show substantial differences in performance on MRCP(UK) Part 1, Part 2, and PACES examinations. BMC Medicine 2008, 6:5. © BioMed Central Ltd.

How to find out more

There are many factors that determine whether a particular medical school makes your shortlist (p. 86). Some of these are easy questions with easy answers such as basic eligibility criteria. But a lot of what you are looking for is more subjective—you are, after all, searching for the ideal medical school *for you*. Making this decision requires good resources and the right questions.

Visiting Unless distance makes travelling impractical, there is no excuse for not visiting the university at least once before you apply. Otherwise it is difficult to make an informed decision as to whether each university justifies a space on your UCAS form.

It is worth contacting university admissions offices or checking their websites in advance to find out practical details such as when the medical school is open and parking arrangements. If you are travelling by public transport, plan the route in advance to avoid wasting time on the wrong bus out of town. Note that some medical schools may not be where you expect them to be (e.g. Warwick is in Coventry and Durham is in Stockton-on-Tees) so it is well worth checking exactly where they are found before setting off. Occasionally universities provide guest rooms that you can book if you decide to stop overnight.

Some medical schools restrict access, which is why you are best visiting on an open day. If you've missed it, ask a friend who studied there or get a contact from your sixth-form college. A friendly medical student might be willing to give you a guided tour if you ask nicely.

Gauging the atmosphere Visiting the medical school and attending the open day is the best way to appreciate the character of the medical school. Is it a team-spirited environment or a constant battle of wits? Were the staff open and approachable or cold and distant? There are more similarities than differences between medical schools but you will often develop a 'feeling' for each institution's ethos when visiting. Speak to as many different students as possible to judge for yourself whether you would fit in. Remember that medical schools like to impress candidates at open days, and so if you have reservations on the day, things may be even worse in reality.

The open day Open days are organized by medical schools and provide an opportunity to talk to students, tutors, course organizers, and other applicants.

Your first priority should be finding the date of the next open day for medical schools you are interested in. Telephone the admissions office to verify the date and time of the open day and to confirm your place. Book early as there is often a limited number of spaces available.

Remember to dress and act appropriately whilst visiting the medical school. Open days are not interviews but potential interviewers may be in attendance and you don't want to be remembered for the wrong reasons.

> **Key points** Try not to be influenced by the weather. The campus might look green and beautiful in the middle of June but it will rain there sometimes as well. Environment is important but try not to fall into the trap of 'sunny = good, raining = bad'.

What to ask This is your golden opportunity to clarify discrepancies between information sources and reassure yourself about admissions criteria. Speak to as many people as possible and, if you get on especially well with someone, ask for their email address. Fellow applicants are a good source of support and might be your medical student colleagues in 12 months' time. Questions you may wish to consider asking current medical students include:

- What's a typical day like for you? (NB this will differ between years.)
- How much contact do you have with your tutors?
- What is the pastoral support like for students?
- How much clinical exposure do you get in the first two years?
- What are the facilities like for ...?
- How expensive is it to live in this area?
- How many students passed/failed their exams in your year?
- Where do people live in different years?
- Is it a safe, student-friendly area?
- What was your interview process like?
- Would you apply here again? Why/why not?

Other sources There is very little that a successful open day or friendly telephone call will not be able to answer. But should you experience any difficulties try the following:

- Obtain a copy of the prospectus from a careers fair, open day, admissions office, or via the university website (see p. 107).
- Use the Students' Union/JCR websites for 'unofficial' prospectuses that are often written by students and offer a more informal perspective.
- Utilize contacts acquired from the open day/personal visit.
- Ask your high school for details of successful applicants from previous years and contact them. Social networking sites are a good place to begin.
- Compare notes with colleagues at school who are considering applying for the same course.
- Search the internet for the MedSoc student committee and drop them an email asking for advice. Or try online forums (p. 338) but take everything you read with an extra large pinch of salt.

Key points If all else fails, pay another visit to the university and approach a friendly student around the library or cafeteria. If they can't help, they should be able to point you in the direction of someone who can.

Undergraduate medical schools

Chapter 8

Undergraduate medical schools

Understanding the profiles

Since choosing the right medical school is so important to winning a place (p. 85), the following pages give detailed descriptions of every medical school in the UK. Separate profiles are available for graduate entry courses (p. 228); graduates on standard courses may face different entry requirements (including admission tests). Foundation and access courses follow the same pattern after the first year as described here, although entrance requirements will be different.

The writers To ensure the most accurate information, the profiles have been written in collaboration with one or two medical student representatives from each medical school (see p. ix). A senior member of the admissions team or medical school faculty was also asked to describe what makes their medical school unique and what types of students they are looking for.

Warning!

While every possible step has been taken to ensure the accuracy of this information (including multiple reviews by the admissions teams at each medical school), errors may persist. Furthermore, medical schools are continually striving to improve their courses and methods of picking the best students, so the details may change from year to year. Before you make an important decision based on this information, check the medical school website or contact its admissions team. Double-checking is a good principle to follow when working in the NHS too!

Key to the profiles

To make it simple to compare medical schools the profiles have been written in a consistent format:

University This section gives a broad overview of the structure of the university and how it relates to the medical school and describes some of the facilities available to medical students.

Course Teaching and clinical exposure vary widely between different courses (p. 88). This section outlines the structure of each course, how different stages are taught, and some of the options that students can select.

Lifestyle There is far more to medical school than studying, so this section describes some of the options available for life outside the classroom.

Factoid An interesting snippet or little known fact about the city, university, or course.

Entrance requirements

There is no point in applying to a medical school when you do not meet basic requirements; always check these before submitting your UCAS form. Also bear in mind that:
• Medical school websites offer extensive details on alternative entrance requirements such as Scottish Highers and the International Baccalaureate.
• Not all A-levels are created equal; some combinations will not be accepted (p. 20).

Table 8.1 This sample profile explains the criteria we have collated for each school

Myth	A popular myth about each medical school…
Reality	…and the reality according to the locals
Personality	Personality traits commonly found at each medical school
Best aspects	Why studying there is better than sliced bread
Worst aspects	Why studying there can make your blood boil
Requirements	Admission test, A-level, and GCSE requirements (please take the warning on p. 108 into account)

Course length	Total length of course	Structure	Campus, City, or Collegiate (p. 89)
Type of course	Carbon fibre, Plate glass, Red brick, or Stone (p. 94)	Year size	Medical students per year group
Typical offer	Required A-level grades (AS-levels indicated by lowercase)	Intercalated degree:	Extra degrees available (p. 87)
Applicants	Number of applicants	Student mix:	Proportion of mature (>21 years old) and international students in a year group
Interviews	Number interviewed	% Mature	
Offers	Number given offers (p. 91)	% International	

Competition	All medical courses are highly competitive; this subjective scale aims to highlight how they compare to other medical schools
Living costs	A subjective rating of living costs
Work	All medical courses have packed timetables and intense workloads (expect at least 40 hours/week); this subjective scale aims to highlight how much additional free time you might get compared to other medical schools

Insider's view…

The inside scoop on what the medical school is looking for during the admissions process written by a senior member of the admissions team or medical school faculty.

England

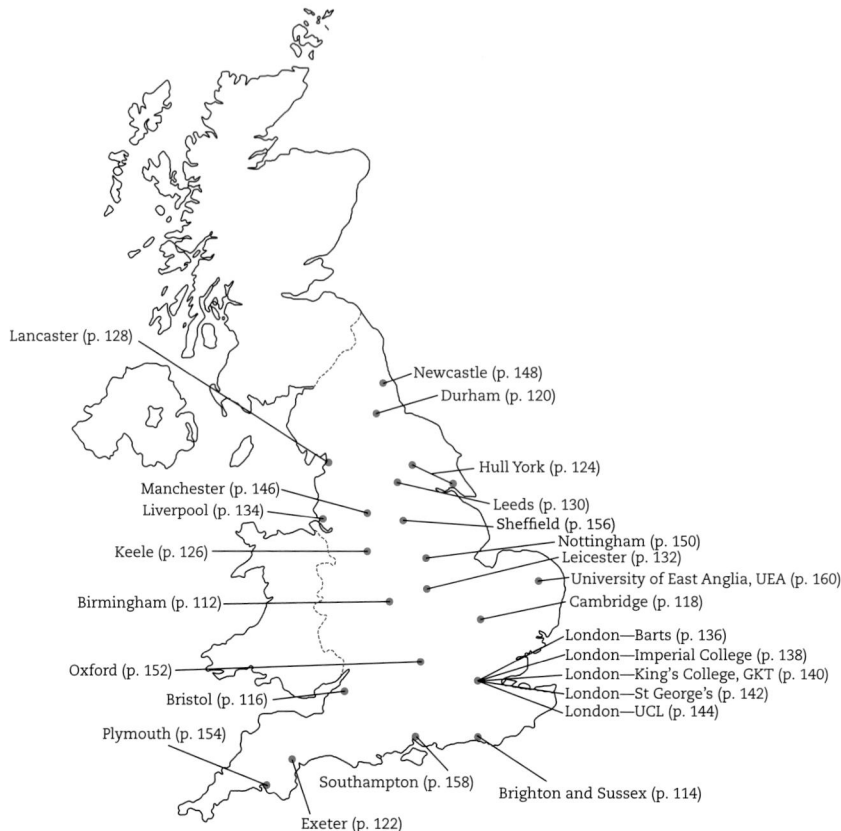

Figure 8.1 Undergraduate medical schools in England

Birmingham

Although the medical school at Birmingham University is over 100 years old, the course and facilities are cutting edge. As the home of five Nobel laureates there is a strong tradition of research that pervades the medical school. Studying at Birmingham makes for a fantastic educational and cultural experience.

University Birmingham has a vast medical school situated on the Edgbaston campus, around a 20 minute bus journey from the city centre. The new Queen Elizabeth teaching hospital is right next to the medical school and is one of 15 hospitals throughout the West Midlands that are used as clinical placements. The wide diversity of patients guarantees Birmingham students meet a broad cross-section of the population and see a plethora of medical problems. There are good public transport links and many trusts have free 'shuttles' between their hospitals; travelling to placements is rarely an issue. Birmingham students can also benefit from their local rail service, as this is the only university in the UK to have its own station!

Course The integrated course incorporates clinical exposure from the first term. The first two years (pre-clinical) are focused on the core sciences. A typical pre-clinical week would consist of four days at medical school in lectures and small group tutorials. Anatomy teaching benefits from a newly refurbished prosectorium, which contains ten ventilated tables and individual flat screens for displaying X-ray and MRI scans. New students will also benefit from improved library and computer facilities. In the pre-clinical years, you receive GP teaching once a fortnight, where you can observe consultations, receive basic clinical teaching, and cover some clinical skills. The clinical years are mainly hospital-based, with a fortnightly GP attachment and occasional lecture at the medical school. Specialist rotations begin in the fourth year, at which point the group sizes get much smaller. A recent development in the course structure has dramatically reduced the number of placements in the final two years which enables students to spend less time changing hospitals and more time integrating with clinical teams. With such renowned research facilities within the medical school, such as the Institute for Cancer Studies, many students choose to intercalate—an option that is available at any stage after your second year. There are a wide range of subjects on offer apart from the usual biomedical and clinical sciences subjects, such as 'international health' and 'history of medicine'. Should you have a burning desire to study a course not offered here, Birmingham Medical School will also allow its students to go to other universities for this year.

Lifestyle There are various catered and self-catering options for first-year campus accommodation, including rooms near the medical school on the Edgbaston campus. This campus is set within 250 acres of stunning parkland, benefiting from its own shops, bars, banks, and even an art gallery!

In the unlikely event that the highly active MedSoc fails to keep you entertained, you're within easy reach of the city's highlights: the Bullring shopping centre (Europe's biggest), four bustling indoor and outdoor markets, hundreds of restaurants offering a range of international cuisine, and of course Broad Street, home to many pubs, bars, and one of the largest and most popular nightclubs around, Gatecrasher. Huge stars regularly perform at the nearby NEC and NIA or, if you prefer something quieter, the Symphony Hall is one of Europe's finest concert halls. Is it any wonder that over 40% of Birmingham students choose to stay here after their studies?

Factoid Janet Parker, the last person in the world to die of smallpox in 1978, contracted the disease while working as a medical photographer in the anatomy department at Birmingham Medical School. See Table 8.2.

Table 8.2 Birmingham

Myth	Old, overcrowded, and lost in a second-rate city
Reality	Successful medics who thrive in one of the greatest places to be
Personality	Sociable, outgoing city people
Best aspects	Lifestyle; the UK's second-largest city offers as much as London, but with fewer crowds and less expense; you will NOT be bored
Worst aspects	Some West Midlands placements are a long way to travel
Requirements	**No admissions test**; **A-level** three A2s including chemistry and biology (or human biology); **GCSE** preference given to applicants offering A* grades in mathematics, English and science subjects, with overall GCSE performance also considered

Course length	5 years	Structure	Campus
Type of course	Red brick (p. 94)	Year size	345
Typical offer	A*AA	Intercalated degree:	BMedSci
Applicants	2736	Student mix:	
Interviews	1069	% Mature	3%
Offers	805	% International	8%

Uncompetitive	🏆🏆🏆🏆🏆	Competitive
Low living costs	💰💰💰💰💰	High living costs
Working really hard		Not working/chilling out

Contact details	University of Birmingham Medical School, College of Medical and Dental Sciences, University of Birmingham, Edgbaston, Birmingham, B15 2TT Tel: +44 (0) 121 414 3481, Web: www.medicine.bham.ac.uk

An insider's view...

We are quite explicit in our selection requirements, which allow applicants to better match their academic profile with our criteria. Selection for interview is based primarily on exam results, though we also consider evidence of commitment to medicine through work experience (voluntary work in the healthcare sector is sufficient). Candidates must have predicted A-level grades of AAA or have achieved A*AA. We give preference to applicants with AAAA from four subjects in Year 12. We also give preference to applicants with A* grades at GCSE in Mathematics, English (Language or Literature), and science (triple or double award). We do use information relating to school performance to select a proportion of interview candidates, which may allow us to reduce these academic requirements. We do not 'score' the personal statement prior to interview and we do NOT use the UKCAT. The interview is composed of multiple 'stations' to assess: motivation for medicine; communication; self-insight; ethical reasoning; scientific understanding, and interpretation of data. At the interview stage, exam results are considered to distinguish candidates with the same interview score.

Dr Austen Spruce, Medicine Admissions Tutor

Brighton and Sussex

As England's smallest medical school, Brighton and Sussex Medical School (BSMS) has a real family feel. Students belong to both the Universities of Brighton and Sussex, yet all study as one cohort on the university campuses, which are next to each other. With full access to the facilities of both universities and located in the cosmopolitan city of Brighton, there is something for everyone!

University BSMS opened its doors in 2003, boasting brand-new state-of-the-art resources. Each campus has purpose-built lecture theatres, seminar rooms, and computer suites. The University of Brighton campus houses a fully equipped clinical skills area for use by all students; they are also one of the few medical schools to have access to a simulator patient (named Meti). The purpose-built medical research centre situated at the University of Sussex ensures that BSMS is at the heart of new developments in all areas of medicine. In years three and four, study is based primarily in the Royal Sussex County Hospital in the centre of Brighton. This means you will never have far to travel and the familiar environment makes clinical study less daunting! In fifth year, placements are further afield but accommodation is provided and all hospitals are linked electronically via the university network.

Course The integrated medical course at BSMS incorporates many teaching methods, including PBL and IT-based; there is an emphasis on small group work with students mixed up in several different groups to ensure everyone gets to know each other quickly. In the first two years a systems-based approach is used to provide students with core scientific knowledge alongside clinical teaching, which begins in week one. Anatomy teaching is aided by both computer-based imaging classes and regular dissection. In the new dissection suite, each group of eight students is allocated a cadaver and dissects the particular system that is being studied at that time. Students are also given the opportunity to direct their learning with student-selected modules offered throughout the course. An intercalated degree is optional between the third and fourth years and can be undertaken at the University of Brighton, the University of Sussex, or elsewhere. The main exams are taken in the third and fifth years, although there are modular assessments throughout the course. A major component of the fourth year is an individual in-depth research project. You are assigned to a BSMS research team with whom you undertake a project on a medically relevant topic of your choice.

Lifestyle First year medical students are guaranteed accommodation at either the Brighton or Sussex campuses, which are next to each other in Falmer, a parkland area four miles from the city centre. The Sussex campus is shared with students from many other subjects, offering a fantastic opportunity to socialize with non-medics! Both campuses have bars, restaurants, libraries (a 24-hour library on the Sussex campus!), and sports/fitness facilities (for a fee). Should you want to escape from it all, there is handy pedestrian access to an area of outstanding natural beauty: South Downs National Park. After the first year, students generally live in Brighton city centre where transport links are very good or they can apply to be 'Residential Advisors' and stay on at the Sussex campus. Brighton is a rich city that will satisfy every personality. The dynamism of the festivals, events, and clubs on offer is tempered by the beautiful Sussex countryside, surrounding historic villages, and relaxing hiking trails. Being by the sea is another bonus—you can't beat a lunch on the beach in between clinics.

Factoid In 2013 BSMS has the most satisfied medical students for the second year running; this is partly explained by being taught on statistically the sunniest university campus in England! See Table 8.3.

Table 8.3   Brighton and Sussex

Myth	'New' touchy-feely medics, more into sun-bathing than studying
Reality	A 21st century course in a relaxed city
Personality	Laid-back, but able to get the job done
Best aspects	The small, family atmosphere in a seaside town makes for a fantastic medical school experience
Worst aspects	An overload of seminars teaching communication skills
Requirements	**UKCAT**; **A-level** three A2s and one AS including grade 'A' in A2 chemistry and biology; **GCSE** at least a 'B' in English and maths

Course length	5 years	Structure	Campus
Type of course	Plate glass (p. 94)	Year size	135
Typical offer	AAA or A*AB	Intercalated degree:	BSc
Applicants	2500	Student mix:	
Interviews	450	% Mature	20%
Offers	230	% International	7%

Uncompetitive		Competitive
Low living costs		High living costs
Working really hard		Not working/ chilling out

Contact details	Brighton and Sussex Medical School, BSMS Teaching Building, University of Sussex, Brighton, East Sussex, BN1 9PX Tel: +44 (0) 1273 643529, Web: www.bsms.ac.uk

An insider's view...

BSMS is committed to modern patient-focused education, with a high proportion of early clinical contact. The medical course has a strong science base benefiting from research-informed teaching, which equips our graduates with the ability to practise evidence-based medicine. The programme is delivered in an integrated systems-based manner using a variety of traditional and contemporary approaches, which we believe enhances the learning experience. The relative small size of BSMS means students and staff quickly get to know each other and the high proportion of small group teaching means all students get the support they need. Student-selected elements are important aspects of the course and our students benefit in particular from a self-organized elective period and engagement with an individual research project in year four. We are therefore looking for enthusiastic and capable students with self-motivation directed to becoming one of tomorrow's doctors.

Prof. Darrell Evans, Associate Dean

Bristol

Home to Banksy, Skins, and Clifton Suspension Bridge, Bristol is a fantastic setting in which to study medicine. Once a major port, Bristol has enjoyed a rich and vibrant history with most of its unique architecture surviving to this day. Bristol also offers a six-year pre-med course for students who did not take science A-levels (see p. 259), and a four-year graduate course for those who have done a medically related degree (see p. 235).

University Most first year students are based at the Stoke Bishop Halls of residence. Stoke Bishop Halls are a 40-minute walk from the medical school and each morning students can be seen migrating across the Bristol Downs for lectures or whizzing by on the new free bus service. The medical school itself features a newly refurbished medical library complete with coffee shops, essential for those late-night cramming sessions. The university also offers students the large, recently redesigned Arts and Social Sciences Library and the Law Library housed in the incredible Wills' Memorial Building. All libraries have computer facilities and the 24-hour Computer Lab is available when these close.

Course The first two years are lecture-based covering topics such as the molecular and cellular basis of medicine, human basis of medicine (including attending GP placements), and systems-based teaching. Cadaveric teaching is held in the anatomy labs every Wednesday morning, which also feature modern computer simulations. The second year includes five weeks of hospital-based activities that begin immediately at the start of term.

At the end of the second year students achieving a high enough grade average may choose to intercalate and work towards a BSc qualification. Around 40% of students intercalate across a range of subjects including anatomical sciences, bioethics, medical humanities, and numerous others.

From the third year onwards all activities are clinically based. Students may be sent to a number of hospitals throughout the South West. The Bristol Royal Infirmary is the main teaching hospital in the city; however, students may be sent as far away as Yeovil or Swindon for eight-week placements. Other hospitals include Royal United Hospitals in Bath, Musgrove Park Hospital in Taunton, Weston General Hospital, and Gloucester and Cheltenham Hospitals.

Lifestyle After their first year, most students live in rented accommodation in the Redland or Clifton areas of Bristol. Nearby campus facilities are excellent and include the Pulse fitness suite and Coombe Dingle sports complex. Both medical and university societies organize student events and Bristol features a vibrant nightlife with the majority of bars and clubs located in the Triangle area or Park Street. The recently constructed Cabot Circus in the city centre features boutique shops, restaurants, and a cinema complex. In addition, Bristol Hippodrome and Colston Hall regularly feature live musical and theatrical performances.

Factoid Famous comedians including Matt Lucas, David Walliams, and Simon Pegg are all Bristol alumni. See Table 8.4.

Table 8.4 Bristol

Myth	West Country bumpkins dressed exclusively in Jack Wills
Reality	A lively mix of hard-working medical students (some of whom wear Jack Wills)
Personality	Confident, relaxed, and keen to learn
Best aspects	Enthusiastic teaching and plenty to do in the great city of Bristol
Worst aspects	Lack of feedback and support during exam periods (although this is getting better!)
Requirements	**No admissions test; A-level** three A2s including grade 'A' in A2 chemistry, as well as A2 biology and/or physics; **GCSE** at least five 'A's including English language, maths, and two sciences

Course length	5 years	Structure	Campus
Type of course	Red brick (p. 94)	Year size	208
Typical offer	AAA	Intercalated degree:	BSc, BA
Applicants	3447	Student mix:	
Interviews	813	% Mature	7%
Offers	344	% International	8%

Uncompetitive		Competitive
Low living costs		High living costs
Working really hard		Not working/chilling out

Contact details	University of Bristol, Senate House, Tyndall Avenue, Bristol, BS8 1TH
	Tel: +44 (0) 117 928 9000, Web: www.bris.ac.uk/medical-school

An insider's view...

The research ethos of the University of Bristol underpins the teaching of the medicine course. With an appropriate core of medical knowledge and understanding, developing cognitive and transferable skills relevant to medical practice, students are prepared for their FY1 and equipped for lifelong learning throughout their careers. Students can intercalate, studying for an additional year towards a second degree in a variety of subjects. Student-Selected Components form a large part of the course, allowing students to pursue specific areas of interest through project-based work. For the final three years of the course, students are immersed in clinical settings benefiting from our unique Academy system, allowing them to experience a diverse variety of hospital environments and patient contacts—from the busy city centre to more rural-based hospitals.

Matthew Holt, Medical Admissions Co-ordinator

Cambridge

The medical course at Cambridge is as traditional as punting on the River Cam or singing in King's College Chapel (p. 203).

University As a collegiate university, Cambridge has no defined university campus. Instead, 31 colleges of varying size and character are dispersed across the whole city, each providing its own students with accommodation, canteens, and libraries. Pre-clinical lectures are mainly at the New Museums site in the middle of town, next to Pembroke College. In the clinical years, the main hub is Addenbrooke's Hospital and many students choose to rent accommodation privately within walking or cycling distance from the clinical school. Indeed, there is nowhere in Cambridge that is more than a short bike ride away and walking and cycling are the predominant modes of transport.

Course In the first two years students are given an intense and thorough grounding in the scientific principles of medicine. Rather than taking a systems-based approach, core medical sciences are explored separately, with anatomy, physiology, and biochemistry in the first year, followed by pharmacology, pathology, reproduction, and neuroscience the following year. Although this gruelling curriculum, delivered primarily through lectures and practical classes, can be a source of frustration for medical students eager to meet their first patients, the solid foundation it provides is ultimately invaluable. The third year is dedicated to a specialist subject in which students earn their BA degree. Most choose to study a scientific discipline and take advantage of being at one of the most renowned research centres in the world by carrying out their own research project. There is also the chance to pursue a non-medical subject, from anthropology to zoology!

The true bastion of the Cambridge educational experience (and the silver bullet to the challenges posed by the rigorous course) is the supervision system. Students receive weekly supervisions in small groups (one to four students) from a specialist in each subject. Supervisors offer the opportunity to clarify and further discuss lecture material and also to deliver feedback on essays.

Most Cambridge medical students currently stay in Cambridge for their clinical studies; the remainder go on to other clinical schools, typically in London or Oxford. Cambridge University hopes to increase the number of clinical places available in Cambridge for 2017. Students proceeding to Cambridge clinical school will have their main clinical teaching base at the large Addenbrooke's Hospital, with a third of the time spent in regional district general hospitals. The bulk of the learning is ward-based, through consultant-designated teaching (and supervisions!), but clinical pathology is taught through lectures and great emphasis is placed on development of communication skills through critical appraisal in small group sessions. The newly built state-of-the-art Deakin Centre offers fantastic facilities for honing practical clinical skills as well as a cafe for your morning coffee fix!

Lifestyle Students are usually offered college accommodation for the entirety of the pre-clinical course. When away on placements in clinical years, free accommodation is provided in district general hospitals, giving the flexibility to commute to/from Cambridge at the weekends. In the first year you will usually have your own room on a corridor with around five other students, who may or may not be studying medicine. Each college possesses its own perks and quirks (p. 208), but all provide the facilities and funding to enable their students to get involved in every conceivable extracurricular activity! College bars and local pubs outnumber a modest selection of nightclubs, but these often suffice after an evening's formal hall with friends.

Factoid The famous end-of-year May ball held at St John's College was rated the seventh best party in the world, according to *Time* magazine. See Table 8.5.

Table 8.5 Cambridge

Myth	Brainy boffins in ivory towers isolated from patients
Reality	Hard-working and enthusiastic students with a desire to improve their clinical competence through scientific understanding
Personality	Intense, competitive, versatile
Best aspects	Receiving personal tuition from some of the top scientists in the world is an extraordinary and once-in-a-lifetime privilege
Worst aspects	The exams—they are just as bad as everyone says, only worse!
Requirements	**BMAT**; **A-level** three A2s with at least two out of chemistry, biology, physics, and maths (though three of these are preferred); **GCSE** at least 'C's in science and maths

Course length	6 years	Structure	Collegiate
Type of course	Stone (p. 94)	Year size	280
Typical offer	A*AA	Intercalated degree:	BA (compulsory)
Applicants	1639	Student mix:	
Interviews	Approx. 1600	% Mature	5%
Offers	293	% International	8%

Uncompetitive		Competitive
Low living costs		High living costs
Working really hard		Not working/chilling out
Contact details	University of Cambridge School of Clinical Medicine, Addenbrooke's Hospital, Box 111, Hills Road, Cambridge, CB2 2SP Tel: +44 (0) 1223 336700, Web: www.cam.ac.uk	

An insider's view...

As expected from a leading international centre for scientific research, Cambridge's medical course is unashamedly scientifically oriented. This might not suit all tastes, but provides a fantastic opportunity for scientifically inclined students to excel. Our philosophy is that medicine progresses through the application of new scientific/technological developments in clinical practice. Medical training at Cambridge therefore differs sharply from elsewhere, retaining a clear division between an initial in-depth grounding in pre-clinical sciences and clinical training. The course is tough and highly competitive: we are looking for the most able students, with a particular interest in and flair for the sciences as well as vocational motivation.

Dr Steve Edgley, Director of Studies, St John's College

Durham

Durham School of Medicine and Health offers a two-year pre-clinical course (Phase I) followed by a three-year clinical course (Phase II) based at Newcastle Medical School (p. 148). When choosing where to study Phase I students can choose to apply to Durham only, Newcastle only, or indicate no preference by completing the 'Campus Code' on their UCAS application. The School of Medicine and Health is based at Queen's Campus in Stockton-on-Tees (about 20 miles south of Durham).

University Queen's Campus was built on the banks of the River Tees, and its main features are the Wolfson Research Institute, the Holliday and Ebsworth teaching buildings, as well as a brand new gym and sports centre, two residential colleges called 'John Snow', and 'Stephenson', and these each have their own college bars and common areas. Other Durham students are allocated to the Queen's Campus according to subject of study (including Psychology and Business). Alongside their modern campus and library facilities, students have access to the historic buildings on the Durham campus. Clinical experience in the first two years takes place at local hospitals (e.g. James Cook University Hospital, Middlesbrough). In the clinical years students are allocated to one of four clinical bases along with the Newcastle students (see p. 148 for details).

Course The case-based course at Durham has identical learning objectives to Newcastle medical school to ensure that students have equivalent knowledge when they come together. Teaching is through a combination of lectures, small-group tutorials, practicals, video, role-play, computer-assisted learning, and self-directed learning. Anatomy is taught innovatively in a variety of ways, including prosections, models, body painting, the computer-based Virtual Human Dissector, and ultrasound. The course is integrated with students meeting patients and learning clinical skills from the outset. The course also includes community placement, for instance with a local charity, unlike the Newcastle course. The small year size and collegiate system make for a friendly atmosphere, good rapport with the staff, and very interactive teaching, as well as endless help and perseverance for students who are struggling with any aspect of the course. At the end of the second year the year group is merged with those at Newcastle to undertake Phase II, including opportunities to intercalate, undertake an elective, and choose special study modules. This is described on p. 148.

Lifestyle Durham has a collegiate system (similar to Oxbridge, p. 203) and students join one of the two close-knit colleges on campus. College accommodation boasts en-suite bedrooms and common rooms along with being within easy walking distance of lectures. It is relatively expensive for the area, but local accommodation for second year and beyond is very affordable. Queen's Campus students have access to a huge range of societies and sports teams because they can choose between those based at Durham, in their college, or within the medical school; there is something to suit every hobby, interest, and ability. The colleges themselves are the social hubs for their students, but medics have the added advantage of a thriving and well-organized MedSoc, as well as other academic and charitable committees such as the Surgical Society and Marrow, which are well subscribed despite the relatively small campus size. Middlesbrough and Yarm are close by for nightlife, as well as there being a free bus connecting Queen's Campus with the city of Durham, which has an enviable and lively student scene!

Factoid Stockton-on-Tees has the world's oldest railway ticketing office (which is appropriate since the 'Stephenson' that the college is named after built the first public railway). It also has the widest high street in the UK. See Table 8.6.

Table 8.6 Durham

Myth	The overspill that couldn't fit into the lecture theatre in Newcastle
Reality	A close-knit community who benefit from small group sizes, interactive learning, and the chance to experience the perks of collegiate life
Personality	Sociable, dynamic, enthusiastic, and prepared to work hard
Best aspects	Long holidays, the chance to get to know everyone on campus personally, and small group teaching of the tricky parts of medicine!
Worst aspects	Short term lengths can make the work feel a little intense at times
Requirements	**UKCAT; A-level** three A2s with at least AS chemistry or biology; **GCSE** at least five 'C's including English, maths, and science; grade 'A' in chemistry or biology if not taking it at A2 or AS-level

Course length	5 years (2 at Durham, 3 at Newcastle)	Structure	Collegiate
Type of course	Stone (p. 94)	Year size	104
Typical offer	AAA	Intercalated degree:	BA, BSc
Applicants	541	Student mix:	
Interviews	303	% Mature	45%
Offers	218	% International	6%

Uncompetitive		Competitive
Low living costs		High living costs
Working really hard		Not working/chilling out

Contact details	Medicine Undergraduate Admissions, Durham University, School of Medicine and Health, Queen's Campus, University Boulevard, Stockton-on-Tees, TS17 6BH Tel: +44 (0) 191 33 40353, Web: www.dur.ac.uk/school.health

An insider's view...

The strong 'family' feel and close links with staff on the integrated campus are greatly valued by many of our students and we know that this is a feature in making the decision to choose the Durham Phase I programme. There are also close links with the community running through our programme, which many find attractive. The School of Medicine and Health at Queen's includes some of the UK's most prestigious health research groupings and there is a particular strength in research into medical education itself, which means our students benefit from state-of-the-art approaches to teaching and learning.

Prof. John C. McLachlan, Associate Dean of Undergraduate Medicine

Exeter

The University of Exeter Medical School was formed in 2013 after the founding universities of Peninsula Medical School (initially opened 2002) decided to build on their success by establishing two separate schools in Exeter and Plymouth. The new curriculum is based on that of Peninsula Medical School. The University is expanding rapidly, especially since being named the 'University of the Year' 2012/13 by *The Sunday Times*.

University Medical students spend their first two years at Exeter before moving to clinical campuses in Exeter, Truro, Barnstaple, and Torbay for years three, four, and five. The medical school is linked with NHS trusts through Devon and Cornwall, each of which has developed resources for medical students meaning a plentiful supply of libraries, IT suites, and other educational resources. There is also an abundance of high quality clinical skills resources (e.g. plastic arms for practising cannulation) as should be expected of a new, purpose-built medical school.

Course The curriculum places a heavy emphasis on patient-focused teaching to make truly holistic doctors. This means early clinical experience and two years of structured small group learning. Group work is supplemented by lectures and clinical skills sessions so students are not left completely to their own devices. Although there is no dissection or prosection, there is heavy use of radiological imaging and living anatomy.

The third and fourth years are organized into 'pathway' weeks. Each week is spent studying a different clinical presentation (e.g. shortness of breath) within a relevant primary care or hospital setting. One potential disadvantage is loss of continuity as students move departments often, but it also means an unrivalled spectrum of patients to learn from. The fifth year is spent rotating (every five weeks) through core specialities, learning how to become a foundation doctor.

Assessment is continuous, regular, and always focuses on clinical application. Examiners are interested in how knowledge is applied, not simply whether one can list twenty causes of atrial fibrillation.

The curriculum encourages students to focus on what will be needed as a junior doctor and also expects students to take responsibility for their learning. This self-directed approach helps many students thrive but others can find the lack of structure frustrating. The selection process is designed to choose those who will benefit most.

Special Study Units (SSUs) take place throughout the five years, ranging from extended clinical placements (e.g. in intensive care) to research and teaching. In year five the SSU takes the form of a traditional elective. An intercalated course from a wide range of options is available for the top 15% of each year, based on medical school exam grades.

Lifestyle Accommodation is easily available and first years are all guaranteed rooms in university halls. Students at Exeter are surrounded by the beautiful Dartmoor countryside and rarely find themselves more than fifteen minutes from a beach. The small cohort size and small town make for a highly cohesive student body. There is a wealth of outdoor activities from kite-surfing to rock climbing; between the sea and Dartmoor most tastes are catered for.

Factoid Harry Potter author JK Rowling used one of her professors at the University of Exeter as the basis for Albus Dumbledore. See Table 8.7.

Table 8.7 Exeter

Myth	BM BS – Bachelor of Mooching, Bachelor of Surfing
Reality	Teaching students to focus on patients from day one... and allow some time for surfing!
Personality	Students need to be highly motivated and able to direct their own learning
Best aspects	Intense focus on patients and the clinical presentations of disease
Worst aspects	Split from Plymouth is likely to create some wrinkles
Requirements	**UKCAT; A-level** three A2s including chemistry and either Biology or Physics; four AS with C in non-A2 subject; biology at least to AS grade C.

Course length	5 years	Structure	Campus
Type of course	Carbon fibre (p. 94)	Year size	129
Typical offer	A*AA-AAA	Intercalated degree:	Various
Applicants	1814	Student mix:	
Interviews	503	% Mature	N/A
Offers	210	% International	N/A

Uncompetitive		Competitive
Low living costs		High living costs
Working really hard		Not working/ chilling out

Contact details	The Student Centre, College House, St Luke's Campus, Exeter, EX1 2LU Tel: +44 (0) 1392 725 500, Web: http://medicine.exeter.ac.uk/

An insider's view...

As part of a Russell Group University and the Sunday Times University of the Year, the University of Exeter Medical School builds on the success of the Peninsula College of Medicine and Dentistry. The course integrates the science and clinical aspects of medicine ensuring an excellent education and student experience. Our students learn in a research-rich environment and our problem-based education model produces doctors who are recognised to be amongst the best prepared to practise medicine.

Professor Steve Thornton, Dean of the University of Exeter Medical School

Hull York

The Hull York Medical School (HYMS) opened in 2003 as a partnership between the Universities of Hull and York and local NHS trusts. It is a modern, purpose-built school with teaching facilities and a curriculum that have been specifically designed to train doctors for 21st century medicine. The curriculum is currently being reviewed to keep the course up to date and relevant for the modern doctor; student feedback has been at the heart of the review to ensure the curriculum meets students' needs.

University Half of the incoming students are randomly allocated to either Hull or York, base campus, which are about an hour's drive apart. Phase 1 teaching takes place at their base campus, either Cottingham Road (three miles from Hull city centre) or Heslington (two miles from York city centre). Students have 24-hour access to many of the medical buildings and both the Hull and York libraries and electronic resources. The four clinical placements in Phase 2 last six months each and rotate between the main HYMS sites: Hull, York, Scunthorpe, Grimsby, and Scarborough. All non-base sites offer free NHS accommodation. Public transport runs to all five clinical sites, but can be infrequent so having a car is helpful.

Course The course is split into three phases. Phase 1 (two years) consists of problem-based learning (PBL), clinical skills classes, biopracticals, resource sessions, plenaries, and a one-day clinical placement each week. Anatomy is taught by prosections, models, and included in PBL; students can opt for student selected component (SSC) modules that involve dissection. Full-time clinical teaching begins in Phase 2 (two years) with eight-week rotations through different specialities (e.g. oncology, cardiovascular) in a variety of healthcare settings (GP, hospital, community clinics, surgery). Phase 3 (one year) is designed to give students as much experience of being an FY1 doctor as possible, often acting as a 'doctor's assistant'; the year includes an eight-week elective and formal work shadowing in general practice, medicine, and surgery.

The course is organized into blocks, each of which set learning outcomes to aid self-directed learning. There is a spiral curriculum meaning topics are revisited with increasing depth as you progress throughout the course. A wide variety of SSCs are available throughout the course including clinical (e.g. plastic surgery), science-based projects (e.g. biomedical science and research), humanities (e.g. sign language), the arts (e.g. drama), and sports (e.g. yoga, sports medicine). Students with a good academic record can opt for an intercalated degree at a wide range of UK universities after the second or fourth year. An intercalated Master's degree is available for students with a prior Bachelor's degree.

Lifestyle Hull and York university accommodation is guaranteed for first years; students are advised to choose rooms in self-catered houses as the medical curriculum terms are longer than the standard university terms. Most students pursue private accommodation for the following years. The cost of accommodation in Hull is amongst the lowest in the country, approximately £60–100 per week; York is slightly more at £80–120 per week. The social life in both Hull and York is fantastic. Hull has an award-winning Students' Union that hosts many well-known bands while York has a collegiate system with socials at each college for all to attend and friendly college rivalry. York has a superb mixture of historic buildings, galleries, and cafes along with a varied and vibrant mix of theatres, bars, and clubs. All sites are surrounded by stunning scenery and make for excellent days out and a nice break in your spare time.

Factoid HYMS has excellent links with the Medical Societies of Hull and York. Student society events are held at their historic society buildings and students are encouraged to attend the prestigious talks. See Table 8.8.

Table 8.8 Hull York

Myth	A northern GP factory valuing patient communication over science
Reality	An exciting course employing the most up-to-date teaching methods in both patient communication and science
Personality	Dynamic, independent, and proactive with good life-experience and excellent communication skills
Best aspects	Having two campuses and enjoying social activities at both, with keen (but friendly) inter-campus competition
Worst aspects	Distance between all sites means quite a bit of travelling, particularly in Phase 2 and 3
Requirements	**UKCAT**; **A-level** three A2s including chemistry and biology and one AS-level; **GCSE** 8 grade A to C including 'A's in English and maths

Course length	5 years	Structure	Split Campus
Type of course	Carbon fibre (p. 94)	Year size	141
Typical offer	AAAb	Intercalated degree:	BSc, MSc
Applicants	1100	Student mix:	
Interviews	475	% Mature	14%
Offers	300	% International	7.5%

Uncompetitive		Competitive
Low living costs		High living costs
Working really hard		Not working/ chilling out
Contact details	Hull York Medical School, University of York, Heslington, York, YO10 5DD Tel: +44 (0) 870 1245500, Web: www.hyms.ac.uk	

An insider's view...

The HYMS course encourages you to develop your skills as an independent, flexible learner. It is designed for those who want a hands-on, interactive course revolving around patients from the outset. The course features early, extensive patient contact and all learning is rooted in clinical situations. HYMS is seeking students with a genuine interest in medicine, excellent communication skills and reasoning ability, and a passion for working with people.

Dr Janine Henderson, HYMS Associate Dean of Admissions

Keele

Keele is the one of the newest undergraduate medical schools in the UK (est. 2003 using the Manchester curriculum). A Keele curriculum has since been designed with the first cohort of students having graduated in 2012. Helping to shape a developing curriculum and using brand-new facilities makes it an exciting time to be a part of Keele Medical School. Keele also offers an additional health foundation year (p. 259) for applicants without the necessary science subjects required for entry into the standard five-year course.

University The brand-new purpose-built undergraduate medical school (which cost £12.5 million) is based on the green and rural Keele campus near Newcastle-under-Lyme. It includes several laboratories, plentiful IT facilities, and a student common room to socialize and study (or sleep!) in. The small year group provides a friendly, caring atmosphere where all students know and support each other. The campus provides some great restaurants, bars, and sports facilities. Two of the three clinical years are spent at the University Hospital of North Staffordshire (in Stoke-on-Trent, within walking distance of most rented accommodation) and the other year either at the Royal Shrewsbury Hospital (35 miles away, accommodation onsite at this hospital is available), or at Stafford General Hospital (16 miles away). Being able to spend time in both teaching and district general hospitals offers students a variety of learning opportunities.

Course Although it is new, the systems-based curriculum is highly rated by its students. The curriculum is a spiral, meaning that topics are revisited several times with increasing complexity throughout the five years. Students are assigned to a group of 12 who take most classes together including the weekly PBL (p. 88) clinical scenario. Alongside PBL there are lectures, seminars, practical classes, and regular tutor contact. Anatomy is taught by a combination of full body dissection with prosections and computer aids. Early clinical exposure starts from the first term with hospital-based placements and clinical skills teaching. The Keele curriculum puts a strong emphasis on the psychosocial aspects of medicine.

The clinical teaching at the hospitals is excellent and the continuing PBL cases help stimulate deeper learning. To accompany timetabled learning there are also opportunities to 'sign up' to placements and get a unique chance to see an area of personal interest or to improve your understanding in an area of weakness. In the third year students return to Keele campus for teaching one day a week, packed with applied sciences, clinical pathology, and ethics seminars to complement clinical learning.

Students in their second or fourth year with an interest in intercalating can do so providing they have passed all exams in the previous years. Students can opt for a one-year intercalated Bachelor's degree after second year or a one-year Master's degree (most universities only offer a Bachelor's) after the fourth year in research or a medical subject.

Lifestyle The large, green campus surrounded by beautiful Staffordshire countryside is a great place to study. Students in the first two years tend to live in university accommodation spread across campus and near the medical school. Clinical students move to rented accommodation close to the hospital for their years in Stoke-on-Trent, Stafford, or Shrewsbury. For urban excitement, Stoke town centre is a short bus journey away while Manchester and Birmingham are easily accessible by train. The medics' social calendar includes staff vs. students sports, awesome nights out (e.g. pyjama pub crawl), and the infamous surgical and KMS balls.

Factoid Keele Medical School was first suggested in the late 1960s; however, it was felt that the university was too small to support it. Not many medical schools can boast such an extensive planning period! See Table 8.9.

Table 8.9 Keele

Myth	An unknown, untested medical school in the middle of nowhere
Reality	A tried and tested course adapted to a beautiful rural setting
Personality	Eager, friendly, sociable, and independent students
Best aspects	The family-like atmosphere fostered by the small size and campus setting; the opportunity to complete an intercalated Master's degree
Worst aspects	Written finals in 4th year can lead to stress about gaps in knowledge
Requirements	**UKCAT**; **A-level** three A2s including chemistry and/or biology plus another science or maths, at least 'B' in AS chemistry if not taking A2; **GCSE** at least four 'A's with 'B's in English, maths, and sciences

Course length	5 years	Structure	Campus
Type of course	Carbon fibre (p. 94)	Year size	129
Typical offer	A*ABb-AAAb	Intercalated degree:	MMedSci
Applicants	1848	Student mix:	
Interviews	501	% Mature	27%
Offers	281	% International	3%

Uncompetitive	Competitive
Low living costs	High living costs
Working really hard	Not working/ chilling out
Contact details	Keele University Medical School, Keele University, Keele, Staffordshire, ST5 5BG Tel: +44 (0) 1782 733642, Web: www.keele.ac.uk/health/schoolofmedicine

An insider's view…

As one of the smallest undergraduate medical schools in the UK, Keele offers a highly supportive learning environment in which students and staff work together to develop the knowledge, skills, and attitudes required by tomorrow's doctors. Our mission is to graduate excellent clinicians and our focus throughout the course is on making learning directly relevant to clinical practice. We welcome applications from students from all backgrounds who have a thorough understanding of the academic, organizational, and personal demands of a medical career. This understanding should be gained through school/university study, participation in health-based or caring work, and activities involving teamworking.

Dr Gordon Dent, Director of Admissions (Undergraduate Medicine)

Lancaster

Situated in the North West of England and at the heart of Red Rose country, the historic city of Lancaster began life as a Roman fort in 80 AD; it still has a lot to offer. Lancaster is surrounded by a diverse mix of city, coast, and countryside, with the Lake District and Morecambe Bay just a stone's throw away. The university is a vibrant place to study, with a top ten UK ranking for both research and teaching, and a 91% student satisfaction rating.

University Lancaster is one of only a few remaining collegiate universities in the country. Each college has its own unique atmosphere and encourages a strong sense of identity amongst its students. The medical school is on the main campus, which has 360 acres of parkland just three miles from Lancaster; it is also one of the safest campuses in the UK. More than £450 million has been invested into the campus since 2002, including the new state-of-the-art £20 million sports centre that opened in the summer of 2011.

Course Lancaster is the newest medical school in the UK, with the first cohort of students graduating in 2011. Students initially received their degree from Liverpool University (and used the same curriculum), however, from September 2013 the course has been independent from Liverpool.

The course has a PBL (problem-based learning) format, with only one or two lectures a day, and students are expected to engage in plenty of independent study. They are assisted by a wide range of facilities to help them do this, including the Clinical Anatomy Learning Centre (CALC) on campus and the clinical skills labs at each local hospital. Much emphasis is placed on communication skills, including regular sessions with 'simulated patients,' played by actors.

Clinical teaching begins in first year, with weekly practical skill sessions (e.g. cardiovascular examinations, venepuncture). Clinical placements begin at the start of year two, with students spending two days a week in medicine or surgery placements in the Morecambe Bay hospitals (Royal Lancaster Infirmary, Furness General Hospital, and Westmoreland General Hospital). In the third year students rotate through five specialities, (e.g. paediatrics, obstetrics and gynaecology) supplemented by PBL and clinical teaching. Final exams are at the end of fourth year, and are followed by a five-week long elective. On their return students enter the clinically-intensive fifth year to prepare them for becoming junior doctors. Students also complete four special study modules, carrying out research in an area of their choice; 10–20% of students continue their research interests by intercalating between the fourth and fifth year.

Lifestyle The majority of first year students live in halls of residence on the main university campus, whilst most students move into private rentals in one of the student areas surrounding the city from the second year. Since Lancaster is so compact, just about wherever you choose to live lies within walking distance of the town centre. All students spend half their fourth year living in Barrow-in-Furness; however, free hospital accommodation is provided. Lancaster University has a massive number of societies and sports teams to get involved with to keep you busy, and with the nine college bars on campus and the infamous university nightclub 'the Sugarhouse' in town, evenings will definitely not be quiet. The medical society also organizes regular social events, including the fresher's and winter balls, annual trips to other medical schools, the medic pantomime, and inter-year sporting tournaments.

Factoid James May, Andy Serkis (Gollum), and Jason Queally, Olympic gold medal winning cyclist, all graduated from Lancaster University. See Table 8.10.

Table 8.10 Lancaster

Myth	An untried and untested medical school
Reality	A brand new and exciting opportunity to study medicine in a thriving university
Personality	Friendly, sociable, and driven
Best aspects	With only 50 in each year group, there are rarely more than six other students in any small teaching group
Worst aspects	Placements in a few local hospitals may limit the opportunity to observe more complex clinical cases
Requirements	**No admissions test; A-level** three 'A's, two of which must be in biology and chemistry, and one B in AS-level; **GCSEs** at least 15 points from nine GCSEs (A*/A = 2 points, B = 1 point), with at least 'B' in English, maths, and science

Course length	5 years	Structure	Campus
Type of course	Carbon fibre (p. 94)	Year size	50
Typical offer	AAA	Intercalated degree:	BSc, MSc
Applicants	519	Student mix:	
Interviews	168	% Mature	16%
Offers	112	% International	0%

Uncompetitive		Competitive
Low living costs		High living costs
Working really hard		Not working/ chilling out
Contact details	Lancaster Medical School, Furness Building, Lancaster University, LA1 4YG. Tel +44 (0) 1524 5 94547, Web: www.lancs.ac.uk	

An insider's view...

At Lancaster Medical School, students learn through problem-based learning and extensive clinical experience, with an emphasis on effective communication skills and medicine in the community. The first clinical placement occurs in year 1 and students are on the wards and in GP practices from the beginning of year 2. The admissions process consists of three stages: (1) Academic aptitude: only applicants who meet the academic entry requirements progress beyond stage 1; (2) Non-academic criteria: the personal statement is assessed to determine those who most ably demonstrate the required non-academic criteria; and (3) Multiple mini interview (MMI): interviewees are ranked according to their MMI score and offers are made to the highest scoring applicants.

Dr Karen Grant, Deputy Director of Medical Studies and Director of Admissions

Leeds

With one of the largest student populations in the country, Leeds has a lively and vibrant feel with a highly respected nightlife. Medicine at Leeds is progressive and adaptable, yet remains uniquely traditional. Leeds offers the integration of basic science and clinical teaching, early patient contact, and anatomy taught using cadaveric dissection (one of the last UK medical schools to do so). There is a strong emphasis on clinical research—the new RESS strand (Research, Evaluation, and Special Studies) runs throughout the course, incorporating student-selected components, elective experience, and an 18-month final project.

University Less than one mile north of the city centre, the main university campus houses the medical school including the well-equipped Health Sciences Library (HSL). A brand-new, cutting-edge undergraduate library is opening in September 2014, which should alleviate demand on the HSL. The other excellent facilities of the university are only two minutes away, including The Edge (a brand-new gym and pool complex) and Leeds University Union, which, with an excellent selection of shops, cafes, bars, and clubs, has consistently been voted one of the best student unions in the UK.

A new, multi-million pound Clinical Practice Centre at St James's Hospital provides the ideal venue for learning and revising clinical skills.

Course The refreshed curriculum evolves in response to student feedback and the ever-changing role of the doctor. The first two years are a mixture of lectures, web-based, problem-based, and small group learning, with early clinical exposure. Anatomy is taught by full body, cadaveric dissection in small groups over the first two years, and examined by regular spot tests. The last three years of the course are clinically based and consist of five-week placements rotating through medical and surgical specialties. Each placement is preceded by a week of preparatory lectures. Most clinical placements are at the Leeds General Infirmary (LGI) on campus or St James's University Hospital (Jimmy's) two miles away. A few placements are in nearby district general hospitals (e.g. Harrogate). e-Learning is a major component of the course, with fourth and fifth years receiving Apple iPhones pre-loaded with medical textbooks and apps for assessment during placements. Students take an 8–10 week elective at the end of the fourth year.

Students are well supported throughout the course with regular personal tutor meetings (with academic staff in the first two years, and clinicians thereafter). Leeds has a strong research focus, with the Leeds Undergraduate Research Enterprise programme offering early research experience and mentorship to its scholars. RESS projects throughout the course allow students to focus on fields of research and practice that most interest them. Many students intercalate a BSc or BA between third and fourth year.

Lifestyle The majority of students live in university halls on or near the campus for their first year then move to privately rented houses in the student area northwest of campus (Hyde Park, Woodhouse, or Headingley). Leeds has an excellent public transport system and many people cycle, although having a car is a bonus for the clinical years later. The social life is superb with an endless variety of both university and medical school societies and sports teams. Leeds University Union organizes some of the best club nights in the city. Outside the university, Leeds is a hub for music, arts, and theatre; there are also excellent opportunities for climbing, walking, cycling, and camping in the beautiful Yorkshire Dales nearby.

Factoid The first hand transplant in the UK was performed by Professor Simon Kay of Leeds School of Medicine in December 2012. See Table 8.11.

Table 8.11   Leeds

Myth	A medical school that doesn't teach pharmacology, in a bleak industrial Yorkshire city
Reality	A dynamic medical school with a strong research record, based in a large and lively city, with excellent social and cultural offerings
Personality	Friendly, lively, and outgoing
Best aspects	Early clinical contact; flexibility to pursue topics of interest
Worst aspects	Unattractive campus, the quality of private student housing in Hyde Park
Requirements	**UKCAT; A-level** three A2s including an 'A' in chemistry; **GCSE** six 'B's including English, maths, and sciences

Course length	5 years	Structure	Campus
Type of course	Red brick (p. 94)	Year size	243
Typical offer	AAA	Intercalated degree:	BA, BSc
Applicants	3500	Student mix:	
Interviews	500	% Mature	13%
Offers	415	% International	9%

Uncompetitive						Competitive
Low living costs						High living costs
Working really hard						Not working/chilling out

Contact details	Leeds School of Medicine, Room 7.09 Worsley Building, University of Leeds, Leeds, LS2 9JT Tel: +44 (0) 113 343 7234, Web: http://www.leeds.ac.uk/medicine

An insider's view …

Leeds already offers one of the best undergraduate medicine courses (the 'MBChB') in the United Kingdom, but we are currently undergoing a programme of review to the MBChB course to provide an even better undergraduate course that will prepare you for a successful transition to working as a doctor and to give you a great start to your career. In addition to the many strengths of our existing course, such as our integrated wet anatomy teaching, clinical placements, and SSC programme, Leeds students will be able to see patients at every stage of their career on the course, with a range of experience in hospitals, the community, and GP surgeries. We are mapping skills for success as a new doctor (career development, patient safety, leadership) through the course, taking our students from the start of their university course to graduation as a doctor.

Helen Mistry, Curriculum Support Officer

Leicester

Situated at the heart of England, Leicester is known for its ethnically diverse population, superb curry houses, and an orange-coloured cheese (Red Leicester). The university has a proud tradition of high quality research and teaching at both undergraduate and postgraduate levels and is a vibrant place to study.

University The medical school building is based on the main university campus, which is a short walk from Leicester city centre. The campus has just finished an extensive refurbishment including the Union building (complete with cafes, shop, and nightclub) and a new library. There is also a large park east of the campus (and a large cemetery to the south to help motivate you in your medical studies!). In the clinical years about half the time is spent in Leicester's three large hospitals (Royal Infirmary, General, and Glenfield) while the other half is spent at affiliated hospitals that range from 30 miles (Kettering) to 65 miles away (Boston). Free accommodation is provided at all of these hospitals and with smaller teaching groups the standard of teaching is very high. Needless to say, having a car (or friends with cars) is a big asset in the later years.

Course Leicester follows a lecture and systems-based course complemented by seminars, laboratory practicals, and dissection. There is a strong emphasis on integrating clinical teaching from an early stage in the curriculum, including communication skills, history taking (using actors as simulated patients), and clinical examination; it is no surprise that Leicester graduates are known for their bedside manner! Along with the core teaching there are seven student-selected modules to teach you more about areas that interest you the most. The Phase 2 course begins half way through the third year and is composed of 12 placements in hospital and community settings, each lasting seven weeks. Each placement builds on Phase 1 teaching with workbooks and seminars to supplement the clinical work. Placements are spent in a mixture of closely related specialities such as peri-operative care (anaesthetics, ITU, general surgery) and cancer care (oncology and palliative medicine). After finals there is a seven-week elective, studying in any medical setting (usually overseas).

About 10% of students spend a year in research towards an intercalated BSc after the second or third year. Following the BSc, some students may take another two years away from the standard medical course to complete a PhD (MBPhD).

Lifestyle The majority of first year students live in one of the university halls of residence. These are situated in Oadby, a leafy suburb with regular bus links to the city and campus three-and-a-half miles away. In later years most medical students rent houses in one of the student areas surrounding the university and within a gentle walk of campus; the most popular of these is Clarendon Park. The social life is excellent with numerous university societies and teams; the medical society is also very active with regular socials including the famous 'Pyjama Pubcrawl' at the start of each year. Since students account for over 12% of Leicester's term-time population the city centre has developed accordingly, giving it a nightlife that is hard to beat. Recent redevelopments include the Highcross shopping centre and a new cultural quarter. Being in the centre of the country, the city is very accessible, with great train and road links (via the M1, M69). For the outdoorsy types Rutland Water and the Peak District are within 50 miles.

Factoid Sir Alec Jeffreys discovered DNA fingerprinting at Leicester in 1984. See Table 8.12.

Table 8.12 Leicester

Myth	Students learn more about communicating with patients in foreign languages than they do about medical science
Reality	A culturally rich and redeveloped city centre university campus with a medical school proud of both its science and communication teaching
Personality	A sociable bunch, as good at communicating with each other as they are with patients
Best aspects	Relaxed atmosphere, regular small-group teaching, and a highly structured course
Worst aspects	Some of the 'award-winning' campus architecture is hard to appreciate
Requirements	**UKCAT**; **A-level** three A2s including chemistry and four AS subjects including chemistry and biology; **GCSE** 'C's in English, maths, and sciences

Course length	5 years	Structure	Campus
Type of course	Plate glass (p. 94)	Year size	162
Typical offer	AAA	Intercalated degree:	BSc, MA
Applicants	2200	Student mix:	
Interviews	980	% Mature	6%
Offers	350	% International	7.5%

Uncompetitive	🏆 🏆 **🏆** 🏆 🏆	Competitive
Low living costs	💰 💰 💰 💰 💰	High living costs
Working really hard		Not working/chilling out

Contact details	Leicester Medical School, Maurice Shock Building, University of Leicester, PO Box 138, Leicester, LE1 9HN Tel: +44 (0) 116 252 2969, Web: www.le.ac.uk/sm/le

An insider's view...

Leicester Medical School prides itself on its friendly and caring approach to students. Leicester's results in the National Student Survey confirm that it is an excellent place to study. The integrated course structure of Phase 1 builds knowledge and skills in a logical manner providing an excellent basis for full-time clinical attachments. The entire course emphasizes a patient-centred approach and our graduates are well equipped to cope with the demands of the Foundation Programme. The course is demanding but students find plenty of time to enjoy their social lives through the medical students' society and many other groups.

Dr Kevin West, Admissions Tutor

Liverpool

Liverpool's School of Medical Education is a welcoming, supportive, and progressive place to study. The teaching methods are innovative and it is one of the most affordable places to live as a student. As the Beatles sang, 'Don't pass me by'.

University The medical school is on the city side of the main campus by the Royal Liverpool University Hospital, about five minutes from the city centre. It has some excellent resources including the internationally renowned Human Anatomy Resource Centre (HARC), two 24-hour libraries, and the Centre for Excellence in Developing Professionalism (CEDP) that aims to develop and improve medical education. During the clinical years most of the attachments are within the city and those further away are mostly accessible by public transport. Fifty students in each year are based at Lancashire University with clinical attachments at the University Hospitals of Morecambe Bay; students specify which course they are applying to by the UCAS code. The university's support services are extremely helpful with immediate access to financial and pastoral assistance. There is a dedicated career advisor for students studying medicine who can provide one-to-one support.

Course Problem-based learning (PBL) is at the heart of Liverpool's pioneering medical education programme and has been designed to encourage independent thinking and clinically relevant learning. Sessions take place with a facilitator in groups of six to eight. First-year teaching includes biological sciences and basic clinical and communication skills; anatomy is taught in the HARC using prosection, state-of-the-art models, computer programs, and student-led sessions. Years two to four are focused on learning to diagnose and manage illness through a combination of hospital, community (e.g. GP), PBL, and lecture-based teaching. Students will have the opportunity to go on placements to specialist regional trauma, burns, neurology, and paediatrics centres. There are five special study module options in the first four years that allow students to tailor the course to their interests. There is a five-week elective in the third year, which is often spent overseas; the timing of this is ideal since it is before the summer holidays, allowing for some well-deserved travelling! Around twenty students will be in Blackpool Victoria hospital for their fourth year placement and can live in hospital accommodation there for the year.

At the end of year four students take their finals and can choose to take an intercalated degree. For those with suitable language skills there is also an option to spend 16 weeks studying aboard in Europe during the fifth year, via the Erasmus scheme. The whole of the fifth year comprises five seven-week placements with the aim to prepare students for their FY1 job (p. 10). For the community attachment in the fifth year, students can chose to go to Llandudno in Wales, which provides free accommodation.

Lifestyle The relatively cheap living costs and lively nightlife makes Liverpool an exciting student city. There are also a lot of places to explore outside the city such as the Knowsley Safari Park and Formby beach. Most students live in university halls of residence for their first year, allowing easy access to a wide range of social and sports events. During term-time there is also a student bus providing access to the city centre. From year two most students live near Smithdown Road (rents around £75 per week), which has easy access to buses, supermarkets, and cosy cafes. Nearby Sefton Park is Liverpool's equivalent of Central Park—it is stunning in summer, with community music and food festivals. Liverpool is easily accessible by train to other parts of the country; it takes just a little over two hours to London. The John Lennon Airport has flights to over twenty countries for those who fancy a weekend away.

Factoid Set up in 1874, the Liverpool Medical Students' Society pre-dates the founding of the University. See Table 8.13.

Table 8.13 Liverpool

Myth	PBL—Playstation-based learning		
Reality	PBL allows the relevant science to be learned in the clinical context and encourages communication and social skills		
Personality	Genuine, open-hearted, and supportive; the course experience is cooperative, not competitive		
Best aspects	Hands-on clinical experience from day one provides an important holistic view of the patient: you will become a well-rounded doctor		
Worst aspects	Long hours in hospital in the fifth year, including up to four night-shifts in A&E		
Requirements	**No admissions test; A-level** three 'A's, two of which must be in biology and chemistry, and one B in AS-level; **GCSEs** at least 'C' in nine separate subjects		
Course length	5 years	Structure	Campus
Type of course	Carbon fibre (p. 94)	Year size	292
Typical offer	AAAb	Intercalated degree:	BSc, MSc
Applicants	3000	Student mix:	
Interviews	1000	% Mature	10%
Offers	550	% International	8%
Uncompetitive			Competitive
Low living costs			High living costs
Working really hard			Not working/chilling out
Contact details	Admissions Enquiries, School of Medical Education, Cedar House, Ashton Street, Liverpool, L69 3GE Tel: +44 (0) 151 795 4370, Web: www.liv.ac.uk/medicine		

An insider's view . . .

Liverpool medical graduates are excellent teamworkers with highly developed communication skills and the knowledge and understanding required of any doctor entering foundation training. The final year at Liverpool is recognized as being excellent preparation for FY1 and beyond, while the problem-based learning approach to the curriculum develops appropriate skills in lifelong learning. Liverpool graduates leave university with the professional attitudes recognized as important by the NHS in the 21st century. We consider candidates from all backgrounds. Applicants are expected to be motivated, thoughtful, caring, and compassionate individuals with the academic potential necessary to complete the programme.

Dr John Smith, Director of Medical Studies

London—Barts and The London

BL is a medical school with centuries of tradition, producing graduates such as William Harvey, Robert Winston, and *Monty Python* actor Graham Chapman. It is part of Queen Mary University of London and is situated in East London, enabling students to benefit from 'the city' experience and the cultural diversity of the East End; this offers a unique opportunity to treat diseases rarely seen in the rest of the UK.

University The medical school occupies two main sites: one in the City and the other in the East End (25-minute tube ride away). The West Smithfield site (next to Barts Hospital) is steeped in historical beauty, only a short walk from St Paul's Cathedral. The pathology museum holds hundreds of specimens to aid your learning experience, and the nearby Doniach Museum houses the skeleton of the elephant man, Joseph Merrick. The Royal London/Whitechapel site has a state-of-the-art clinical skills lab and simulation centre along with modern library facilities (in a beautiful setting of a renovated church).

Course A major emphasis is placed on small group PBL (p. 88) and communication skills. The first two years are organized into modules by systems of the body; each module teaches the appropriate anatomy (with prosections), physiology, pathology, and relevant practical procedures at the new clinical skills centres. PBL is used to reinforce lectures on basic science. The spiral curriculum means that each body system is visited at least twice during the five-year course. Patient contact begins from the first term with students working in a community setting, covering a range of diverse populations with varying healthcare needs. From the third year students rotate between different hospital specialities. BL students have a choice of hospitals, both 'in-firms' and 'out-firms'. The in-firm hospitals include Barts Hospital (a tertiary cancer centre), the London Chest specialist cardiac and chest unit, and The Royal London, home to the air ambulance on BBC's Trauma. The out-firms extend into Greater London and Essex, but are all easily accessible via public transport and have accommodation available.

Over five years, students take 13 'Student Selected Components' (SSC) making up approximately 20% of the course. There are 800 to choose from, including the opportunity to fly with the London air ambulance services! Although intercalation is not compulsory, a wide range of degrees are offered after years 2, 3, and 4. The intercalated degree in Sports and Exercise Medicine is particularly popular.

Lifestyle Most first years live in university halls at Mile End or Charterhouse Square before moving to privately rented accommodation in the surrounding areas. BL has a fantastic sense of camaraderie that is felt from the first day through your adopted 'family'. The BL Students' Association at the Whitechapel site (autonomous from the Queen Mary's Students' Union) is at the heart of this close-knit community, organizing many of the fantastic student events, clubs, and societies available. During RAG charity week, medical schools throughout London compete to raise money with various activities (including the legendary toga party). BL has consistently triumphed as top collector, nearly always raising over £100,000 a year. Barts also has a wide range of sporting activities on offer; in 2012, Barts and The London Rugby Club won the United Hospitals' Challenge Cup (the oldest rugby tournament in the world). Outside the university some of the trendiest areas in London are on the doorstep so there is always something to do or see, whatever your taste.

Factoid Barts and The London is a union of the oldest medical school in the UK (London Hospital Medical College) and the oldest remaining hospital (Barts Hospital) founded in 1123. See Table 8.14.

Table 8.14 London—Barts and The London

Myth	The 'soft' option of London medical schools
Reality	We produce 'the best doctors in London' according to the General Medical Council during their recent visit
Personality	Incredibly friendly and always eager to get involved!
Best aspects	Sense of community; strengthened by the BL Students' Association and the fantastic pastoral system
Worst aspects	London is expensive (but special grants/loans are available and East London is less costly than other areas of the capital)
Requirements	**UKCAT** (minimum of 2400); **A-level** three A2s and one AS including two sciences at A2 (including chemistry and/or biology), 'B' in AS chemistry or biology if not taking A2. **GCSE** AAABBB or above to include biology, chemistry (or dual award), English, and maths

Course length	5 years	Structure	City/Campus
Type of course	Carbon fibre (p. 94)	Year size	271
Typical offer	AAAb	Intercalated degree:	BMedSci, BSc
Applicants	2089	Student mix:	
Interviews	862	% Mature	18%
Offers	500	% International	10%

Uncompetitive		Competitive
Low living costs		High living costs
Working really hard		Not working/ chilling out

Contact details	Queen Mary, University of London, Barts and The London School of Medicine and Dentistry, Student Office, Garrod Building, Turner Street, London, E1 2AD Tel: +44 (0) 207 882 2243, Web: www.smd.qmul.ac.uk

An insider's view...

Barts and The London is dedicated to producing doctors able to meet the challenges of 21st century medicine. We are looking for students who are able to work hard and who are self-directed and enthusiastic to learn, but who are also willing to immerse themselves in the abundant extracurricular activities within the school. There are opportunities to work with world-class scientists, as well as being exposed to some of the best clinical medicine in Britain. BL is the 'Olympic medical school', being sited three miles from the 2012 Olympic stadium and park; do you have what it takes to be part of it?

Dr Adam Feather, Member of the admissions panel

London—Imperial College

Imperial College is one of the largest, most competitive, and prestigious medical schools in the country. It was formed from several mergers including Imperial College and the medical schools of St Mary's and Charing Cross. Its reputation has grown dramatically since, both in the UK and across the world.

University Like many universities in London, the facilities are widely distributed. Pre-clinical teaching is split between the South Kensington and Charing Cross (Hammersmith) campus. The central library in South Kensington has an extensive medical library that is open 24 hours a day; libraries are also available at the teaching hospitals. Clinical years are divided between 16 hospitals in the North West Thames Deanery including the teaching hospitals of St Mary's, Hammersmith, Chelsea and Westminster, Charing Cross, and Northwick Park. Most of the hospitals are readily accessible by underground train or bus, so a car is rarely necessary, and accommodation is provided at sites that are further afield.

Course The six-year systems-based course includes a compulsory BSc. The two pre-clinical years consist of lectures, seminars, and practicals alongside PBL (p. 88) and interactive e-learning. Anatomy is taught by a mixture of dissection, lectures, living anatomy seminars, and online videos. Throughout the course lectures are available online, which complement the learning objectives and aid revision. Clinical exposure begins in year one along with teaching in communication skills and an introductory three-week hospital placement in the second year. An influx of Oxbridge students join the year as the clinical phase begins in year three; this is hospital-based with general medical and surgical placements

The fourth year is devoted to the BSc, consisting of lectures and a three-month research project or specialist module. While most of these are systems-based (e.g. immunology), Imperial also offers a popular BSc in Management at its Business School, and a BSc in Pharmacology. There are opportunities to pursue a three-year PhD. Fifth year begins with a lecture-based pathology course followed by rotations through the major clinical specialities, which continue into the final year. Year six also includes a seven-week elective, special studies modules, and professional work experience in preparation for graduation.

Examinations are held at the end of each academic year with little in course assessment with the exception of the BSc year. Examinations are paper-based, with additional practical exams in the clinical years.

Lifestyle The social scene is busy; in fact Imperial has a separate Union devoted to medical students with its own buildings, bar, sports teams, and societies. Together with the main Students' Union there are over 300 clubs and societies. Whether you are drawn to museums, galleries, bars, bands, or sports you will find that you have far more options than you have time for given the excellent location of Imperial's campuses and hospitals. Students also get free membership to Ethos, a modern sports centre on the Kensington campus complete with rock climbing wall and pool.

Factoid Sir Alexander Fleming (discovered penicillin), David Livingstone (African explorer), and Lord Ara Darzi (surgeon and former Minister for Health) all spent time at the institutions that make up Imperial College School of Medicine. See Table 8.15.

Table 8.15 London—Imperial College

Myth	The training ground of arrogant male surgeons
Reality	A multicultural and international mix of friendly students who are proud of Imperial and the career opportunities it offers
Personality	Hard-working, sociable, able to cope in a big medical school
Best aspects	Ability to explore your artistic side with languages and humanities courses; over 300 societies and a huge Students' Union
Worst aspects	Expectations are high and the end-of-year workload is heavy; yearly summer exams are tough and re-takes not uncommon
Requirements	**BMAT** roughly 4.9 in Sections 1 and 2, and 2.5C in Section 3; **A-level** three A2s including two sciences (including chemistry and/or biology) and one 'B' in AS chemistry or biology (if not taking A2); **GCSE** 'AAABB' from double/triple award sciences, English, and maths

Course length	6 years	Structure	City
Type of course	Stone (p. 94)	Year size	283
Typical offer	AAAb-AAAC	Intercalated degree:	BSc (compulsory)
Applicants	2168	Student mix:	
Interviews	575	% Mature	5%
Offers	399	% International	6%

Uncompetitive	🏆 🏆 🏆 **🏆** 🏆	Competitive
Low living costs	💰 💰 💰 💰 **💰**	High living costs
Working really hard		Not working/ chilling out
Contact details	Imperial College Medical School, Sir Alexander Fleming Building, South Kensington, London, SW7 2AZ Tel: +44 (0) 20 758 95111, Web: www1.imperial.ac.uk/medicine/ teaching/undergraduate	

An insider's view...

In short, we want the very best who will become superb doctors and leaders in their chosen field. Competition to gain entry remains fierce. We want our students to have a very good basis in, and understanding of, the scientific principles that underpin medicine. These are often the key principles that medical professionals return to when dealing with difficult problems. Thus, the emphasis on science, and the opportunity that every student has to obtain a BSc, is entirely appropriate. I am not, however, looking for 'anoraks'. I am looking for well-rounded individuals who have the ability to communicate well, become great clinicians, and make a real contribution to the future of the profession.

Prof. Jenny M. Higham, Dean of Undergraduate Medicine and Director of Education

London—King's College

The jewel of King's College London School of Medicine is the teaching provided by the world-famous Guy's, King's, and St Thomas' Hospitals (now working together as King's Health Partners Academic Health Sciences Centre).

University The main hub of the medical school is based at the Guy's Campus, south of the River Thames next to London Bridge. For pre-clinical students, the vast majority of teaching is based at Guy's. On site, there is one main library open for the majority of the day, as well as a 24-hour library for the night-owls. At Guy's there is also the Gordon's Museum, one of the largest pathology museums in the world, which has a collection of 8,000 pathological specimens going back to 1608. Students can relax on campus in 'The Spit' or Guy's Bar.

Course The integrated medical curriculum is divided into five phases, with phase I lasting a single term and introducing students to the major systems. Phase II focuses on basic science in a clinical context with a new clinical scenario presented every week and each scenario is grouped into systems areas. In the pre-clinical years, medicine is taught through lectures, tutorials, and group sessions with lab work. Anatomy is taught in the dissecting lab supported by the largest UK medical anatomy museum. In the clinical years (phases III to V), students may be allocated anywhere in the South East from the three main hospitals—Guy's, St Thomas', or King's College Hospital to the outer reaches of Kent such as Canterbury and Margate. Ward teaching is combined with lectures on clinical pathology, public health, and health promotion and there is a strong emphasis on developing communication and patient skills. Students also have access to the Chantler Clinical Skills Centre, the largest centre of its kind in the UK, where students can practise their clinical skills on anatomical models.

Student-selected components (SSCs) are offered throughout the course and an optional BSc is available after years two, three, or four, with 23 degree programmes at King's and the chance to intercalate elsewhere if your choice of course is not available. During the ten-week elective, students can apply to explore various specialties in world-leading hospitals linked with King's such as Johns Hopkins in the USA.

Lifestyle The vast majority of medical students live around campus. This includes halls at Wolfson House and Great Dover Street (a ten-minute walk from campus). After the first year, you could either re-apply for halls and become a senior student or rent accommodation around London. King's has an abundance of societies which you can join, ranging from writing for the *GKT Gazette* (established 1872!), mentoring school children through the SHINE programme, or even getting involved with organizing shows or plays. Volunteering also plays a big role in the student life at King's, with opportunities locally and globally. If none of these takes your fancy, then playing sport for the medical school might appeal; it can involve competing to win the Macadam Cup (the annual competition between the medical school and the university itself). The MSA (Medical Students' Association) and the Students' Union put on plenty of socials and formal balls throughout the year.

Factoid The Colonnade gardens on Guy's campus have the world's only life-size statue of the 19th century poet (and surgeon apprentice) John Keats, who studied medicine here. See Table 8.16.

Table 8.16 London—King's College

Myth	'Too big'—a large and faceless London medical school
Reality	A large London medical school with ample student support
Personality	Practical and hard-working
Best aspects	The highly resourceful Virtual Campus (online learning resource) keeps students up-to-date with the latest notifications as well as providing access to lectures, revision videos, and past exam papers
Worst aspects	Living and housing expenses are among the highest in the country
Requirements	**UKCAT**; **A-level** three A2s including chemistry and/or biology with AS chemistry or biology if not taking A2; **GCSE** 'B' in English and maths (unless taking AS/A2)

Course length	5 years	Structure	City/Campus
Type of course	Red brick (p. 94)	Year size	330
Typical offer	AAAb	Intercalated degree:	BSc
Applicants	3599	Student mix:	
Interviews	1100	% Mature	22%
Offers	653	% International	11%

Uncompetitive	Competitive
Low living costs	High living costs
Working really hard	Not working/chilling out
Contact details	Student Admissions Office, King's College London, Hodgkin Building, Guy's Campus, London Bridge, London, SE1 1UL Tel: +44 (0) 20 7848 6501, Web: www.kcl.ac.uk/study/ug

An insider's view...

Undergraduate medical students at King's College London School of Medicine study in an institution with research excellence while gaining a broad clinical experience in a very diverse community within London. King's Health Partners is a pioneering collaboration between the Medical School, King's College, and three of London's most successful NHS Foundation Trusts. The partnership aims for excellence in clinical medicine, research, and education through a new Education Academy. These links give medical students access to extensive clinical experience and active translational research. This is seen in the very broad programme of student-selected components (SSCs), where students can choose from a range of over 800 SSCs from languages and humanities to research and careers, the elective programme, and the opportunity for self-designed attachments.

Prof. John Rees, Dean of Undergraduate Education

London—St George's

St George's, University of London (SGUL) is one of the oldest medical schools in the UK. It is less traditional than other London medical schools and ideally suited to students wanting 'something different' in a central location.

University St George's is a specialist medical college of the University of London. You will find student physiotherapists, nurses, midwives, pharmacists, and paramedics training here as well. In fact the only students at SGUL are those studying biomedical science or healthcare-related degrees. This is an opportunity to learn alongside the colleagues you will be relying on as a doctor in years to come. Perhaps unsurprisingly the university is much smaller than most others, with only around 3,500 students. Its small size may explain St George's reputation as a friendly, caring community of student clinicians.

St George's boasts a rich history of contributions to medicine with alumni including Henry Gray (of *Gray's Anatomy* fame), Edward Jenner (the father of vaccination), and Harry Hill (comedian and television presenter). Originally located next to Hyde Park Corner, the university, since 1980, shares a site with St George's Hospital in the cosmopolitan area of Tooting in South London.

Course The entire course is a 'spiral' curriculum, where students will cover the material repeatedly throughout the entire MBBS course in ever-increasing detail. The first two years are pre-clinical years: semester one covers all the bodily systems and semesters two to four (spread across the two pre-clinical years) cover each system again in more detail. In the third year, the standard undergraduate MBBS5 course merges with the graduate MBBS4 course, spending half the year in PBL and the other half of the year in clinical attachments. Years four and five are both clinical years with five- to six-week attachments. Intercalating is optional, and can be taken anytime between years two and four.

Lifestyle St George's Students' Union is smaller than many others but you're still unlikely to get bored. As well as the usual array of societies and sports clubs, St George's has a particularly strong selection of community and charity projects. It raises more money for charity per student than any other London medical school. Although Tooting is in zone three (ideal for those worried about London prices), the centre of London is only 20 minutes away by underground and convenient to access major rail stations such as Wimbledon, Clapham Junction, and Waterloo.

In any event, London has plenty to keep students entertained: world-famous sights, huge shopping centres, international cuisine, bars and restaurants of every variety, and peaceful parks. Transport is easy since the whole city is connected by a single tube system and it helps that the hospital and medical school are found on the same site.

Factoid St George's is the second-oldest university in the UK to train doctors formally, only beaten in age by Oxford. It was founded in 1733 and has trained quite a few doctors since! See Table 8.17.

Table 8.17 London—St George's

Myth	Students with phenomenal social skills, mostly developed from socializing
Reality	A whole university dedicated to healthcare—the ideal training ground for new doctors
Personality	Laid-back for London medical students!
Best aspects	A small, friendly community in a large, vibrant city
Worst aspects	Everyone is a healthcare student, so there is a real danger of becoming institutionalized
Requirements	**UKCAT; A-level** three A2s including chemistry and/or biology and one AS in chemistry or biology if not taking A2; BBCb will be considered if this is 60% higher than your school/college's average performance—see website; **GCSE** average of 'A' in top eight subjects, 'B' in English

Course length	5 years	Structure	City
Type of course	Plate glass (p. 94)	Year size	135
Typical offer	AAAb-BBCb	Intercalated degree:	BSc
Applicants	1033	Student mix:	
Interviews	398	% Mature	0%
Offers	249	% International	7%

Uncompetitive	🏆 🏆 **🏆🏆🏆** 🏆🏆 🏆🏆	Competitive
Low living costs	💰 💰 💰 💰 **💰**	High living costs
Working really hard	🧍 🧍 **🧍** 🧍 🧍	Not working/ chilling out

Contact details	St George's, University of London, Cranmer Terrace, London, SW17 0RE Tel: +44 (0) 20 8672 9944, Web: www.sgul.ac.uk/courses/undergraduate/mbbs5

An insider's view...

SGUL provides education and training to more than 3,500 medical and healthcare students on one site. On our main campus we share a site with St George's Healthcare NHS Trust, one of the busiest in the NHS, which sees on average half a million patients annually. This allows us to offer students unrivalled diversity at the sharp end of clinical practice. St George's is also renowned for its pioneering widening participation schemes to increase access to medicine for people from all backgrounds. These have helped increase the proportion of students joining St George's from state schools from 53% nine years ago to more than 80% today.

Gordon Coutts, Press Officer

London—University College (UCL)

UCL Medical School (UCLMS) offers world-class, research-led medical teaching in the heart of London. The medical school emerged from the amalgamation of the Middlesex, University College, and Royal Free Hospitals, combining a rich history of science and medicine into a single institution.

University UCL is the oldest and largest constituent college of the University of London, opening its doors as early as 1828. It was the first non-secular university in Britain and the first to admit women on equal terms with men, whilst the Royal Free was the first to admit women for training in medicine specifically.

The Medical School spans three London campuses incorporating the three teaching hospitals of the Royal Free in Hampstead, the Whittington in Archway, and the new University College Hospital in Bloomsbury. In addition to the three medical libraries, the university also has a renovated main library and science library and great IT facilities (including cross-campus WiFi).

Course The MBBS programme, which was updated in 2012, is designed to integrate early clinical experience with the basic sciences. In the first two years, teaching is largely lecture and tutorial based, with lab sessions and cadaveric dissection (~8 students/cadaver) alongside clinical skills teaching and clinical exposure in general practice and hospital medicine (through shadowing a junior doctor). The third year consists of the intercalated BSc, which is compulsory for students who don't already hold a degree. UCL has one of the widest ranges of BSc in the country, from anatomy and neuroscience to philosophy and international health. For those particularly interested in research, there is also the MB/PhD programme, providing an opportunity for students to complete their MBBS, a BSc, and a PhD in eight years.

Professional development is emphasized throughout the programme so that students develop the background, skills, and attitudes necessary to practise medicine, and a comprehensive selection of science and non-science student-selected components are also provided throughout the course.

Years four and five enable the student to transfer their basic science knowledge into clinical practice through a range of clinical attachments in teaching hospitals, district general hospitals, and within general practice and the community. This experience is further refined in the final year of the programme. These three years draw extensively on the facilities of leading partner healthcare institutions such as Great Ormond Street Children's Hospital, Moorfields Eye Hospital, and the National Hospital for Neurology and Neurosurgery at Queen's Square. Most of these sites are within close proximity to the main UCL campus, although the further placements can involve longer journeys, with free accommodation provided at these. Students go on an eight-week elective in their final year, with most taking the opportunity to study overseas in a contrasting healthcare environment.

Lifestyle All first year students are offered accommodation in halls of residence. Much-needed breaks from studying can include anything London has to offer as the UCL campus is just minutes from the West End and Oxford Street. UCL's Students' Union has over 190 clubs and societies run by students, as well as its own theatre: the Bloomsbury Theatre. The medical students' society, RUMS, also has its own sports teams and social events, so there will be something for everyone! Transport around central London is easy to negotiate—just grab an Oyster card and enjoy the underground and 24/7 bus service. If all else fails, it rarely hurts to walk. However, driving in London is not recommended.

Factoid UCL's MBBS programme has been rated the best in London, and ranked sixth in the world in recent league tables! See Table 8.18.

Table 8.18 London—University College

Myth	Posh, white rugby players who hate King's College London
Reality	An eclectic mix of students with a healthy streak of competitiveness towards their fellow London medics, receiving research-led teaching in the heart of a vibrant metropolis
Personality	International students through to Londoners born and bred; our reputation and location attract a wide range of students wanting to work and play like no other!
Best aspects	Medicine you might never see outside of London: malaria, TB, and Crimean-Congo Haemorrhagic Fever!
Worst aspects	The costs of living in central London
Requirements	**BMAT; A-Level** three A2s and one AS with chemistry and biology at A2, preference given to those offering a 'contrasting' third A-level or AS-level (e.g. humanities); **GCSE** 'B's in maths and English and a 'C' in a Modern Foreign Language

Course length	6 years	Structure	City
Type of course	Red brick (p. 94)	Year size	330
Typical offer	AAAc	Intercalated degree:	BSc (compulsory)
Applicants	2500	Student mix:	
Interviews	700	% Mature	9%
Offers	550	% International	7%

Uncompetitive	Competitive
Low living costs	High living costs
Working really hard	Not working/chilling out

Contact details	Medical Admissions Office, UCL Medical School, UCL, Gower Street, London, WC1E 6BT Tel: +44 (0) 20 7679 0841, Web: www.ucl.ac.uk/medicalschool/undergraduate

An insider's view . . .

We want students who are academically gifted, good communicators, and willing to join proactively in the academic, clinical, and social life of the medical school and university. Our course has the best features of a modern integrated course whilst maintaining traditional components where appropriate. There is a strong emphasis on scientific excellence and the translation of science into clinical practice. We wish to train the clinical leaders of the future, producing doctors prepared for practice in the NHS, for the forefront of medical science, and for the wider global health community.

Dr Paul Dilworth, Sub Dean Careers

Manchester

Manchester may conjure images of football, curry, and rain, but it has a medical school with one of the most innovative courses in the UK. The emphasis on enquiry-based learning (EBL) allows for a flexible lifestyle and those with a background in European languages can continue learning them and study abroad.

University The medical school building is in the heart of the university campus and includes a comprehensive medical library and purpose-built PBL rooms perfect for group study. Clinical teaching is split between four base teaching hospitals: Central Manchester, South Manchester, Salford Royal, and Lancashire (Preston). Each base has several smaller hospitals attached, which students rotate around, and accommodation is often available at the more distant sites. All students spend time at The Christie, a world-renowned specialist cancer hospital right on our doorstep!

Course The new Manchester curriculum is a hybrid between problem-based learning (PBL), clinical experience, and traditional lecture-style teaching. The aim is to provide both the basic medical AND clinical knowledge needed to become a junior doctor. EBL is structured around clinical cases and organized by systems (e.g. gastrointestinal). For the first year EBL sessions are in groups of 12 with a weekly case supported by relevant lab work, lectures, and anatomy tutorials, including full-body dissection with one cadaver and one teaching clinician per group. Patient contact begins from the first semester and increases during the 'intermediate' phase starting at year two.

About 100 St Andrews students join for Phase 2 and 3 (years three to five), as the EBL approach continues in smaller groups (around six to eight students) randomly assigned to a specific 'base' hospital. All Phase 2 students are given an iPad for use in clinical teaching, ward attachments, and online teaching resources via the sophisticated 'blackboard platform'. The university has even developed some its own 'apps' and 'iBooks' for its students to use.

Throughout the course, student-selected component blocks allow students to develop their interests, including an 11 week project option in year four and an eight week medical elective in year five.

Manchester has a huge research centre and many students choose to take an intercalated bachelor's or master's degree after year two, three, or four. There is also a European Option programme (students with A-level standard French, German, or Spanish study the language over four years and spend 16 weeks at a European partner hospital in the fifth year) leading to a Diploma in Global Health.

Lifestyle University accommodation is guaranteed for all first year students and most of it is in Fallowfield, about ten minutes from campus by bus. Most students move to private accommodation in Fallowfield or neighbouring Withington from the second year onwards. Students based in Preston for Phase 2 and 3 (years three to five) live there, as it is 50 miles away.

The university has invested greatly in improving the campus, including computing resources, sporting facilities, theatres, a concert hall, museum, and gallery. The large student population means that there are a wide variety of charity, student, and sporting clubs, including numerous medics' societies that organize regular socials. The city itself also has a lot to offer including the internationally renowned music and club scene (see the film '24 Hour Party People') as well as fairly well-known football teams. When you've had enough of city life, the Lake District and Peak District are easily accessible for a spot of fresh air.

Factoid With over 60,000 students, most of whom live near the Oxford Road, it is unsurprising that this is the busiest bus route in Europe. See Table 8.19.

Table 8.19 Manchester

Myth	DIY medical teaching allows students to effectively communicate their lack of real knowledge
Reality	Truly well-rounded students who learn to think like a doctor from day one
Personality	Self-directed study attracts outgoing, determined, and mature students able to take responsibility for their learning
Best aspects	Case-based PBL is engaging and allows you to pursue interests; studying in small, close-knit groups helps form strong friendships
Worst aspects	Unmotivated students can struggle with PBL
Requirements	**UKCAT**; **A-level** three A2s with 'A' in chemistry and at least one other science or maths; **AS-levels** at least four subjects are expected; **GCSE** at least seven GCSEs, five 'A*'s or 'A's, and two others of at least 'C'; at least 'B' in English, maths, and dual award science

Course length	5 years	Structure	Campus
Type of course	Carbon fibre (p. 94)	Year size	380
Typical offer	AAA	Intercalated degree:	BSc, MSc
Applicants	2520	Student mix:	
Interviews	925	% Mature	11%
Offers	630	% International	8%

Uncompetitive						Competitive
Low living costs						High living costs
Working really hard						Not working/ chilling out

Contact details	Manchester Medical School, Stopford Building, Oxford Road, Manchester, M13 9PT Tel: +44 (0) 161 306 0460,Web: www.mms.manchester.ac.uk/undergraduate

An insider's view...

Applicants are expected to demonstrate high standards in both academic and clinical achievements. They will have a strong ethical framework; a strong sense of responsibility (for patients and communities); an empowering sense of fairness (needs of a diverse society, both locally and internationally); and the ability to become a leader and agent of change. They will also need to demonstrate caring work experience, commitment, communication, and teamworking skills. The enquiry-based learning course offered will use flexible learning methods, lectures, dissection, seminars, skills laboratories, and clinical learning in hospitals and community settings, which will be delivered from the start of the course.

Linda Harding, Admissions Co-ordinator

Newcastle

Despite Newcastle being one of the largest medical schools in the country, it retains many aspects of smaller schools because undergraduates are divided between two teaching sites for the Phase I pre-clinical teaching (years one and two): approximately 220 students go to Newcastle University and 100 students attend the quieter Queen's Campus of Durham University (see profile p. 120). Applicants can apply to a specific site or indicate no preference by completing the 'Campus Code' on their UCAS application.

University In contrast to many other universities, Newcastle's campus and medical school is in the centre of the city. Located near the leafy Leazes Park and Town Moor, it is within easy walking distance of all the shops and restaurants that Newcastle has to offer. The one downside of this arrangement is that finding parking near the campus can be difficult; however, most students live within walking distance. The campus is well equipped with libraries and computer clusters (many with 24-hour access) along with good sporting facilities. Clinical placements are split between four clinical bases: Tyneside (Newcastle and surroundings), Teeside (Stockton and surroundings), Wearside (Sunderland, south of Newcastle), and Northumbria (a large area north west of Newcastle). Many of these placements require driving or car sharing with other students. Some of the hospitals further afield offer accommodation and they all have libraries and computing facilities for students.

Course Phase I (pre-clinical) is an integrated systems-based (p. 88) course taught using lectures, seminars, and laboratory practicals. Anatomy is taught in small groups using prosections and computer-based models rather than dissection (although there are opportunities for dissection in the fourth year). The curriculum has a spiral structure (subjects are repeated with increasing complexity), with clinical exposure from the beginning. Phase II (clinical) begins at the start of year three. Newcastle and Durham students are assigned to one of the four clinical bases (see **University**) and rotate through the different clinical specialities. All students are based in Newcastle for the fourth year, which begins with a term of lectures followed by three student-selected components. Each component lasts six weeks and can include clinical placements anywhere in the country. The year ends with an eight-week elective followed by two weeks of holiday. Fifth year follows a similar pattern to third year, but at a different clinical base. It is possible to undertake an intercalated BSc after the second year or, unlike most medical schools, an MRes after the fourth year.

Lifestyle University accommodation in Newcastle is mostly hall-based and spread out across the city at varying distances from the campus (from a five-minute walk to a three-mile bus ride). After the first year, virtually all students live in privately rented accommodation, usually in Newcastle; however, those in the Tees-based unit for year three or five may choose to live closer to hospitals while on placement there. Newcastle offers some of the cheapest accommodation in the country and the general cost of living is low. Outside of medicine, there's plenty to keep you busy, with numerous university societies and sports teams as well as all the nightlife that Newcastle is famous for. Getting around the city is easy thanks to the metro, a light rail system, which can also take you to the beach in Tynemouth if you ever want to get out of the city.

Factoid Newcastle University owes its existence to the medical school. The medical school, established in 1834, joined Durham University in 1851. In 1937 it became King's College, Durham, which then became Newcastle University in 1963. See Table 8.20.

Table 8.20 Newcastle

Myth	Only good for hen nights and stag parties
Reality	A successful medical school in a fantastic city, with an excellent record in teaching and research, as well as an amazing nightlife
Personality	Lively, fun grafters
Best aspects	Living in a great student-friendly city while studying medicine in a wide variety of geographical and socio-economic areas
Worst aspects	Having clinical attachments outside of Newcastle can mean a long commute each day; the (lack of) parking on campus
Requirements	**UKCAT**; **A-level** three A2s with at least AS chemistry or biology; **GCSE** 'A' in chemistry, biology, or dual science if not taking AS/A2

Course length	5 years	Structure	City/Campus
Type of course	Plate glass (p. 94)	Year size	206
Typical offer	AAA	Intercalated degree:	BSc, MRes
Applicants	1897	Student mix:	
Interviews	900	% Mature	7%
Offers	411	% International	9%

Uncompetitive		Competitive
Low living costs		High living costs
Working really hard		Not working/ chilling out

Contact details	Newcastle University, Claremont Road, Newcastle upon Tyne, NE1, 7RU Tel: +44 (0) 191 222 6000, Web: http://www.ncl.ac.uk/ undergraduate/degrees/a100

An insider's view ...

The case-based integrated approach that our curriculum follows means that in the 'pre-clinical' years all teaching is delivered in the context of clinical cases and all content has clinical relevance. The pure science elements of the curriculum are de-emphasized and so our admissions policy does not require applicants to have studied science at A-level. Our clinical training is not based on the traditional '-ologies' but rather focuses on core competencies and knowledge that will enable successful transition to FY1, and is achieved in close partnership with our regional NHS trusts. Selection is aimed at finding bright, motivated individuals who want to develop into doctors willing to view their patients as members of society and not just as a collection of symptoms.

Dr David Kennedy, MBBS Degree Programme Director

Nottingham

Nottingham combines the academic rigour of a traditional medical course with extensive early clinical experience and a strong emphasis on communication skills and ethics. The course includes an obligatory intercalated degree (BMedSci), but unlike other medical schools this is squeezed into year three of the five-year course.

University The large and green main university campus is a ten-minute bus ride away from the city centre, with the medical school, based in the Queen's Medical Centre (QMC), a short walk from campus. The recently constructed and eco-friendly Jubilee campus is about 15 minutes' walk away, with a regular university bus service between them. The majority of the first two years are spent in the QMC lecture halls, seminar rooms, dissection room, and laboratories, with access to the dedicated medical library, 24-hour computer room, student cafes, and purpose-built clinical skills centre.

Clinical placements are largely undertaken at the QMC, Nottingham City Hospital (20 minutes by bus), Royal Derby Hospital (40 minutes by car or bus), and Kings Mill Hospital, Mansfield (40 minutes by car, accommodation provided). Additionally, a few students are also placed at Lincoln or Boston which are roughly 90 minutes away and provide accommodation.

Course The first two years of this systems-based course are mainly taught by lectures, with some seminars and laboratory practicals, and optional modules available in year two. Students learn anatomy by full-body dissection in small groups supported by lectures and seminars. There is a strong emphasis on patient contact right from the beginning, with regular sessions spent in the hospital or GP surgery during the first two years. Students are taught to appreciate medicine from the patient's point of view by regular contact with the same patient over an 18-month period in the Community Follow-up Project. The first six months of year three are dedicated to a research project for the BMedSci with a broad range of options available. Halfway through year three, students start the clinical phase of the course alongside the graduate entry medical students with a 16-week block comprising of medicine and surgery. The fourth year comprises a total of 40 weeks covering paediatrics, obstetrics and gynaecology, psychiatry, ENT, ophthalmology, dermatology, care of the elderly, and four weeks dedicated to a student-selected module.

The final year is dedicated to the ACE (Advanced Clinical Experience) module consisting of 36 weeks covering medicine and surgery, musculoskeletal disease and disability, primary care, critical illness, and medical assistantship. Finals take place in March followed by a nine-week elective to recover!

Lifestyle First year students are guaranteed a place in university accommodation, most of which is on the main or Jubilee campus. Each hall has its own common room, bar, library, social events, and sports teams, giving a strong sense of community. In later years most students move into private accommodation in neighbouring Lenton or Dunkirk; the campus atmosphere is preserved because all your friends will be within walking distance. The Students' Union offers over 200 societies, teams, and social events and if that's not enough there are medics' societies and social events too. Nottingham city centre is large enough to have a wide range of shops, restaurants, pubs, and clubs but small enough that it's very easy to get around, especially in view of the developments to the tram network. Transport links are excellent by train or car and the Peak District is just a short drive away.

Factoid The piano in the lobby of the medical school was acquired in April 1982 by Dr Stanley Monkhouse, an anatomy instructor and founder of the Medical School Music Society. Some years later Dr Monkhouse retired from the Society, medical school, and the medical profession to become a vicar! See Table 8.21.

Table 8.21 Nottingham

Myth	The unoriginal choice after the Medlink, Medisix, or Medsim courses
Reality	The right choice for applicants looking for a solid grounding in research and clinical science
Personality	Work hard, play harder!
Best aspects	The stunning University Park and futuristic Jubilee campus, against a backdrop of rolling hills and lakes; intercalated degree without adding an extra year to your studies
Worst aspects	The January exam sessions can ruin Christmas
Requirements	**UKCAT**; **A-level** three A2s at grade A including chemistry and biology, third A-level in any subject except general studies and critical thinking; **GCSE** six 'A's including sciences, 'B's in English and maths

Course length	5 years	Structure	Campus
Type of course	Red brick (p. 94)	Year size	249
Typical offer	AAA	Intercalated degree:	BMedSci (compulsory)
Applicants	2750	Student mix:	
Interviews	750	% Mature	1.5%
Offers	380	% International	10%

Uncompetitive ▢▢▢▢▢	Competitive
Low living costs ▢▢▢▢▢	High living costs
Working really hard ▢▢▢▢▢	Not working/chilling out

Contact details	Faculty of Medicine and Health Sciences, University of Nottingham Medical School, Queen's Medical Centre, Nottingham, NG7 2UH. Tel: +44 (0) 115 823 0000, Web: www.nottingham.ac.uk/mhs/undergraduate-courses

An insider's view...

Nottingham has a high number of applicants and so attracts outstandingly able students onto both its A-level and graduate entry course (p. 244). The interviews are designed to select the best communicators and most vocationally motivated students. Our teaching philosophy is to put the patient at the centre of the student's learning with clinical experience from week one. The integrated BMedSci degree provides an opportunity for the more scientifically minded student to excel. Although our course is tough and very competitive, Nottingham is a friendly place of learning, nurturing the lifelong skills required to be a good doctor.

Miss Brigitte E. Scammell, Admissions Sub-Dean

Oxford

If you're going to study medicine, where better than the place where doctors first discovered the living cell, understood the circulatory system, and treated patients with penicillin.

University Medicine at Oxford goes back over 700 years so they must be doing something right. In fact, the university as a whole has been ranked highest in the UK every year since 2003 by *The Times Good University Guide*, and is now ranked the best medical school in the world by them too! As a collegiate university its medical students are taught by both individual colleges and the medical school. In the first three years you will feel as if you have two homes: your room in college and the Medical Sciences Teaching Centre. The latter is an uber-modern complex with lecture theatres, laboratories, and even computer suites. This alone dispels the myth that Oxford is as resistant to change as *Staphylococcus* is to antibiotics. The jewel in the Oxford crown is weekly meetings with your college tutor in which essays are used as the basis of discussion. You'll have no trouble writing these as Oxford boasts the second-largest library in the UK, as well as more than 40 other college/faculty libraries for your use.

Course The pre-clinical course unashamedly focuses on the scientific basis of medicine and there is little patient contact. The course has not yet capitulated to the PBL craze embraced by other medical schools and teaching still comes from lectures, practical classes, and college tutorials. Pre-clinical disciplines such as physiology, anatomy, and pathology are each individually examined by short-answer and essay papers. Anatomy is taught using prosected specimens but there are full-body dissection opportunities as well. The third year revolves around a research project, which students choose, and leads to a BA (Hons) degree in Medical Sciences.

After the third year, entry to the clinical course is competitive. Although everyone continues with medicine, you cannot guarantee staying in Oxford and about 15% of students finish clinical training in London. In Oxford, teaching is based at the John Radcliffe Hospital and surrounding district general hospitals and GP practices. The medical elective is three months long, longer than most medical schools, although by this time you'll feel as if you've earned a placement in the sun!

Lifestyle Oxford has every society known to mankind and a few others (korfball, anyone?!). The collegiate system means that you can pursue an activity casually at college level, or more seriously as part of the university team. Most students try rowing and there are dedicated novice events to help them give it a go. Osler House, the clinical students' club, offers support to students and lots of socializing opportunities. Most medical students live in colleges (spread around Oxford) but many choose to rent houses closer to the hospital in later years. Driving is almost impossible as parking is scarce but nothing in Oxford is more than a short cycle ride away.

Factoid Medicine at Oxford is packed with traditions. In the first year you'll be treated to 'Dissection Drinks', i.e. drinks disguised as bodily fluids, while clinical medics put on an annual pantomime in which the star is invariably a pink elephant named Rita. Honestly. See Table 8.22.

Table 8.22 Oxford

Myth	Geeks safe from skin cancer as they rarely leave the Oxford spires to see daylight
Reality	Three science-intense years followed by three patient-centred years—the best of both worlds
Personality	Gifted musicians, varsity sportsmen, student journalists, world debaters, or just students interested in science ... anything goes!
Best aspects	The third-year project where students research an area of interest for a whole year, an unrivalled opportunity to pursue research at a high standard and even sometimes get published!
Worst aspects	First and second year exams are awful, but almost all students pass
Requirements	**BMAT**; **A-level** three A2s at A*AA with chemistry and one other science or maths; **GCSE** at least 'C' in biology, physics, or maths if not taken to a higher level

Course length	6 years	Structure	Collegiate
Type of course	Stone (p. 94)	Year size	150
Typical offer	A*AA	Intercalated degree:	BA (compulsory)
Applicants	1468	Student mix:	
Interviews	425	% Mature	1%
Offers	154	% International	1%

Uncompetitive		Competitive
Low living costs		High living costs
Working really hard		Not working/chilling out

Contact details	Medical Sciences Office, John Radcliffe Hospital, Headington, Oxford, OX3 9DU Tel: +44 (0) 1865 221689, Web: http://www.medsci.ox.ac.uk/study/medicine

An insider's view...

The course is intended for students with a particular enthusiasm for the science that supports medicine and its continuing advancement. It provides more in-depth knowledge than you will immediately need for the clinical stage of your training and is designed to provide you with an understanding and enthusiasm for science and scientific method that will serve you well both now and later in your career.

Prof. William James, Sir William Dunn School of Pathology

Plymouth

Plymouth University Peninsula School of Medicine was formed in 2013 after the splitting of the Peninsula Medical School (opened in 2002), between the University of Exeter and Plymouth University. The new curriculum is based on that of Peninsula Medical School, but with refinements to fit with Plymouth University's values and the distinctive local clinical opportunities.

University For the first two years medical students are based in the purpose-built Portland Square at Plymouth University's main campus near the city centre. Derriford, one of Europe's largest hospitals, is the main base for the students in years three to five and is a 15-minute bus journey from the city centre. It's a great place to see a wide range of specialties, including many only found at the largest hospitals including neurosurgery and transplant surgery, as well as being Devon and Cornwall's major trauma centre. There is also an abundance of high quality clinical skills resources, as is to be expected of a new, purpose-built medical school.

Course The first two years at Plymouth (and Exeter) are unique in being structured around the human life-cycle (i.e. conception to old age) considering the normal physiology in year 1 and abnormal pathology in year 2. A wide range of teaching styles are used, including lectures, workshops, clinical skills sessions, small groups and self-directed learning (SDL), with a heavy emphasis on patient-focused teaching and early clinical experience. The curriculum integrates clinical and science learning structured around clinical cases (years one and two), trigger presentations (years three and four), and indicative presentations (year five). In years three to five there is extensive exposure to the clinical environment, providing plenty of patients to base one's learning on.

From year three, students are extensively immersed in the clinical environment. Just like being a doctor, the curriculum is based on presentation of illness (e.g. shortness of breath) rather than being disease-based (e.g. heart failure or pneumonia). Each presentation is studied for a week, including relevant primary care, hospital-based care, and patient-centred/ethical issues. This last component is excellent training for the Situational Judgement Test that forms a key component of FY1 applications. Students move departments frequently, but gain an unrivalled spectrum of patients to learn from. The fourth year is the most intensive and exam-filled year of the course. This relives the pressure for the fifth year, where students rotate through core specialities every five weeks, essentially learning the job of a foundation doctor. The chance to study for an intercalated BSc/MSc between years four and five is offered to the top-graded 15% of each year.

Lifestyle University accommodation is readily available with priority given to first years. Students at Plymouth are surrounded by the beautiful Dartmoor countryside and are never more than 15 minutes from a beach. It's not unusual to wake up in the morning, smell the sea air, hear the seagulls, and think 'I'm on holiday'. There is an active MedSoc run by students which organizes various socials and balls throughout the year, as well as making the most of the beautiful countryside by organizing horse riding on Dartmoor—so don't miss out!

Factoid Driving 15-minutes north will take you to the wilds of Dartmoor, while south will take you to a beach suitable for surfing, sunbathing, and barbequing! See Table 8.23.

Table 8.23 Plymouth

Myth	The single parent of a university divorce
Reality	A fresh, new, innovative medical school, not afraid to train doctors a little differently
Personality	Self-motivation is a quality shared by every doctor who qualifies from Plymouth—you will not survive the course if you expect to be spoon-fed
Best aspects	Being taught by doctors, not scientists—everything you learn is clinically relevant
Worst aspects	The location is a double-edged sword; quite far away from the rest of the UK
Requirements	**UKCAT**; **A-level** three A2s including chemistry and then either biology or physics; and biology at least to AS; one AS-level at grade A–C; **GCSE** seven 'C's including English, maths, and science

Course length	5 years	Structure	Campus
Type of course	Carbon fibre (p. 94)	Year size	86
Typical offer	A*AA or AAA	Intercalated degree:	BSc, MSc
Applicants	1066	Student mix:	
Interviews	270	% Mature	10%
Offers	120	% International	7.5%

Uncompetitive		Competitive
Low living costs		High living costs
Working really hard		Not working/ chilling out
Contact details	Plymouth University Peninsula School of Medicine, The John Bull Building, Tamar Science Park, Research Way, Plymouth, PL6 8BU Tel: +44 (0) 1752 437 333, Web: www.plymouth.ac.uk/peninsula	

An insider's view...

Plymouth offers an exciting and challenging undergraduate medical programme, which is forward-thinking and focused on patients and improving health. It offers an integrated, clinically led, and patient-focused curriculum that promotes meaningful interactions with patients from an early stage. The curriculum emphasizes activity-based, structured, small-group learning methods, and learning in the clinical environment and from patient encounters, coupled with extensive support for independent learning. Students develop an integrated knowledge and understanding of the sciences, clinical, communication, and leadership skills, and personal and professional values that underlie safe and effective medical practice.

Prof. David Bristow, Associate Dean, Teaching and Learning

Sheffield

Once a bleak industrial city famous for its steel but also for its smog, Sheffield has cleaned up its act to become a thriving and cosmopolitan place to live. The balance of city life with its many parks (earning it the title of 'greenest city') has drawn 60,000 students to study at its two universities and the medical school at the University of Sheffield has a long-earned reputation, training doctors since 1828.

University Whilst some teaching takes place at the city's Northern General Hospital, the vast majority of lectures and seminars take place in the newly refurbished facilities at the Royal Hallamshire Hospital, near to the main university campus and student accommodation. As part of the refurbishment, the health sciences library has been transformed into a modern working environment complete with a cafe and the main university library is open 24/7. Most of the peripheral hospitals used for placement are easily within commuting distance, allowing students to live in Sheffield all year round. Lift sharing to these hospitals is common, so having a car is an easy way to become popular!

Course Content is delivered system by system and is usually pinned to clinical examples to show how theory becomes practice. The course starts with a pre-clinical block, with teaching focusing on the underlying medical sciences. Fortnightly Integrated Learning Activities break up the lectures with PBL-style tutorials, and anatomy is taught mainly by full-body dissection, a real highlight of the course. During this time students are introduced to history taking and clinical skills with actors and mannequins. There is also the opportunity to get hands on with a two-week clinical placement in the first year, and a research attachment in the second year. Students then move onto the wards, putting these new skills and knowledge into practice with placements across the different hospital specialties and in GP practices. Sheffield offers not one but two elective periods, of six and seven weeks respectively. There are a range of intercalations available: students can take a year out to study a Master's in Law (LLM) or Public Health (MPH) or, most commonly, perform some research leading to a BMedSci. Pre-clinical exams are a mixture of short answer and multiple choice papers, and a spotter exam (another multiple choice paper based on anatomy and histology specimens). Clinical exams are much the same but with the spotters replaced by Objective Structured Clinical Examinations (OSCEs).

Lifestyle Like any medical school, there is much work to do. However, there are plenty of opportunities to let your hair down. The student-run Medical Society provides a number of sports teams (running timetable-friendly training sessions), societies, and nights out, including the epic yearly fancy dress social which attracts more than 1,000 people. Sheffield itself has a lot to offer, with plenty of bars and restaurants to visit, the Meadowhall shopping centre just up the road, and the Peak District National Park not far away either. The city is very laid back and the locals are extremely friendly, with many students choosing to make Sheffield their home after university.

Factoid At four per person, Sheffield has more trees per capita than any other European city—a reflection of its many parks and proximity to the Peak District. See Table 8.24.

Table 8.24 Sheffield

Myth	An average university in an average city
Reality	High quality medical education, with a social scene to match
Personality	Simply banterful
Best aspects	Full-body dissection and the opportunity to go on elective twice!
Worst aspects	Navigating Sheffield's hills just to get home
Requirements	**UKCAT**; **A-level** three A2s including chemistry and at least one of biology, physics, or psychology; at least ABBB at AS-level; **GCSE** six 'A's including at least a 'C' in English, maths, and the sciences (dual awards accepted)

Course length	5 years	Structure	Campus
Type of course	Red brick (p. 94)	Year size	244
Typical offer	AAA	Intercalated degree:	BMedSci, MPH, LLM
Applicants	996	Student mix:	
Interviews	595	% Mature	7%
Offers	434	% International	8%

Uncompetitive						Competitive
Low living costs						High living costs
Working really hard						Not working/ chilling out

Contact details	The Medical School, University of Sheffield, Beech Hill Road, Sheffield, S10 2RX. Tel: +44 (0) 114 271 3349, Web: www.shef.ac.uk/medicine/ prospective_ug

An insider's view...

The Sheffield curriculum has undergone a series of changes over the last decade through a process of refinement and revision of the course. We feel that integration of medical sciences and clinical medicine is important in successful learning and we promote the acquisition of basic clinical skills from the very beginning of the course through contact with patients. We have a very well-developed programme that utilizes patients as educators and this is founded on the belief that patients are valid and reliable assessors of students' professional behaviours and clinical skills. We combine traditional teaching methods of lectures and bedside teaching with a longitudinal thread of problem-based learning.

Mike Jennings, Admissions Tutor

Southampton

If you want sun and sea on the south coast, you would be wise to consider Southampton. Although the medical school spans decades rather than centuries, it has a solid reputation for the atmosphere and interactive nature of its course.

University The medical school recently moved to Southampton General Hospital where facilities include two large lecture theatres, smaller seminar rooms, a large library, clinical skills rooms, numerous computer suites, and a cafe. Students are based in the separate South Academic Block, but proximity to the wards means students are exposed to hospital life from day one. Some lectures are taught on the main university campus, which is within walking distance. Campus facilities include the Hartley Library and the Jubilee Sports Centre.

Course Southampton is renowned for pioneering an interactive, hands-on approach to medical education. Medical students meet patients from the first few weeks of the programme. The course begins with two pre-clinical years of systems-based learning with a strong focus on the basic sciences. Students can also select modules to learn about medical humanities, teaching, and research. One afternoon each week is spent with a hospital consultant or GP. Teaching is a mixture of lectures, seminars, tutorials, and prosection anatomy practicals.

In year three students undertake a research project in a chosen area of interest. Most students choose to remain in Southampton, but there are opportunities to do projects elsewhere in the UK or abroad. This year leads to a BMedSci and many students also go on to publish or present their research, giving Southampton students a competitive edge. In addition, many students choose to pursue an intercalated degree between the third and fourth years.

The main clinical component of the course begins in the fourth year. As is the case in many medical schools, Southampton students are sent far and wide, to cities as diverse as Portsmouth and Winchester. This means the student/doctor ratio remains low. In year five students take part in further full-time clinical attachments in hospitals spanning the entirety of Wessex, including Jersey.

Southampton has recently pioneered an exchange programme with the University of Kassel, Germany. This exciting project gives Southampton students the opportunity to undertake part of their third and fourth years in Germany as part of an exchange programme. This is the first project of its kind, providing an opportunity for intercultural exchange.

Lifestyle The medical student cliché 'work hard, play hard' is certainly apparent in Southampton. The university provides many opportunities to partake in sports (from kite surfing to extreme ironing!), volunteer work, and theatrical and musical groups. Some medical students find their timetables are not always compatible with these activities, hence the creation of unique medical clubs. These include everything from medics' netball, hockey, and rugby to the choir, Medsin, and a host of other volunteer groups. Medic groups are a great opportunity to meet students from other years, compete against other medical schools, and take time out from life on the wards. If you're looking for places to escape to, how about half an hour's drive to 375 square kilometres of New Forest National Park or a short ferry ride across to the Isle of Wight?

Factoid In the latest assessment by the Quality Assurance Agency, which monitors standards of teaching in the UK, Southampton University was awarded the highest level of achievement for the standard of its teaching and education. See Table 8.25.

Table 8.25   Southampton

Myth	A student beach holiday, funded by the taxpayer
Reality	A structured, time-intensive course, with no rules against studying on the beach!
Personality	Fun, friendly, and balanced
Best aspects	Patient contact from day one—daunting but the best way to learn
Worst aspects	A very exam-oriented course
Requirements	**UKCAT**; **A-level** three A2s including chemistry or grade 'A' chemistry and biology at AS; **GCSE** seven 'B's including English, maths, and science

Course length	5 years	Structure	Campus
Type of course	Plate glass (p. 94)	Year size	202
Typical offer	AAA	Intercalated degree:	BSc
Applicants	3000	Student mix:	
Interviews	Mature non-graduates	% Mature	10%
Offers	350	% International	Unknown

Uncompetitive	🏆 🏆 🏆 **🏆** 🏆 (4th of 5 filled)	Competitive
Low living costs	💰 💰 **💰** 💰 💰 (3rd of 5 filled)	High living costs
Working really hard	(4th of 5 filled)	Not working/ chilling out

Contact details	Southampton General Hospital, Tremona Road, Southampton, SO16 6YD Tel: +44 (0) 2380 796 586, Web: www.southampton.ac.uk/medicine

An insider's view . . .

The School of Medicine is committed to the highest quality of provision in pursuit of excellence in biomedical sciences and clinical research. We have a reputation for academic excellence in all aspects of teaching and research. Should you wish to study basic science or clinical research, the School of Medicine in Southampton will give you a great environment in which to develop your skills and provide the foundation upon which to build an exciting research career.

Dr Chris Stephens, Director of Education

University of East Anglia (UEA)

While Norwich Medical School at the University of East Anglia (UEA) is relatively new, it is already well established as a highly reputable medical school.

University The university is located about two miles west of Norwich city centre, on a small campus famous for its beautiful broad, open parkland and concrete buildings, including the iconic ziggurats. It takes about 20 minutes to walk across the campus, which houses everything from lecture theatres, seminar blocks, student accommodation, and the union bars to a renowned art gallery (the Sainsbury's Centre) and world-class sports facilities at the 'Sportspark'. The medical school has its own building, which contains fully equipped seminar rooms, a student social space and computer area, and staff offices. The main teaching hospital is the Norfolk and Norwich University Hospital, which is a 15-minute walk from the campus across the university sports fields. The main clinical skills teaching area is in the NNUH and has 24-hour access for students. Clinical attachments also take place at three peripheral hospitals and GP surgeries throughout Norfolk and Suffolk, and transport is provided from campus to these placements.

Course The course is systems-based with an emphasis on problem-based learning (PBL). Each module covers one or more system and its associated specialities. Approximately two-thirds of each module is spent on the campus in lectures, seminars, and PBL, learning about relevant physiology, pathology, and social sciences. The other third of the module is spent in a GP surgery, gaining clinical experience. PBL consists of a group of ten students discussing a weekly clinical scenario guided by a tutor. At the end of the week, the group presents this work to each other to consolidate what has been learnt. The weekly trips to the GPs allow patient contact from the first week, and are a huge benefit of the course. Other areas in which the Norwich course excels are communication skills, which are taught regularly using professional actors as practice patients; anatomy, which has the option of dissection; and research methods, which are taught via regular lectures and an audit project in the fourth year. Teaching is excellent, with 91% of students satisfied according to the 2012 national student survey. However, to succeed in PBL, you must also be happy to undertake plenty of self-directed learning in addition.

Lifestyle Self-catered accommodation is provided for the first year of study and is excellent. Most students rent nearby private accommodation from the second year. The centre of campus is 'The Square', which consists of the student union and its bars, as well as various food outlets, a post office, and banks. The student night club, the LCR, is also sited here and is known for cheap and messy nights, as well as a fantastic live music venue (which has hosted bands such as Coldplay, the Killers, and Calvin Harris). The university sports teams are a huge part of campus life, with the on-campus 'Sportspark' (one of the largest indoor sports centres in Britain) the perfect training site. The Sainsbury's Centre for Visual Arts is another on-campus asset and holds famous works by Henry Moore and Francis Bacon. Norwich city centre is ten minutes away by a regular 24-hour bus. The city is super-safe and super-cool, with a great variety of nightclubs, independent bars, restaurants, and shops. The med school also has its own social scene, including a newspaper, sports teams, and a fab MedSoc, which regularly organizes nights out, charity events, and balls.

Factoid Sir Paul Nurse of UEA was awarded the Nobel Prize in 2001 for his work on regulators of the cell cycle, central to our understanding of cancer. See Table 8.26.

Table 8.26 University of East Anglia

Myth	'Teach yourself medicine' course
Reality	A new, well-structured course which produces doctors who cure and care
Personality	Friendly, caring, team players
Best aspects	Patient contact from week one; highly integrated course structure
Worst aspects	Frequent assessments throughout the year
Requirements	**UKCAT**; **A-level** three A2s at grade A including biology and one other science; one further AS-level at grade B or above; **GCSE** six passes at 'A' or above including English, maths, and two science subjects

Course length	5 years	Structure	Campus
Type of course	Carbon fibre (p. 94)	Year size	166
Typical offer	AAAb	Intercalated degree:	BSc, MRes
Applicants	1528	Student mix:	
Interviews	608	% Mature	30%
Offers	299	% International	8%

Uncompetitive		Competitive
Low living costs		High living costs
Working really hard		Not working/ chilling out

Contact details	Norwich Medical School, Faculty of Medicine and Health Sciences, University of East Anglia, Norwich, NR4 7TJ Tel: +44 (0) 1603 591515, Web: www.uea.ac.uk/medicine

An insider's view...

UEA provides one of the most integrated courses in the world. The whole course is delivered in system-based modules that combine the basic sciences with clinical practice across all five years. The psychosocial and population sciences receive as much emphasis in teaching and assessment as the biological sciences. One day a week is spent in primary care from first year through to fifth year and one-third of each module is spent in hospital placements. Particular emphasis is placed on consultation skills, analytical skills, and research methods. All students are required to carry out a research or audit project in the fourth year.

Prof. Sam Leinster, Dean of School of Medicine

Northern Ireland

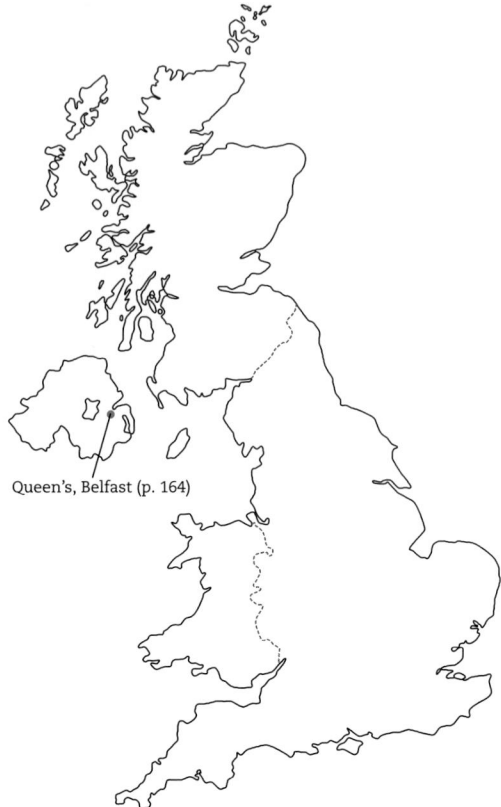

Queen's, Belfast (p. 164)

Figure 8.2   Undergraduate medical schools in Northern Ireland

Queen's, Belfast

Belfast is a small city with a big personality and Queen's University Belfast (QUB) is one of its cornerstones. It is a progressive university with strong leadership and vision for the future, so much so that it was awarded 'Entrepreneurial University of the Year' in 2009 and the 'Queen's University Prize' for innovation in cancer research in 2011. Building on a complex history of division and conflict, QUB's mission statement is 'equality, tolerance, and mutual respect' and their students come from Northern Ireland, the rest of the UK, the Republic of Ireland, and a diverse range of countries overseas.

University The first two years are based at the Medical Biology Centre (MBC) on the university campus, which is a 15-minute walk from the city centre. The MBC includes a cafe, library, and large computer suite. The campus itself has numerous facilities including a new library and a refurbished Students' Union with a not-for-profit shop, various cafes, bars, a pharmacy, and a book store. Clinical teaching takes place at 14 different hospitals; six of these are within ten miles of the university and the others (19 to 83 miles from campus) all offer free accommodation. The majority of hospitals can be reached by bus; however, most students in the clinical years do have a car. Hospital allocations are performed with a ranking system to keep it fair. There's an emphasis on helping students fulfil their personal and professional potential; this includes an Enterprise Students' Union to inform students about the many opportunities to improve their skills.

Course The first two years are pre-clinical, which is taught with an integrated, systems-based curriculum (p. 88). Anatomy is taught by dissection in groups of six to eight with some input from prosections. From the beginning of the course there is an emphasis on clinical and communication skills, which includes GP and hospital-based teaching. Clinical teaching begins in year three, which is split between hospital placements and self-directed learning from an extensive online learning facility and learning DVD, which includes every lecture along with self-assessment opportunities. The final two years are full-time clinical attachments with students rotating through major specialities. Students are encouraged to fully integrate themselves into the healthcare team and to learn practical skills. There is a six-week elective at the start of the fifth year followed by a four-week holiday allowing for a period of travel. The university has a bursary scheme to help fund elective periods. There are many student-selected components including sports physiology, teaching CPR in primary schools, history of neuroscience, and sign language. All students can apply for research-based intercalated degrees between the second and fourth years at either Bachelor's or Master's level.

Lifestyle First years usually live in the main halls of residence called 'Elms Village', just 20 minutes' walk from the MBC. Each hall has its own shop, bar, and cafe, and accomodation-some of the lowest accommodation fees in the UK. From the second year most students move to cheap privately rented accommodation in one of three student areas, which are about 20 minutes from campus. The social life is good with plenty of student bars and a brilliant live gig venue on campus, as well as more upmarket places in the city centre. Belfast is surprisingly easy to get to, being just an hour's flight from any UK airport. There are also hundreds of beautiful places to visit in Northern Ireland (NI) or a short drive away in the Republic of Ireland.

Factoid Students Working Overseas Trust (SWOT), a charity run by QUB medical students, raises over £30,000 a year, which is taken to hospitals in the developing world by students on their electives. See Table 8.27.

Table 8.27 Queen's, Belfast

Myth	Narrow-minded locals who aren't adventurous enough to study further from home
Reality	QUB offers every possible opportunity for adventure and broadening your horizons, regardless of how far you are from home!
Personality	Friendly students who never take themselves too seriously but always apply themselves when the crucial time comes
Best aspects	Exposure to patients from early on in the first year; the long holidays
Worst aspects	Large tutor groups (eight to ten students) and frustratingly the clinical tutors don't always turn up when they are supposed to
Requirements	**UKCAT**; **A-level** three A2s including chemistry and at least one other science or maths; at least one AS including biology; **GCSE** six 'A*'s, 'C' in English; **Graduates** require a minimum of a 2:1 in their degree

Course length	5 years	Structure	Campus
Type of course	Red brick (p. 94)	Year size	261
Typical offer	AAAa	Intercalated degree:	BSc, MSc, MRes
Applicants	1365	Student mix:	7%
Interviews	1365	% Mature	10%
Offers	500	% International	

Uncompetitive		Competitive
Low living costs		High living costs
Working really hard		Not working/chilling out

Contact details	Centre for Medical Education, Queen's University Belfast, Whitla Medical Building, 97 Lisburn Road, Belfast, BT9 7BL Tel: +44 (0) 289 097 2450, Web: www.qub.ac.uk/mdbs

An insider's view...

Queen's University Belfast is unique in that it is the only medical school in Northern Ireland. Although it has educated doctors who work on all five continents, many of its alumni work within the health service in NI. As a result there is a strong family atmosphere with good relationships between hospital doctors, general practitioners, and the medical school. These deep loyalties facilitate and ensure that our students are welcomed and well taught and as a consequence many of our students complete their foundation training in NI. Students who are outgoing, flexible, keen to participate, embrace the experiences offered, and who can balance work and social life adapt well to our course.

Dr Keith Steele, Director of Admissions

Scotland

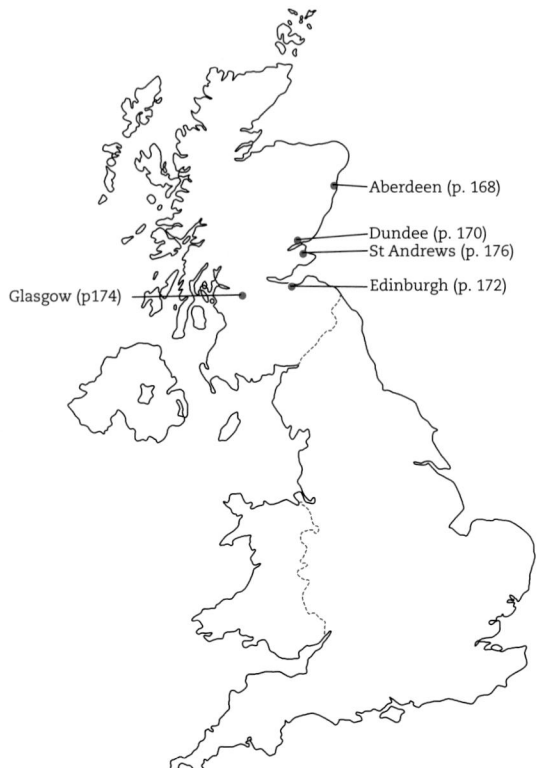

Figure 8.3 Undergraduate medical schools in Scotland

Aberdeen

The University of Aberdeen can honestly claim to be a well-established and highly regarded medical school, in a rich and breathtaking city.

Univeristy The first three years of teaching will take place in the newly constructed Suttie Centre, which houses a lecture theatre, IT suite, anatomy teaching area, and simulated ward space for clinical teaching. This is located on the Foresterhill site, approximately two miles from the centre of Aberdeen. Neighbouring the Foresterhill site is the Aberdeen Royal Infirmary, Aberdeen Maternity Hospital, Royal Aberdeen Children's Hospital, Royal Cornhill Hospital, and Woodend Hospital, where clinical attachments take place. Aberdeen is also one of the few medical schools to provide the option of a 'Remote and Rural' placement, with close liaisons with Raigmore in Inverness, the Highlands, the Western Isles, and even Orkney and Shetland!

Course After a term of lectures in basic sciences and clinical skills, the systems-based course begins, using clinical cases to enhance student learning. The relevant prosectional anatomy, physiology, and biochemistry of each system is taught, allowing students to begin to recognize symptoms, perform clinical examinations, and appreciate what investigations and treatments to use. The community course also begins in the first year, introducing General Practice, Public, Mental, and Child Health, Environmental and Occupational Health, and Care of the Elderly. Student-selected components are integrated into the course and this allows students to work in small groups on a chosen topic. In the third year, students are given the opportunity to study medical humanities, which encompasses a wide range of subjects, from history of art to economics. Aberdeen also offers students the chance to take an intercalated BSc after the third or fourth year.

Lifestyle Halls of residence are available for all first year students, but by the second year most tend to rent flats that are about 20 to 30 minutes' walk from the hospital.

Aberdeen is a compact coastal city with a thriving local economy that can satisfy every cultural taste. Here you will find a vibrant shopping quarter, museums, art galleries, concert halls, and the popular Lemon Tree venue, with its cafe-bar atmosphere, which attracts an exciting mixture of contemporary theatre, dance, stand-up comedy, and music. There are fantastic transport links with the rest of the UK and London is around an hour away by plane.

The university boasts over 50 sports clubs and over 25 societies. The medics at Aberdeen also have their own community with the official MedSoc, and many additional common-interest groups, such as Marrow, the Ogston Surgical Society, and WildSoc. Sports enthusiasts can benefit from the full-size indoor artificial-grass football pitch, a water-based hockey pitch, and both indoor and outdoor athletic training facilities. For those who prefer the great outdoors, you will be spoilt for choice, with popular activities including hill-walking, mountaineering, and skiing in the Cairngorms mountain range; kayaking on the River Dee; wind-surfing on the North Sea; or just relaxing on the beach!

Factoid Aberdeen holds the oldest English-speaking Medical Chair in the world and has one of the largest clinical complexes in Europe. See Table 8.28.

Table 8.28 Aberdeen

Myth	Off the map and even further off the radar
Reality	Easily accessible via car, train, or plane…and worth getting to
Personality	Welcoming, dedicated, and motivated
Best aspects	Being able to spend time learning in locations throughout the entire north east of Scotland
Worst aspects	Dark winter mornings
Requirements	**UKCAT**; **Highers** five S5 at AAAAB, at least 'B' in chemistry, plus two from biology, maths, and physics; **A-levels** three A2s including chemistry and at least one of biology, maths, or physics

Course length	5 years	Structure	Campus
Type of course	Stone (p. 94)	Year size	175
Typical offer	Highers: AAAAB A-level: AAA	Intercalated degree:	BSc
Applicants	2357	Student mix:	
Interviews	600	% Mature	10%
Offers	350	% International	7%

Uncompetitive		Competitive
Low living costs		High living costs
Working really hard		Not working/chilling out

Contact details	Medical Admissions, University of Aberdeen, Polwarth Building, Foresterhill, Aberdeen, AB25 2ZD Tel: +44 (0) 1224 554975, Web: www.abdn.ac.uk/ medicine-dentistry/medical-dental

An insider's view…

The School of Medicine and Dentistry is a vibrant part of the university with distinction in research and an impressive reputation for its teaching. The medical curriculum has been recently updated and provides a high quality learning experience, with integration of science and clinical teaching from year one. The new Suttie Centre for Teaching and Learning located on the joint university/hospital campus provides our students with state-of-the-art facilities for learning clinical skills and anatomy. As the most northern medical school in the UK, we have a special interest in remote and rural healthcare and our students have the option of following a 'Remote and Rural' track in the fourth and fifth years, with clinical attachments scattered across the Highlands and Islands. The Aberdeen programme also features a six-week student-selected option in medical humanities in year three, giving students the chance to broaden their horizons outside of medicine. Our graduates are well prepared for life as junior doctors and we take considerable pride in their progress and achievements.

Dr Rona Patey, Head of Division of Medical Education

Dundee

Dundee Medical School was ranked as the top medical school in the UK in 2008 and 2009 and has remained ranked in the top five since. It has an exceptional research record, is world renowned for medical education, and has just undergone a multi-million pound refurbishment and extension. Being coastal it is Scotland's sunniest and warmest city and in 2012 the university was ranked first in the UK for best student experience.

University The medical school is located within Ninewells Hospital, about 30 minutes' walk from the main university campus and a ten-minute bus journey from the city centre. The medical school has superb facilities including a refurbished medical library, laboratories, social areas, cafes, and shops. There is a multitude of space for both individual and group study, with Wi-Fi throughout. Being located inside the hospital, wards and clinics are nearby for regular clinical teaching. Technology is at the forefront of teaching, with a considerable investment in a web-based virtual learning environment with subject-specific study guides, and all teaching materials provided in advance to empower students' learning. The highlight is the first-class clinical skills centre and the newly designed surgical skills centre, both of which include simulated patients. In the later years, students can choose placements in other Tayside hospitals and further afield in Scotland; however, most teaching takes place in Ninewells, creating a truly close-knit community of students from first to fifth year.

Course The course is divided into three phases: the initial phase lasts eight weeks, combining key scientific principles with regular early patient contact and clinical skills. The next phase runs from November of the first year to the end of the third year and is called 'Systems in Practice'. These years involve system-based teaching, combining full-body dissection in an award winning department, lectures, small-group tutorials, clinical skills, and regular ward-based teaching revolving around an individual topic such as cardiology or respiratory medicine. These years also include three month long 'student-selected components' (SSCs); these can be self-proposed on any topic at any location in the country, from cardiology in London or academic research in Dundee. Clinical experience continues throughout, via both the Clinical Skills Centre and regular patient contact.

The final phase, 'Preparation in Practice', takes place in years four and five with generalist (medicine, surgery, and general practice) and specialist (e.g. paediatrics) rotations. Finals take place at the very beginning of the fifth year, allowing time for further specialization, the elective, and foundation shadowing.

The Dundee course is very flexible with the ability to choose which hospitals you study in (including rural or island GPs for those interested). There are also a wide variety of optional intercalated degrees to choose from, between the third and fourth year, ranging from anatomy to applied orthopaedic technology and teaching in medicine.

Lifestyle First years generally begin in one of the newly built student villages on the main campus. These surround a brand-new institute of sport and gym facilities and a five-floor Students' Union complete with a swimming pool, library, and IT suites. From the second year, students live in privately rented accommodation, which is affordable even in the centre of the city. Dundee is a small but lively place; it is easy to get around by foot, bike, or bus. It is a great place to study, with a huge student population for a city of its size and low living costs. There are a multitude of societies covering all sports and activities from football to skydiving; the medical school has its own teams, with practises and matches arranged around the busy timetable.

Factoid Dundee University Medical School is the origin of the internationally used, and widely feared, Objective Structured Clinical Examination (OSCE). See Table 8.29.

Table 8.29 Dundee

Myth	Dundee students do more self-reflecting than their bathroom mirror
Reality	A course that teaches you to manage patients and symptoms, not just pathology and disease
Personality	Enthusiastic, outgoing, strong team players
Best aspects	The freedom to focus on what you love in addition to what you need to know; a small medical school where you will recognize everyone in your year
Worst aspects	The challenging fourth year including a research project and upcoming finals
Requirements	**UKCAT**; **Highers** five at S5 including chemistry and another science; **A-level** three A2s including chemistry and another science; **GCSE** 'B' in biology if not taking A2

Course length	5 years	Structure	Campus
Type of course	Red brick (p. 94)	Year size	147
Typical offer	Highers: AAABB / A-level: AAA	Intercalated degree:	BMSc
Applicants	1800	Student mix:	
Interviews	600	% Mature	15%
Offers	300	% International	7.5%

Uncompetitive		Competitive
Uncompetitive	🏆🏆	Competitive
Low living costs	💰💰	High living costs
Working really hard		Not working/chilling out

Contact details	Medical School Undergraduate Office, Ninewells Hospital and Medical School, Dundee, DD1 9SY Tel: +44 (0)1382 384 697, Web: http://medicine.dundee.ac.uk

An insider's view...

Dundee has a leading international reputation in medical education. It is home to the world-famous Clinical Skills and Cuschieri Surgical Skills Centres, both of which provide integrated skills programmes from expert clinical tutors in the undergraduate curriculum. The medical school is part of the College of Medicine, Dentistry, and Nursing, giving students the chance to learn with and about other professions working in the healthcare sector. Dundee was one of the first medical schools to work with the NHS to involve medical students in learning about patient safety. We want students from a wide variety of backgrounds who want to excel in medicine and who want to work with the school to ensure that they are aware of their own professional limits.

Dr Jean S. Ker, Director of Clinical Skills Centre

Edinburgh

Edinburgh's prestigious medical school is set in the heart of the beautiful capital of Scotland in the shadow of Arthur's Seat. Its long history, excellent reputation for medical education and research, innovative course, and outstanding facilities make it a wonderful place to live and study medicine.

University Edinburgh consistently ranks very highly in the UK and in the world, particularly for medicine. The medical school buildings span three centuries; the oldest, Teviot, is mainly used for pre-clinical teaching, while the newly built Chancellor's Building attached to the Royal Infirmary is mainly for clinical teaching. The Edinburgh Electronic Medical Curriculum (EEMeC) is a web-based learning resource including lecture notes, a virtual clinic, exam question-banks, and staff–student forums; it is used by all years and is an award-winning website. The three main hospitals for clinical experience are the New Royal Infirmary, the Royal Hospital for Sick Children, and the Western General, and all have excellent facilities. There are libraries within each hospital and a newly redeveloped central library with a 24-hour computer lab overlooking the popular Edinburgh Meadows. The Anatomy Resource Centre and cadaver specimens are also available for private study. A few senior students can be attached to more distant peripheral hospitals which offer free accommodation and provide excellent teaching. Edinburgh also has its own Royal College of Surgeons and Royal College of Physicians which allow additional training opportunities for students in the city.

Course The two pre-clinical years follow a systems-based approach taught by lectures, problem-based learning (PBL), and tutorials that amount to two to five hours of teaching per day. Anatomy is taught using dissected prosections. Alongside the medical sciences there is teaching on ethics, communication skills, and psychosocial principles. Contact with patients begins in the first year, developing history-taking skills, before clinical examinations and more history taking in the second year. The second year timetable is less demanding than the first year with more self-directed learning. Students have the option to intercalate from a wide range of medical subjects before undertaking their clinical years.

Clinical teaching also follows systems-based attachments in the third year and then a speciality-based approach (e.g. paediatrics, psychiatry) in the fourth and fifth years. The teaching is a mixture of clinics and ward-based learning and lectures, as well as EEMeC. Throughout the course there are student-selected components including a 14-week research project in the fourth-year and an eight-week elective in the fifth year (often spent overseas).

Lifestyle Most first year students live in university accommodation including Pollock Halls of Residence and self-catered flats spread across the city. From the second year most students move into privately rented flats in the student districts of Newington, Marchmont, and New Town. Public transport networks are widespread, cheap, and easy to use with trams arriving soon. There is a strong community spirit within the course and the social life is very good. Wednesday afternoon is set aside for sports if you so choose and the Medics have a very strong rugby team, as well as basketball, hockey, netball, and football teams.

Outside of the university, Edinburgh has a renowned cultural highlife, including castles, theatres, bars, clubs, and, of course, the world's biggest arts festival, the Fringe. The surrounding area is also stunning with beaches, hills, mountains, and even skiing.

Factoid Infamous body-snatchers Burke and Hare dug up graves and even killed local Edinburghians and sold their freshly deceased bodies to Edinburgh Medical School in the early 19th century. Ironically, Burke's body was donated to the medical school after his hanging and his skeleton is still on show today. See Table 8.30.

Table 8.30 Edinburgh

Myth	Little England—only posh English folk get into Edinburgh
Reality	A great mix of pleasant students from throughout the UK and across the globe
Personality	Professional, competitive, but always helpful and fun
Best aspects	The EEMeC online learning platform, and the beautiful city itself
Worst aspects	Variable level of feedback on exam performance
Requirements	**UKCAT; Highers** five at S5 including chemistry and two from biology, maths, or physics; chemistry and biology recommended as Advanced Highers; **A-level** three A2s including chemistry and one of biology, maths, or physics, AS biology minimum; **GCSE** 'B' in English, maths, biology, and chemistry (or 'BB' in dual award)

Course length	5/6 years	Structure	Campus
Type of course	Stone (p. 94)	Year size	240
Typical offer	Highers: AAAAB A-levels: AAAb	Intercalated degree:	BSc, BMedSci
Applicants	2750	Student mix:	
Interviews	Graduates only	% Mature	10%
Offers	360	% International	7.5%

Uncompetitive		Competitive
Low living costs		High living costs
Working really hard		Not working/chilling out
Contact details	College of Medicine and Veterinary Medicine, University of Edinburgh, The Chancellor's Building, 49 Little France Crescent, Edinburgh, EH16 4SB Tel: +44 (0) 131 242 6407, Web: www.mvm.ed.ac.uk	

An insider's view...

Edinburgh—as all UK medical schools—is required to select those with the greatest aptitude for medical studies from those with high academic ability. It measures academic ability through not only examination grade achievements but also the UKCAT aptitude test and gives equal weighting in selection for appropriate personal qualities, career exploration, and all other forms of non-academic achievement.

Dr Donald Thomson, Director of MBChB Admissions

Glasgow

Glasgow Medical School is a particularly Scottish institution, almost as famous as deep-fried Mars Bars and Auld Lang Syne.

University Glasgow is the fourth oldest university in the English-speaking world and also a member of the Russell Group. The award-winning Wolfson Medical School Building is set in the heart of Glasgow's vibrant West End, boasting its own library, teaching rooms, clinical skills suite, communication skills areas, seminar rooms, and canteen. Medical students have access to the building 24 hours a day—ideal for last minute cramming before exams!

Clinical teaching takes place at 26 teaching hospitals and nearly 200 GP practices throughout the west of Scotland. Most students make use of Glasgow's extensive public transport network over the first few years of the course, but as finals draw nearer many get a car, though this is not a necessity. Summer 2015 will see the official opening of Glasgow Southern General Hospital, which will be the largest teaching hospital in Europe.

Course In 1996 Glasgow boldly opted to end its traditional medical course and embark on an innovative problem-based learning (PBL) curriculum, which was further updated in 2010. The first two phases (years one and two) consist of twice weekly PBL sessions, complemented by lab classes, lectures, podcasts, dissection classes, and clinical skills teaching. The first two years also include weekly vocational studies sessions in which GPs lead tutorials so students learn the communication skills, attitudes, and values expected of them as doctors. Phase 3 (the first half of year three) consists of a week based on each system, with Case-Based Learning sessions twice a week with a clinical tutor, as well as one day per week at a hospital or GP. Phase 4 (until medical finals) is based at local hospitals and GPs, with occasional dedicated teaching weeks on campus, as students' progress through ten five-week clinical attachments.

There are three five-week student-selected components in which students spend time researching a subject that particularly interests them. This can range from rock-climbing to major incident planning; students can also propose their own. Glasgow medical students are the only students in the UK to enjoy two electives (four weeks each), in the summers of years three and four. Half of all Glasgow students travel abroad for their elective and numerous bursaries are also available. Intercalated degrees are available between the third and fourth years though entry is competitive, based on a personal statement and academic performance. Glasgow has an international reputation in clinical and scientific research with state-of-the-art facilities, including the BHF Glasgow Cardiovascular Research Centre and neighbouring Glasgow Biomedical Research Centre.

Lifestyle Students mainly live in the city's West End, where they can enjoy the city's great food, music scene, and nightlife. In their first year, most students live in halls of residence (catered or self-catering), which are shared with students from other faculties. Glasgow has two Students' Unions, each with its own style. The university sports centre is on campus and the building of a new £13.4 million sports and social facility which will be completed by the end of 2014. Currently, just £50 buys students unlimited access to state-of-the-art facilities, 48 sports clubs, and over 40 exercise classes per week. If only the curriculum left more time to enjoy them....

Factoid Joseph Lister, the pioneer of antiseptic surgery, was a Professor of Surgery at Glasgow University and chart-topping singer-songwriter Emeli Sandé previously studied medicine at Glasgow. See Table 8.31.

Table 8.31 Glasgow

Myth	Ginger-haired, haggis-loving, incomprehensible		
Reality	An eclectic mix of competitive and well-rounded students at an excellent institution providing a modern research-led curriculum		
Personality	Sociable hard-workers with a great sense of humour		
Best aspects	Small groups are great for making friends. Glasgow was voted 'friendliest city in the UK', and second only to London for shopping		
Worst aspects	You can rarely leave home without an umbrella		
Requirements	**UKCAT**; **Highers** 5A or 3A3B at S5 with chemistry, biology and maths/physics or AB in 2 Advanced highers in S6; English at SG Grade 2 or Intermediate 2; **A-level** AAA in chemistry and biology, maths, physics at A2; A in biology AS; **GCSE** 'B' in English		
Course length	5 years	**Structure**	Campus
Type of course	Carbon fibre (p. 94)	**Year size**	227
Typical offer	Highers: AAAAA/ AAAABB A-levels: AAA	**Intercalated degree:**	BSc
Applicants	1750	**Student mix:**	
Interviews	550	**% Mature**	18%
Offers	350	**% International**	7.5%

Uncompetitive		Competitive
	🏆 🏆🏆🏆🏆🏆	
Low living costs	💰💰💰💰💰	High living costs
Working really hard		Not working/chilling out

Contact details	Wolfson Medical School Building, University of Glasgow, University Avenue, Glasgow, G12 8QQ Tel: +44 (0) 141 330 2000, Web: www.gla.ac.uk/schools/medicine

An insider's view . . .

The University of Glasgow Medical School has a unique brand that reflects the exposure of medical undergraduates to leading researchers and teachers in clinical and basic science. Our students have the opportunity to experience a diverse mixture of clinical attachments that range from National Tertiary Referral services to single-handed rural General Practice. Our Medical Graduates are highly regarded for the breadth of their undergraduate experience and ability. We aspire to train medical graduates who are highly sought after in every branch of medicine, equipped for postgraduate training in the UK and in other healthcare systems, and who are equipped for a career in medicine in the 21st century.

Rachel Kelly, Admissions Administrator for the College of Medical, Veterinary and Life Sciences

St Andrews

The golfing greens at St Andrews aren't the only courses that are world-class.

University As the oldest university in Scotland, St Andrews is steeped in tradition, with a long record of providing excellent medical education. Students can now benefit from the new medical school building, which lies in the heart of the science campus in North Haugh. The university is closely integrated with the town, so you are never more than a short walk away from teaching facilities, your accommodation, or the town centre. The medical school building houses all the teaching facilities you will need for your three years at St Andrews. A huge range of medical models and dissection specimens are available and enthusiastic staff are on hand to discuss any questions that you might have. Attachments to the local community hospitals, local district hospitals, and GPs are another part of the course, which allow you to gain a great deal of interaction with patients before entering your clinical studies.

Course The curriculum is an integrated one using a mixture of teaching methods including around eight to ten lectures per week along with tutorials, clinical skills sessions, and dissection sessions. St Andrews has a strong emphasis on the medical sciences and cadaveric dissection is a major component, which really sets it apart from many others. Our online curriculum delivery system, Galen, is an incredibly helpful resource, providing weekly timetables, lecture handouts, practice tests, and a lot more. Up to 40% of a week can be clinical skills and all lectures and teaching have a strong theme of clinical medicine.

The last term has a strong emphasis on independent learning, offering the chance to conduct a research or library project in an area of your interest. Furthermore, the Applied Medical Science module allows you to enhance your professional thinking skills and integrate major topics and gives you the opportunity to consolidate your clinical skills and patient examination techniques.

Your medical degree will not finish at St Andrews. Instead, after three years here you will graduate with a BSc Honours in Medicine, and you will then be able to continue your studies at any of the other Scottish medical schools (or Manchester—p. 146). This is nothing to worry about—simply tick a box on applying and the universities do the rest. You will then complete your training at your chosen medical school, earning an MBChB.

Lifestyle St Andrews is officially the world's only little big town. One in three of the population has something to do with the university, so you soon get the feel of a tight-knit community when walking through St Andrews. St Andrews also has lots of crazy traditions to keep things interesting. Whilst the town is slightly limited in its social offerings, the highly active student populace more than compensates for this. With well over 100 student societies, from AstroSoc to ZooSoc, extreme Frisbee to Tunnocks teacake appreciation, there's plenty to keep you busy. The Bute Medical Society is one of the largest and oldest societies in St Andrews and is a strong part of a medic's life. With regular social events, balls, charity events, and cheese and wines, there is sure to be something to suit your taste. Transport to St Andrews is good with regular buses running to Glasgow and Edinburgh and train links are only five minutes out of town.

Factoid The new medical school building is one of the most sustainable and environmentally friendly buildings in the UK! See Table 8.32.

Table 8.32   St Andrews

Myth	Privately educated toffs who've never seen the inside of a hospital
Reality	Diverse group of students, keen to learn, and sharing a thirst for knowledge
Personality	Friendly with a slight crazy streak
Best aspects	Close-knit student community and lifestyle
Worst aspects	Having to leave after three years
Requirements	**UKCAT**; **Highers** five at S5 with an 'A' in chemistry and one of biology, physics, or maths; **A-level** three A2s with an 'A' in chemistry and one of biology, physics, or maths; **GCSE** 'B' in maths, biology, and English if not offered at AS/A2

Course length	6 years	Structure	City
Type of course	Stone (p. 94)	Year size	136
Typical offer	Highers: AAAAB A-level: AAA	Intercalated degree:	BSc (compulsory)
Applicants	1159	Student mix:	
Interviews	546	% Mature	5%
Offers	200	% International	20%

Uncompetitive		Competitive
Low living costs		High living costs
Working really hard		Not working/chilling out

Contact details	School of Medicine, Medical and Biological Sciences Building, St Andrews, KY16 9TF Tel: +44 (0) 1334 463599, Web: medicine.st-andrews.ac.uk

An insider's view...

The programme at the Bute Medical School offers the chance to obtain two degrees for the price of one in offering everyone a BSc in Medicine as well as an MBChB at the end of the course. This is the only medical school in Scotland to do this, offering a distinct choice for students wishing to study in Scotland. By definition it offers a course strong in the basic medical sciences and one that is based on research–teaching linkages in all its aspects. Evidence base informs what is taught and students learn research skills as part of their coursework. All students undertake a research project in their final year and the teaching in the school is informed by medical education research undertaken by the staff. The school has been praised by the GMC for the strength of its anatomy teaching, which is done by full-body dissection. The school consistently comes at the top of the student satisfaction tables, which reflects the highly supportive and interactive programme on offer. The school strives to achieve the feeling of being part of one big family, which is helped by being a school of modest size based in a small country town on the east coast of Scotland.

Prof. Simon Guild, Vice-Dean of Medicine and Head of Teaching

Wales

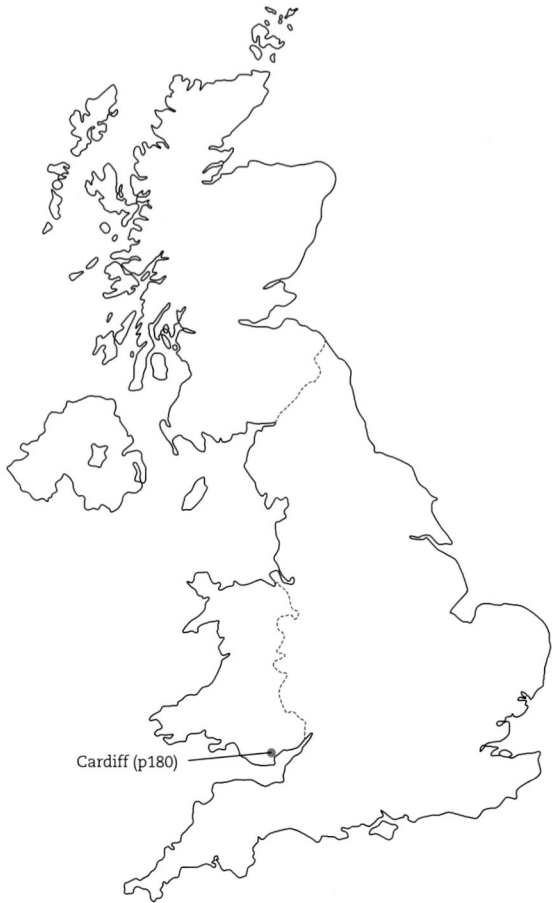

Cardiff (p180)

Figure 8.4   Undergraduate medical schools in Wales

Cardiff

Cardiff is home to the only undergraduate medical school in Wales. It is based in a thriving cosmopolitan city just a short drive from the Brecon Beacons and the beautiful Welsh coastline.

University Cardiff is widely considered to be the most prestigious university in Wales; and with over 30,000 students, it is one of the largest academic institutions in the UK. It is also one of the largest medical schools, accepting over 300 students every year.

The medical school has recently invested in a new, purpose-built medical education facility (the Cochrane Building) at University Hospital Wales. The Centre's facilities include a Clinical Skills Centre, a high-technology medical simulation centre, and a new healthcare library. The building is named in honour of Dr Archie Cochrane—the founding father of the evidence-based-medicine movement.

Course The course is based on a new curriculum that places care-based learning at its heart, including clinical placements from the first term. During the first two years, students are taught on the main campus, just five minutes from Cardiff city centre, with an excellent library, study, and computer facilities. Basic sciences are structured around major body systems and delivered through small-group tutorials, lectures, seminars, group work, self-directed learning, and e-learning. There is an emphasis on teaching in a clinical context, which allows you to see how what you are learning applies to how you will practise as a doctor. Anatomy is taught using full-body dissection (up to 12 students/table), prosections, post-mortem pathology sessions, plastinated specimens, and models. For the clinical years students are initially allocated placements in south-east Wales then across the entirety of Wales in the fourth and fifth years, giving a wide range of medical experiences.

The clinical course also includes lectures taught at the University Hospital of Wales.

Intercalated degrees are available to academically successful students after the third or fourth year. Options include a range of subjects at Cardiff and Bangor University, including the opportunity to intercalate externally. The elective period takes place during the final year.

Due to the significant transition from student to FY1 doctor, final year medical students take part in a Harmonization scheme where students take part in apprenticeships, integrating into a hospital team and gaining hands-on experience. This is a valuable opportunity to learn how to be successful on the ward.

Lifestyle Students live in halls of residence in the first year and usually rent privately in subsequent years. Most students live in Cathays, near the main campus; accommodation is comparatively cheap at about £55 per week. There are many clubs and societies, with particularly successful teams in netball and rugby. There is opportunity for students to choose to play sports for the university teams or to join a medic's team, which plan training around medical students' busy timetables! Cardiff offers an excellent range of facilities, as befitting a capital city. These include the usual shops, theatres, galleries, concert venues, and nightlife. There is a wonderful atmosphere on Rugby International days, especially when Wales play at home in their famous Millennium Stadium—definitely worth a visit! Cardiff offers all the benefits of a capital city with the countryside a short drive away.

Factoid In 2007 Professor Sir Martin Evans at Cardiff was awarded the Nobel Prize in Physiology of Medicine for his contributions to the field of stem cell research. See Table 8.33.

Table 8.33 Cardiff

Myth	An old-school establishment favouring Welsh students
Reality	A dynamic and constantly evolving course with a broad mix of students like any other, but a friendly Welsh charm like no other
Personality	Very approachable, with a strong sense of community
Best aspects	Great lifestyle living in a capital city; friendly staff and students; low living costs
Worst aspects	Students can be sent anywhere in Wales for placements from the fourth year, which can increase your travel costs
Requirements	**UKCAT**; **A-level** AAA in at least two sciences out of biology, chemistry, maths, and statistics (one of which must be biology or chemistry) and a minimum of a 'C' in a fourth AS-level (grade 'A' if biology or chemistry); **GCSE** maths 'B', English 'B', and sciences 'AAB' or 'AA' (double award)

Course length	5 years	Structure	Campus
Type of course	Red brick (p. 94)	Year size	300
Typical offer	AAAc	Intercalated degree:	BSc
Applicants	2700	Student mix:	
Interviews	900	% Mature	10%
Offers	450	% International	9%

		Competitive
Uncompetitive	🏆 🏆 **🏆** 🏆 🏆	Competitive
Low living costs	💰 **💰** 💰 💰 💰	High living costs
Working really hard		Not working/ chilling out

Contact details	Cardiff University School of Medicine, Cardiff University, Cardiff, Wales, CF14 4XN Tel: +44 (0) 29 2074 2020, Web: medicine.cf.ac.uk/ medical-education/undergraduate

An insider's view...

These are exciting times for Cardiff University School of Medicine. The new Cochrane Building (opened in 2011) provides state-of-the-art clinical skills, simulation, and library facilities for our students. And investment in new support staff and academic appointments leaves us better placed than ever before to meet the demands placed on us by students, funders, and the NHS.

Prof. Paul Morgan, Dean of Medicine

Overseas

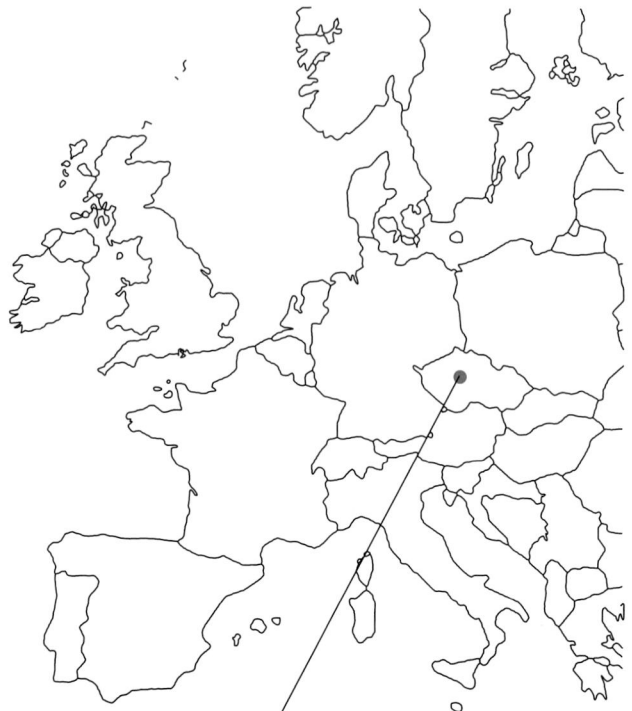

Charles University, Prague (p. 184)

Figure 8.5 Undergraduate medical schools overseas

Charles University, Prague

Applying to Charles University has become a relatively common consideration for UK students, hence its inclusion in this book. Since the Czech Republic is part of the EU, graduates of the medical school can register with the GMC without taking additional exams; however, you are not guaranteed a job and an overseas medical school could count against you in competitive specialities.

University The First Faculty of Medicine is based in the heart of Prague, half an hour's drive from the main airport. Charles University has faculty buildings and teaching hospitals spread across the city, all of which are within walking distance or easily accessible via the incredibly reliable (and cheap) public transport network.

Course The first three years of the course are dedicated to the basic sciences of medicine. Subjects are taught separately rather than being systems-based (including everything from pathophysiology to Latin terminology!), through formal lectures and practical classes. Students at Charles are encouraged to pursue independent learning; nevertheless tutors in each subject are always available to clarify any problems that you may encounter. The Charles medical course offers cadaveric dissection to assist in anatomy teaching and now students can benefit from the brand-new clinical skills area. The renovated faculty library provides a fantastic work space beside the ever-helpful Student Affairs Department (which is a constant source of support for administrative matters). The pre-clinical course also includes a Czech language course, which although not essential for daily life in Prague is extremely helpful for communicating with patients during the clinical years.

The Erasmus programme offers an exciting opportunity during any of the first five years to study medicine abroad and experience the lifestyle, culture, and university life of another country in Europe. If you do not want to spend a whole semester or year abroad, you can choose to do an International Federation of Medical Students' Association (IFMSA) placement, which is a month in one of 20 countries: mainly European, African, Asian, and South American. It can be undertaken pre-clinically (research based) or clinically (hospital/clinic-based placement).

Most subjects end with an oral examination, which is particularly useful for professional qualifications later on in your medical career.

Lifestyle University accommodation is available for the whole medical course, but most students choose to move into private accommodation in the city after the first year; if you share an apartment in the city, just a few minutes away from the campus, you can expect to pay around €450/month. Much to the surprise of many first-time visitors, the country is quite a progressive EU nation. The beautiful hills of the countryside surrounding Prague contrast with the historic quarters, which boast some of the most attractive architecture in the world. As the capital city there is something to suit all tastes: pubs, restaurants, nightclubs, cafes, opera, ballet, and theatres, all at a fraction of the price in the UK. Whether sightseeing along Charles Bridge, shopping in the markets of the Old Town Square, or enjoying a walk along Petrin Hill, there's never a dull moment. Being in Central Europe also gives easy access to visit neighbouring Vienna or Berlin for weekends or enjoy some skiing on the local slopes.

Factoid Jan Purkyně, of the Purkinje fibres of the heart and Purkinje cells in the cerebellum, graduated from Charles in 1819 and became the Head of Physiology. See Table 8.34.

Table 8.34 Charles University, Prague

Myth	The last resort for those who fail to get the grades for a real medical school
Reality	An internationally renowned medical faculty, producing doctors who go on to practise in whichever country they choose
Personality	Adventurous and open-minded
Best aspects	The degree allows registration with the GMC; the opportunity to live and work in one of the finest cities in Europe
Worst aspects	You are not guaranteed an FY1 job in the NHS; the air tickets and €13,000/year course fees make Prague an expensive option
Requirements	Passing an admissions exam set by the university

Course length	6 years	Structure	City
Type of course	Stone (p. 94)	Year size	120
Typical offer	Charles University entrance exam	Intercalated degree	No
Applicants	800	Student mix:	
Interviews	200	% Mature	60%
Offers	140	% International	100%

Uncompetitive	🏆 🏆 🏆 🏆 🏆	Competitive
Low living costs	💰 💰 💰 💰 💰	High living costs
Working really hard	🧑‍💻	Not working/chilling out

Contact details	Charles University—First Faculty of Medicine, Kateřinská 32, 121 08, Praha 2, Czech Republic Tel: +420 224 961 111, Web: www.lf1.cuni.cz/en

An insider's view...

The First Faculty of Medicine is one of the original four faculties of Charles University, established in the 14th century. It is the biggest and most prestigious faculty in the Czech Republic, with over 3100 students studying medicine. They are taught by more than 650 pedagogical and/or scientific experts. Studying medicine in Prague is not only a chance to study in a beautiful and historical city that is, according to many people, the most beautiful metropolis in Europe; it is a chance to get an MD degree that is accepted in both the US and EU.

Student Affairs Department

Perfecting the UCAS form

Chapter 9

Perfecting the UCAS form

The UCAS application form

All applications to British medical schools are handled by the Universities and Colleges Admissions Service (UCAS), including those to graduate entry courses (p. 216). UCAS only permits online applications so it is important to become familiar with the website (www.ucas.com) as early as possible.

Your passport to an interview

Your UCAS form *is* your application. It is one of the major hurdles you have to overcome to get an offer from a medical school, along with A-levels (p. 19), admission tests (p. 69), and the interview or assessment centre (p. 262). Until you are invited to interview, all the medical schools know about you is what is written on your UCAS form and your admission test results. There is limited space to make *your* application stand out so you have to make the most of every box and word.

> Key points The UCAS form is the culmination of all your hard work: school reference (p. 190), predicted A-levels, GCSE and AS grades, work experience, and extracurricular activities. Every word needs to support the case that you will make an excellent doctor.

Some general tips

- Deadlines Applications for medicine (and dentistry, veterinary science, and Oxbridge) have an earlier deadline. This is usually 15 October but check the UCAS website to be certain.
- Courses Although there are five spaces on the UCAS form, you can only apply to four medical schools. The other space can be used as a back-up option (i.e. a non-medical course).
- Deferred entry If you wish to defer your entry for a gap year (p. 30), you can indicate this on your application but check with medical schools before doing so. Some have policies on deferred applicants and others require agreement beforehand.

> Key points The UCAS deadline for medicine is earlier than for other courses, usually 15 October. Start early and try to finish before this date to avoid the risk of last-minute technical problems.

Mechanics of the form

The online UCAS form is quite simple to use, but there are a few things to note.

- Registration This takes less than ten minutes. Keep a careful note of your username, password, and personal ID.
- Email confirmation You will need to confirm that you have provided a valid email address. Use a professional-looking address as this is seen by medical school admissions staff. Create a new account (e.g. www.gmail.com) if necessary.
- Payment The application fee is £23 if you are applying to two or more courses. This is paid online by debit/credit card.

UCAS Track

An online system called UCAS Track is provided to manage and follow your application. This means you can expect to see offers/rejections shortly after decisions are made. You can also use UCAS Track to update personal details and add course choices. Be aware that it is only usually final decisions (e.g. offers/rejections) that appear on UCAS Track. Medical schools will communicate with you directly (e.g. by post) about interview arrangements.

Non-medicine courses

Most applicants can apply to five university courses per year through UCAS, but only four can be medical schools. This means one space is left over and some applicants fill these with other courses they might want to study. Although most choose a related discipline (e.g. biomedical science), this is by no means necessary.

A student's experience...

I applied to a law course in addition to four medical schools, and was worried the law school would think I was uncommitted given my medicine-orientated personal statement. The law course agreed to accept a letter explaining my unusual choice of courses. I explained that I really wanted to work in a profession where I could use my skills to solve problems that make a difference to people. Both medicine and law provided these opportunities. I relied on some legal work experience, which probably helped, and ended up with offers from the law course and two medical schools. The challenge now is to choose!

- **Choose carefully** Even if you don't want to study a non-medicine subject, think about this additional choice. There is little to gain from choosing options you could never imagine accepting.
- **Don't rush** Although medical school applications are required by the early UCAS deadline this is not necessary for many other courses. If you leave the spaces blank you can add more courses through UCAS Track up to the standard deadline.
- **Nothing to lose** There is nothing to lose from choosing a non-medicine subject. They will not prejudice your medical school application; universities cannot see where else you applied until after making offers.
- **Justifying your personal statement** One obstacle is that your personal statement should be written for medicine. Admissions tutors for other courses might struggle to assess your suitability (and commitment) for their subject. Don't be afraid of writing separately to these courses explaining your reasons for applying in this way.

Key points If you think you want to go directly into higher education then use the remaining UCAS space. You can always take the graduate route (p. 216) into medicine later on if that is what you want to do. Only leave these options blank if you want to avoid the temptation to study something else instead.

Your school reference

Every applicant knows their grades and personal statement are fundamental to winning a place. But few think hard about their school reference. For this reason, the reference presents an opportunity to set your application above the competition.

Is the reference important?

The answer to this question is that 'it depends'. It depends on your application and on the medical school. A bad reference will almost certainly have a negative impact. Although most courses require a *satisfactory* reference, there are a number of ways that a *strong* reference could help your application.

- **It may contribute to your application score** Some medical schools include the school reference as part of the overall application score, while others simply use it to filter out applicants with bad references.
- **It subjectively influences the assessor** Admissions staff are human. If they read a glowing personal reference, it will be difficult for them to separate this from the rest of your application. Even if it is not assigned points, the assessor could mark other elements higher as a consequence.
- **You are a borderline candidate** The reference could tip the balance if you are on the cusp of being invited to interview. Similarly, if you miss your offer and need to convince the school you are a strong candidate your whole UCAS application could be reviewed a second time.

> Key points Referees almost always want to write good references but don't know what to say. They often have many to write at the same time. As a result they produce bland, factual statements that don't tell medical schools very much beyond what they can already see from your UCAS form.

Explaining negative elements

If there is a negative element to your application that needs explaining, this should appear in your school reference. This might include unexpectedly low grades (e.g. due to illness or bereavement). Firstly, you do not have space in your personal statement to explain away potential negative aspects. Secondly, this type of explanation is more credible when written by someone other than the applicant. In this case it is particularly important that you meet with your referee so they have all the facts available and can ensure the reference is otherwise very positive.

Bad references

It is rare for applicants to receive a bad reference, but it can happen. Bad references are usually framed in vaguely positive terms but assessors can read between the lines. A bad school reference will often result in a rejected application.

> Key points Anxious about asking to see your school reference? There is no harm in asking so long as it is done politely. If they don't want to share, that doesn't mean they aren't writing nice things about you!

What is a good reference?

Compare the two references below and remember they could be written about the same person. Most applicants receive something closer to the first one and you don't need to be an admissions tutor to spot the difference. The second reference is personal, enthusiastic, and unreserved. It includes specific details and provides objective evidence (e.g. the letter from St Mary's Hospice) to support its claims. The second reference also comments on qualities specific to would-be doctors.

Reference 1

Tim has been a student at John Paget's School since 2002. He achieved mostly 'A*' grades in his GCSEs and some 'A's. His particular strengths are maths and science, which he is now studying at A-level. I do not think he will have a problem achieving your typical offer of 'AAB'. Tim is a pleasant young man who works hard and has lots of friends. He would be a very suitable candidate for your course.

Reference 2

Tim is one of the brightest students I have ever had the pleasure to teach. He consistently achieves 'A' grades and will almost certainly achieve straight 'A's this year. His coursework is always completed to a high standard and shows a depth of knowledge and understanding far beyond the A-level curriculum. In addition, Tim is extremely mature and personable. He interacts well with his peers and teachers alike. His academic ability and superb communication skills make him a natural candidate for medicine.

The manager of St Mary's Hospice, where Tim has volunteered for two years, has written very strongly in support of his medical school application. I have no hesitation in joining her to commend Tim for a place at medical school. He will make a fantastic doctor.

Guaranteeing a strong reference

- **Get to know your teachers** A personal reference is more convincing than a bland, factual statement. Stay on the right side of your teachers so they can genuinely support your UCAS application.
- **Keep a portfolio** Make a note of your achievements and work experience. If someone you work alongside seems particularly impressed by you, ask for a brief reference that you can use later on. A couple of enthusiastic letters of support could be incorporated into your school reference.
- **Choose the right person** It's worth noting that enthusiastic, outgoing people are more likely to write enthusiastic, outgoing references. If you get the chance to choose a referee then pick someone who won't hold back.
- **Provide information** Meet with your referee before they start writing. Ask outright whether they will support your application with a good reference. Take a list of medical school qualities and explain how you meet them.
- **Ask to see the reference** Although references are traditionally confidential, it is increasingly common for applicants to be shown their reference. This provides an opportunity to correct errors and/or provide further information. Don't be afraid to ask (politely) if you can see yours.

The personal statement

While it is natural to feel anxious about the personal statement, you should see it as an opportunity to set yourself apart from a pool of applicants with identical grades.

Some general rules

The personal statement is extremely important. It may take multiple drafts and several weeks to perfect, but this is time well spent.

- **Don't waste space** You have 47 lines or 4,000 characters, whichever you reach first. Every word must be chosen carefully so that you can convey as much information as possible in clear and concise English.
- **Do not copy** All UCAS forms are electronically checked for plagiarism. Do not consider copying even part of a sentence as you will get caught (p. 200).
- **What have you learned?** Listing experiences is not enough; every time you describe an experience you should describe what you learned from the experience and what personal qualities this demonstrates (p. 58).
- **Seek help** While it must be your own work, it is vital to seek advice and criticism from parents, teachers, and friends (who you trust not to copy). Act on the comments they make and do not be afraid to make major changes.
- **Save your work** Write the personal statement in a Word document and save it regularly. This makes it easier to save, print, edit, and check than writing it online in the UCAS form.
- **Think of your reader** The marker may have hundreds of personal statements to go through. Make their life easy by using clear and concise English, avoiding long 'waffly' sentences or vague statements.
- **Be convincing** If you make a claim that is unusual for a student finishing their A-levels then back it up with evidence.

> **Key points** Start early and make multiple drafts. From start to finish it should present a clear argument about why you will make an excellent doctor, backed up by personal experiences and the ability to reflect on and learn from these experiences.

Qualities and skills of a doctor

The qualities that medical schools look for come from two documents published by the General Medical Council (GMC) called *Tomorrow's Doctors* and *Good Medical Practice*. Both are available online at www.gmc-uk.org. They include:

- Honesty
- Communication skills
- Teamwork
- Integrity

- Caring
- Leadership
- Ability to learn
- Dedication

- Decision making
- Moral awareness
- Awareness of limitations
- Respect for others

How is it marked?

While the specifics vary between medical schools, the following are consistent:

- **Fixed marking criteria** Markers are given clear instructions of what to look for and how to score it so that marking is fair and reproducible.
- **Marking criteria are easy to predict** Although few medical schools publish their marking criteria, they will be based on finding applicants with the academic and personal abilities to complete the course. An example of a mark scheme is shown in the box.

Many mark schemes reward reflection on experiences. For example, writing 'I attended a multi-disciplinary team meeting, which taught me the value of effective communication between healthcare professionals' is likely to score better than 'I attended a multi-disciplinary team meeting, which included physiotherapists, occupational therapists, and community nurses'.

All candidates must meet minimum requirements: predicted/actual grades 'AAB'; minimum grade 'A' in chemistry; satisfactory school reference.

- **Commitment** (*max 10*): Valid reasons for studying medicine; relevant work experience; enthusiasm for medicine.
- **Insight** (*max 10*): Demonstrates understanding of qualities, knowledge, and attitudes required of a doctor; shows learning from personal/work experience.
- **Suitability** (*max 10*): Varied interests; achievement beyond educational work; ability to relax.
- **Academic ability** (*max 10*): A-level subject choices; predicted/actual grades; number of subjects; prizes won; other academic distinctions; very strong school reference; high grades despite personal adversity and/or struggling at school.

Key points Make the marker's life easy—clearly state what you have learned and what qualities of a doctor this demonstrates.

How is it used?

The personal statement serves two purposes:

- **Selection for interview** The statement is used to identify candidates who are likely to perform best at interview. The UCAS applications will be ranked, with the applicants above a certain threshold being invited for interview.
- **Material at interview** Your personal statement may be used to structure the interview. Make sure that you can justify every statement that you make.

Some medical schools disregard the UCAS form as soon as the interview lists are drawn up. At these schools all candidates invited to interview have an equal chance of winning an offer. At others the UCAS score can help balance poor performance at interview. Check the websites of medical schools you are applying to (p. 107), since some of them clearly state how they use this information.

What to include

Your personal statement should be a clear and logical statement explaining why you would make an excellent medical student and doctor. It should describe all your main achievements and experiences whilst emphasizing that you have the necessary qualities (p. 192) and ability to learn.

Why do you want to be a doctor?

This is a surprisingly complicated and involved question. There is no single correct answer; as you describe your reasons it is important to be aware of the implications of, or responses to, common answers:

- **To help people** This is a noble intention and it should be true for all doctors. However, it is also true of nurses, midwives, physiotherapists, and many professions outside of health-care. If altruism is really your main objective then charity work or politics may allow you to help more people. What is it about helping people *as a doctor* that appeals to you?
- **The love of science** Most doctors do enjoy learning about science, but again so do many in other professions. If science is your main interest then why not take a science degree and become an academic? Furthermore, medicine is not always that scientific; many patients leave hospital with no formal diagnosis or understanding of what caused their symptoms. Why does *medical* science in a *clinical* environment appeal to you?
- **The profession** There are many aspects of the medical profession that may appeal, including teamwork, contact with people, making important decisions, leadership, status, daily challenges, the salary, and social responsibility. If you describe the aspects that appeal to you the most, it is important that they make you appear in a positive and non-selfish light. What are the *positive* aspects of being a doctor that are not found in other professions?
- **A logical exclusion of alternatives** Hopefully you have considered numerous careers alongside medicine. While it is important to exclude these yourself, it is not enough to say that medicine was the only career left. Medical schools want students with a burning enthusiasm for medicine and being a doctor, and this needs to come across in your personal statement. Why is medicine the best possible use of your skills and qualities?
- **The challenge** There are many challenges in medicine: coping with limited resources, diagnosing diseases, communicating with patients, ethical dilemmas, emotional turmoil, etc. Which challenges of the profession attract you and what evidence do you have that you will be able to cope with them?

> **Key points** Your answer is likely to include a combination of these reasons, backed up by personal experience and a demonstration that you know what the job is like. Try to come up with arguments against the reasons you have written, then rewrite the section including evidence to answer these arguments.

What experience do you have?

Along with stating why you would make a good doctor, you must also describe the extracurricular activities (p. 41), work experience (p. 49), voluntary work (p. 60), employment (p. 62), or research (p. 64) that you have undertaken. If you are applying for deferred entry you should also outline your gap year plans (p. 30). Some people also include significant life events (e.g. severe illness) if this portrays them in a positive light (p. 196).

Personal statements that simply list such experiences can make extremely dull reading and risk a poor score, even if the experiences are incredible. It is better to use this information to back up any claims or statements that you make (along with how the experience taught you to further your learning).

Most interesting experience If there is something about you that really makes you stand out from other applicants then describe it in the first paragraph. Make sure you can describe why this experience is relevant to applying to medical school (e.g. 'While winning a gold medal in the Olympics was exhilarating, I became aware that I wanted more from life than simply being the fastest cyclist . . .').

Why you want to be a doctor While describing your personal reasons (see p. 194), use your work experience to demonstrate that you are aware of the role and challenges of being a doctor. Make sure you clearly state where the work experience was (hospital cardiology ward, GP clinic, etc.) and, if the length of work experience was impressive, include the duration too. What inspired you? What *exactly* did you find interesting? Take the opportunity to reflect on the situation; is there any further insight that you can demonstrate?

Academic suitability While there is no need to repeat your exam results, you should mention any other academic achievements. You can also mention particular academic interests supported by relevant experiences (e.g. reading *New Scientist*) or researching a medical topic well beyond the A-level curriculum (make sure you are ready to answer challenging questions at interview on this topic). What have these academic interests taught you?

Professional suitability You need to demonstrate that you have the qualities necessary to be a member of the medical profession (p. 192). To do this you can use a wide range of experiences, not just those in a healthcare setting.

Commitment to medicine Demonstrate your commitment to medicine using examples of long-term voluntary work or employment. Describe any challenges you faced and what these taught you. If these experiences were in a healthcare setting then use examples of where you interacted with a patient to demonstrate your communication skills and your ability to learn from situations.

A student's experience . . .

I wrote my whole personal statement based around my explanations for wanting to study medicine. I described my personal experience of being a patient, then my work experience and how it helped consolidate my ambition to become a doctor. I discussed my own qualities, with evidence from my hobbies and part-time work, in the context of what I'd seen of life as a doctor during my time in hospital. In this way I was able to fit in all the essential elements while articulating my reasons for applying.

What to avoid

It can be difficult to spot your own mistakes when writing a personal statement so you should always seek the advice of others before submission (p. 192). The following examples should help you avoid some of the most common personal statement blunders.

> Key points The personal statement needs to be extremely concise and clear. Keep two maxims in mind: 'keep it simple' and 'less is more'. Always display yourself in a positive light and make sure you describe a range of experiences.

Inappropriate use of experiences

Poor description of experiences can lose you marks; common mistakes include:

- **Lack of reflection** Simply describing your experiences is insufficient. The markers want to know that you gained insight from experiences and have the ability to learn from them. Highlight how your experiences increased your awareness of, and strengthened your desire for, studying medicine.
- **Exhausting one example** Breadth is crucial to demonstrating commitment. While one experience may be particularly informative, if you use it repeatedly it suggests that you have not done anything else. Try to include a variety of experiences including work experience, voluntary work, and extracurricular activities.
- **Listing experiences** There is also a risk of including too many experiences so that the personal statement reads like a list. Be selective and use the space to describe a few of the best experiences thoroughly.
- **Out-of-date examples** Avoid using experiences from many years ago unless they are especially relevant. A month in hospital as a child is worth including, but joining the Boy Scouts for a year at the age of 12 is not.
- **Inappropriate examples** Consider what experiences say about your personality. If they show a lack of honesty, good judgement, or common sense they should be left out regardless of the outcome.
- **Keep it positive** Focus on the positive aspects of a situation (see box).

> Avoid 'I spent a lot of time caring for my ill grandmother over the last year, which led to my lower than expected AS-level results (the time was very stressful and, whilst I tried to study, it was not always easy to do so).'
>
> Instead 'Having cared for my grandmother, who had severe Parkinson's disease, I learned about the difficulties experienced by family carers first-hand. I have resolved to always consider the holistic support available when managing patients with chronic illness.'
>
> NB If this applicant had communicated with their referees (p. 190) the school reference could describe the difficulties faced at length and justify the lower than expected AS-levels.
>
> Avoid 'I shadowed a GP for two weeks and this showed me that I would really enjoy the challenges of being a doctor. On several occasions I witnessed the doctor encountering difficulties. Watching him overcome these difficulties has inspired me to pursue my medical application.'
>
> Instead 'For two weeks I shadowed a GP serving a diverse local community. I learned the importance of cultural awareness when obtaining a history, especially regarding sensitive issues (e.g. sexual health). The social dimension of medicine is a key reason for my interest in becoming a doctor.'

Other pitfalls

- **Generic statements** You will not score any points by writing your personal statement in vague terms. Be sure to include pertinent details in your descriptions of experiences, unless they detract from the experience.
- **Negative points** The statement provides a relatively short space to sell yourself, so don't waste words explaining poor results or personal weaknesses. Your school reference is the correct place to explain about exam glitches or challenging personal circumstances (p. 190).
- **Gimmicks** It can be tempting to write something extravagant to catch the reader's attention. But writing a mature, reflective personal statement is more likely to impress than employing a literary gimmick.
- **Needless controversy** Another risky way of seeking attention is taking an extreme political or ethical position. You must be very careful if you plan to do this. Although we all have our personal beliefs, doctors should serve patients impartially and without judgement. Your application should reflect this principle.
- **An impossibly wide audience** It is impossible to write an application that will appeal to selectors at every type of medical school (p. 94). For this reason you should be applying to four similar courses (p. 88) and tailoring your application accordingly. For example, you could emphasize your interest in developing your communication skills or highlight your dedication to academic excellence and basic science.
- **Too many words** Long-winded descriptions are tiresome to read and waste valuable space: cut the waffle, stay away from needlessly long words, lose irrelevant details, and avoid repetition.

Key points As you write, try to eliminate any unnecessary words. This will make the writing clearer and allow you to fit in more experiences. Be ruthless with your statement from the beginning and you'll be much happier with the finished product.

Finishing the statement

A strong conclusion is as important as a captivating introduction. It should leave the reader with a good impression of your whole application. Having invested time and effort so far, avoid a trite, over-simplistic, or exaggerated conclusion. By the end of the last sentence, the selection panel must be confident that you are a suitable candidate for their course.

How to conclude

- **Do NOT repeat yourself** Your final paragraph should not be wasted repeating experiences you've already described. You have a finite amount of space and repeating examples only highlights limited experience. You may need to refer to a previously mentioned experience, but leave out the details.
- **Avoid new experiences** The conclusion should summarize what has already been written rather than adding new information.
- **Contextualize** What are the broader implications of your skills and qualities? Perhaps you've alluded to an interest in public health by describing a conversation with hospital doctors about healthcare rationing (p. 274) or the rising incidence of diabetes (p. 276). You may conclude that, having demonstrated an ability to work compassionately and impartially, your skills will be essential for practising medicine in a resource-limited health service. In this way you are describing what you have to offer to medicine.
- **Draw themes together** You may have covered many different topics, using very discrete experiences. The conclusion should identify key 'take home' messages for the reader.

A student's experience...

Having discussed a range of topics in my personal statement, from browsing *Nature* articles to shadowing a hospital doctor, I had several options for how to conclude. I felt it was best to describe how my passion for understanding science would be the driving force behind my future medical career. I also used this as an opportunity to reiterate my suitability for the traditional style of course that I was applying for.

Editing

Once you've drafted your personal statement, start editing. There is *always* room for improvement. You should aim to show your finished version to as many different people as possible and be prepared to alter your text based on their comments. Ask them explicitly to be critical—you will not be helped by twenty readers if all they do is offer reassurance. There are two broad criteria by which you need to assess your personal statement: content and style.

Content

- **Themes** Have you discussed everything you intended to? There are basic elements that you need to include (reasons for studying medicine, insights from work experience, etc.), but what about the additional topics that you wanted to cover? Do they reinforce your application or are they repetitive? Are there any contradictions? Remember, if you raise medical issues, you should be prepared to discuss these at interview.
- **Evidenced statements** Every claim should be supported by a personal experience. For example, anyone can list the ideal qualities of a doctor, but a good applicant will describe how they have demonstrated each one.
- **Clarity** The point of each paragraph should be immediately obvious by the end of it. If there is any doubt as to its meaning, discard it and start again.
- **Representative of you** Whilst you need to remain positive, your statement must be an honest account of you, your experiences, your qualities, and what you can offer to medicine. Any attempt to mislead the selection panel will inevitably be uncovered, often at interview. Make sure you stick to the facts.

A student's experience...

My statement focused on shadowing experiences with a district nurse, GP, and physiotherapist. I also described mentoring junior school pupils. In my conclusion I highlighted my interpersonal and leadership skills, which are essential for a doctor working in our multi-disciplinary NHS in the 21st century.

Style

- **Tone** Your tone should be positive and professional throughout.
- **Unique** It should be immediately obvious that you wrote your statement. Insightful reflection and thought-provoking discussion will only be remembered if they are based on personal experience. Never copy someone else's work, since UCAS automatically checks for this (p. 200).
- **Consistency** This goes for all aspects of your statement, including punctuation and spelling. The use of indented versus spaced paragraphs should remain the same throughout your document.

Key points When writing your personal statement, be sure to save your work regularly under different filenames (which include the date) to allow you to return to older versions should you wish to.

Personal statements

The following section reiterates the importance of keeping your personal statement *personal*, and describes how specific examples may be reviewed.

Example personal statements

WARNING! *Plagiarism in personal statements*

UCAS now uses sophisticated software to check whether any part of your form matches material in other submitted statements. If a match is found, these applications are flagged to medical schools as containing potentially plagiarized material. In 2007, UCAS found that 5% of medical school personal statements contained copied material, including 234 claiming a passion for science after 'accidentally burning holes in [their] pyjamas after experimenting with a chemistry set on their 8th birthday'. Using the internet and this book to gain advice for personal statements is essential, but there is no excuse for copying, even just a sentence. Plagiarism is a severe failure in integrity and almost guarantees immediate rejection.

Avoid Ever since I was a child I have been intrigued by how we work. I believe that there is nothing more wondrous than developing a greater understanding of the human body. This has been supported by my passion for A-level biology.

Analysis The student offers a reasonable reason for wanting to study medicine and tries to show evidence to support this (the passion for biology). However, they do not clearly describe how this interest will make them a good doctor and do not demonstrate how this 'passion' has affected their actions.

Instead My lifelong interest in how the human body functions has developed into a passion for human biology that has led me to read widely beyond the boundaries of the A-level curriculum. Whilst I am excited about continuing these studies at medical school, it is the thought of using this interest to help people that really thrills me.

Avoid Last summer I spent a month designing primers for PCR amplification of single nucleotide polymorphisms (SNPs) around the Cystic Fibrosis Transmembrane Conductance Regulator (CFTR) gene to investigate the effect of these SNPs on transcription. I downloaded the surrounding sequence from the UCSC genome browser, then used Primer3 for design, followed by BLAT and BLAST to ensure they were unique.

Analysis The excessive use of jargon may mean that the reader cannot appreciate what the student did. There is no clinical relevance and it also focuses too much on what they did rather than why they did it or what they learned.

Instead Meeting a patient with cystic fibrosis led me to learn more about this disease. I discovered that a local research laboratory studied cystic fibrosis and, after contacting them, I was offered the chance to spend a month working with a PhD student. The research focused on the regulation of the cystic fibrosis gene, which may allow development of drugs to treat milder forms of the disease. This experience helped me appreciate the role of a doctor as the interface between patients and medical research.

Avoid After spending months trying to find a doctor to shadow, my hard graft paid off! I shadowed a paediatrician for three weeks, watching fairly routine jobs and playing with the children on the wards. Whilst this was amazing fun (despite a few rascals) there was a serious element to it. I learned that playgroups could be used to make developmental assessments and monitor chronic diseases. These experiences taught me a lot about the boring side to medicine, the importance of MDT, and what I want to do in life—paeds!

Analysis The student's writing style is too informal for a personal statement. It fails to demonstrate professionalism, which is fundamental to being a doctor. It dwells on negative aspects that make it sound like the student is complaining or uninterested. The student alludes to fairly difficult themes, but then fails to match them to the relevant experience and reflect further. While working with play therapists as part of a multi-disciplinary approach is important, the applicant is applying for a role as a doctor not a play therapist. The only comment about the paediatrician's role is negative.

Instead Part of my work experience was spent shadowing a hospital paediatrician on the children's ward. I was enthused by the patient contact and fascinated to watch how the paediatrician tailored his style of communication to suit all patients, from infants to adolescents. I later had the opportunity to practise this myself, working with a specialist who was assessing the development of children through play. I learned the importance of a team approach to medicine and that diagnosis and management requires far more than analysing biochemistry reports.

Avoid Working as a head boy with my team of prefects has taught me a lot about myself and confirmed my suitability for a medical career. Beyond the obvious leadership element required for such a position, succeeding both in this role and my studies demanded expert time-management skills. I am certainly ready to take on the professional responsibilities of becoming a doctor and overseeing other hospital staff, whilst maintaining a healthy work–life balance.

Analysis This statement describes many skills and transferrable qualities but they are not clearly demonstrated. It exaggerates the importance of his work as head boy, claiming that this means he is ready to lead hospital staff (a situation that is many years of experience away, if ever). He does not use specific activities or experiences to justify the claims and there is no mention of the importance of teamwork, either in his position at school or within medicine.

Instead As head boy I led a team of prefects in a project to teach study skills to younger students through leaflets, revision timetables, and teaching groups of 30 or more. The project required me to assess and utilize the strengths and weaknesses of the different prefects, maintain the group's focus on our overall goals, and keep to a tight timeline. I learned the importance of teamwork and valuing every member of a group, which is as important in a multi-disciplinary clinical team as in this situation.

Key points There is more to a personal statement than describing your experiences and listing the qualities that you think a doctor should have. Through mature reflection your experiences should demonstrate how you already think like, and possess the important qualities of, a doctor.

Getting into Oxbridge

Chapter 10

Getting into Oxbridge

Oxbridge demystified

Ancient. Wealthy. Exceptional. Inaccessible. Elitist. Intellectual. Competitive. The universities of Oxford and Cambridge attract many colourful descriptions, with varying degrees of truth behind each one. These institutions are often perceived as being impenetrable for all but the greatest minds. Many of the qualities essential for medical school also make you a legitimate Oxbridge candidate, including strong A-level grades (p. 19) and diverse extracurricular achievements (p. 41). The following pages describe some of the key features that set Oxbridge applications apart, including the collegiate system (p. 208), the courses (p. 210), and the interview process (p. 212).

The collective term 'Oxbridge' is used to describe Oxford and Cambridge because of features they have in common. Both were founded over 800 years ago and developed into similar collegiate institutions with reputations for academic excellence. Their similarities mean you can apply to *either* Oxford or Cambridge in a single academic year, but not both.

So what's it all about?

- **The people** The single most important advantage of Oxbridge is being surrounded by exceptional people doing exceptional work. It is a chance to learn from some of the greatest academic talent in the world—many tutors will have conducted research that defines current thinking. Consequently, the university attracts clever and hard-working undergraduates. This creates a unique working environment in which some people thrive. Others grow tired of always feeling in competition with their peers.
- **The opportunities** Unique opportunities are found throughout degrees at Oxbridge: the supervision/tutorial system (see p. 210), libraries, research projects (see p. 87), grants (see p. 205), and well-endowed clubs and societies. A healthy supply of benefactors ensures that Oxbridge students benefit from a wide range of opportunities that other institutions cannot always afford.
- **The reputation** Both Oxford and Cambridge are in the top five universities worldwide; everyone has heard of them and this can only help your career. Being an Oxbridge graduate suggests you are someone who works hard and can achieve results.

What's it not about?

- **Sex, drugs, and rock and roll** While there is a good social life on offer, the balance is tipped further towards academic work than some other medical schools. However, there are still fun, if quirky, times to be had.
- **Large circles** Wherever you study, medical students have a reputation for cliquishness. This is exacerbated by the collegiate structure at Oxbridge. Medical students spend a lot of time with others studying the same course at their college. In smaller colleges this can be as few as two or three other people. Fortunately, most colleges accommodate all students (at least in the first year) in common halls, which offers at least some chance of branching out and meeting new people.

- **Being the best** Whilst the determination to succeed is essential to survive an Oxbridge education, unrealistic expectations can crush the aspirations of former head boys and girls alike. In all likelihood, you should forget about being the best, or at least about getting to the top as easily as you did at school. The bell curve of results (once your best friend) isn't as fun on the peak or at the tail end.

Costs and grants

A commonly held misconception is that you have to be wealthy to get into Oxbridge. Quite the opposite is true as both universities offer a range of grants and bursaries. Basic costs such as tuition fees and books are the same as at other medical schools, with accommodation falling between London and home-county prices. Except for a formal college gown (£30–£50), there are no extras that you will be expected to pay for. Ceremonial college dinners that you are invited to are paid for by the college.

All students can benefit from book, hardship, learning, and research grants. Such financial support is available from both the college and the university itself. Means-tested bursaries are also available for students from the lowest-income backgrounds to help meet living costs. These are offered regardless of which college you attend.

Access schemes

Universities are increasingly aware that some students might have experienced more educational disadvantages than others. Some applicants come from schools and/or families with no tradition of studying in higher education. Others may have had an education disrupted by personal or health problems.

At Oxford, all information about a candidate comes from the UCAS form. Those meeting various 'access' criteria, as well as the usual requirements for a conditional offer, are strongly recommended for interview.

Cambridge also considers this information via the UCAS form, as well as by employing a separate 'Extenuating Circumstances Form' (ECF) that students complete through their school. This is used when a student's education has been seriously disadvantaged or disrupted through health or personal problems. If you perform well at interview and in the pre-admission tests, some students have occasionally been made lower grade offers.

Key points Being part of such a world-class institution like Oxbridge is a hard-earned privilege. However, when you apply for your first job as a doctor the medical school you attended is simply not part of the application process. For this reason, Oxbridge is less of a career advantage for doctors than for other graduates. Think very carefully about what you stand to gain (and potentially lose) by applying to Oxbridge. It's not for everyone.

The Oxbridge experience

The experiences of students attending Oxford and Cambridge are defined by the environment, resources, and people. The following examples offer a glance at life as an Oxbridge medic.

A day in the life of an Oxbridge pre-clinical student...

A typical weekday can begin at 6am for rowing practice, followed by four hours of lectures. A successful morning, falling asleep in fewer than half the lectures, is followed by a quick bike ride back to college for lunch. Afternoon dissection may last two hours, before completing a supervision essay with almost no time to spare before the deadline. The college sometimes runs talks from eminent figures, so I may pop over to the conference centre to see a Nobel Prize-winner in the flesh!

A day in the life of an Oxbridge clinical student...

As a second year clinical student at Cambridge, I am currently based at Addenbrooke's Hospital on my paediatrics rotation.

There is a Special Care Baby Unit ward round that starts at 9am. I follow the clinical team for several hours on a business round, where the ST3 (junior doctor) updates the consultant on the progress of each baby under the team's care. Most of the discussion is far too specialized for me to understand, but a friendly ST2 (a more junior doctor) keeps me on my toes by asking me basic clinical questions and answering any questions that I have.

At lunchtime the clinical school holds a student grand round, where a student presents an audit from their recent orthopaedics student-selected component.

There is also a *New England Journal of Medicine* Club in the afternoon, where one of the consultants discusses interesting cases in the literature that are relevant to junior doctors.

Afterwards, I make a dash for the 2pm haematological oncology clinic, where the consultant sees children with haematological malignancies. It is very specialized, but useful as the consultant allows me to examine each of the patients.

At 6pm, members of my college join me on the wards with a junior doctor who takes us on our weekly clinical supervision. For the next two hours we take histories, examine patients, and discuss management, receiving feedback at every step from our clinical supervisor.

Afterwards I grab a quick bite to eat at the college canteen. I've missed a Tennis Society formal event but join the rest of my team in the college bar later on. We have a pint before escaping to the infamous 'Cindies' for a bit of cheeky dancing.

The Union

The Oxford Union is a debating society and the second-oldest University Union (second only to the Cambridge Union). Both the Oxford and Cambridge Unions are world renowned as debating forums and attract a host of international figures and celebrities. These have included Gerry Adams, Hans Blix, Pierce Brosnan, Clint Eastwood, Stephen Hawking, the Dalai Lama, Michael Jackson, Ronald Reagan, Jerry Springer, and Desmond Tutu. The Unions also hold workshops to help sharpen your debating skills and often field one of the most successful teams at the World Universities Debating Championships.

May week

After the madness of exams, May week (quintessentially for Oxbridge, in June) begins. This is the period of post-exam enjoyment, where your pigeonhole is swamped by invitations for garden parties and formal dinners from societies, colleagues, and friends. After a year of hard work, you have earned an extravagant annual college ball. Lasting from 8pm till 8am, this is a night of fine food and drink, popular live acts, funfair rides, and a spectacular fireworks display. It makes a refreshing change from the cheesy bops/ents (discos) that run throughout the rest of the year.

A similar experience

I think going to Oxbridge is very much like attending any other medical school. The course is a little more theoretical to begin with, but outside of that, you do what appeals to you. I find I have an experience closer to my medic friends at other universities than non-medics in my own college.

Diversity prevails!

As a student from a 'non-traditional' background (p. 255), I applied to Cambridge University with some hesitation at first. My school did not have a history of sending students to Oxbridge and I was the first in my family to study beyond high school. Although I had my own preconceptions about Oxbridge, having experienced the environment first-hand I can reassure those interested in applying that your background need not deter anyone. Despite the stereotypes, Oxford and Cambridge are diverse, multicultural institutions working hard to address any imbalances that remain in their student make-up. If you are a strong candidate then you can compete for a place regardless of your sex, ethnicity, or personal, health, or social circumstances.

The colleges

In the UK the collegiate system is unique to Oxford, Cambridge, Lancaster (p. 128), and Durham (p. 120) medical schools. Medical students at other institutions usually live on a campus or in a city and travel to their teaching centre or hospital each day. A centrally placed Students' Union is found at the heart of their community and most students participate in extracurricular activities at university level.

Oxford and Cambridge differ because they are both made up of over 30 independent colleges. The colleges operate independently despite all belonging to the same university. An Oxbridge student's pre-clinical life outside of lectures and practical sessions is based almost entirely within their college. The college provides key amenities to its students, such as:

- **Accommodation** Some colleges offer accommodation for all three pre-clinical years, either within college or in college-owned properties in town.
- **Dining** There are formal and informal halls, a distinction based solely on strict serving times and whether or not a formal gown and smart dress must be worn.
- **Supervision/tutorials** These are small teaching groups made up of students from the same college (p. 208).
- **Facilities/financial aid** The quality of grants (p. 205), libraries, and even gym facilities varies between colleges.
- **Clubs and societies** Almost all are duplicated at college and university level. The university sports teams play at a much higher standard and consist of the best players from across the colleges. At Oxbridge the 'Students' Union' is replaced by each college's 'Junior Common Room' (JCR) and the bar.
- **Support** Pastoral and academic welfare is provided by two fellows from the college (senior academic figures, who sit on a college's governing body). Your pastoral support will come from a fellow of a discipline other than medicine.

Choosing a college

As well as choosing between Oxford and Cambridge (p. 211) you can also apply to a specific college. Since you will spend so much time in your college this is a decision to consider carefully.

- **Exclusion criteria** First make a list of the colleges that are applicable to you. Be aware that some colleges are single-sex or for graduates only. At Oxford, Permanent Private Halls are often small foundations associated with a particular religious order. They can only award a limited number of degrees.
- **Size** Would you prefer a large college where you meet new people every term or the cosier atmosphere of a small college and familiar faces?
- **Locality** Particularly in Cambridge there can be a 'large' (in Oxbridge terms) distance between central and out-of-town colleges. Avoid the latter if you can't ride a bike and still want to make it to lectures on time.

- Age Colleges range from a few decades to many centuries old and most architectural tastes can be accommodated.
- Facilities/grants Very dependent upon the wealth of each college. This can make a big difference, including book grants worth hundreds of pounds each year, free access to the college gym, and travel grants.
- Culture You can only get an authentic feel for each college by visiting and speaking to current students. Avoid 'rational' decisions based on out-of-date statistics and hearsay.

The choices

Just like universities (p. 89), Oxbridge colleges have their own individual characters. These are shaped by the diversity of students and the unique infrastructure that each has developed over the years. Look at the college prospectus and the 'alternative' (i.e. student-written) prospectus for each college of interest. As well as the college website, the student JCR might provide helpful information online. If you still have questions, each college has an Undergraduate Admissions Office that will be happy to take your call.

The only real way to gain an appreciation is to attend the college open days and speak to people studying medicine at the college. Nevertheless, the 'tasting' guide below might be helpful as an overview of the choices on offer:

- Vintage Burgundy white wine Old and opulent, benefiting from its unique *terroir* in the centre of town. These money houses have a reputation for attracting the rich, croquet-loving public school boys. Despised and envied by the other colleges for their size, wealth, and arrogance. *E.g. St John's (Cam.), Christ Church (Ox).*
- Dr Pepper® Out of town and out of mind for the rest of the university. As a result, the people here have to get along very well and they usually do. If you can find them on a map of the city, you win a place. *E.g. Girton (Cam.), St Hugh's (Ox).*
- Milk These are friendly colleges; genuinely happy places filled with smiley people. Often not as cut-throat competitive as some of the other colleges. *E.g. Clare (Cam.), Corpus Christi (Ox).*
- Iced tea You don't choose them, they choose you. Either single-sex or graduate colleges. *E.g. Newnham (Cam.), Harris Manchester (Ox).*

Open applications If you really can't make your mind up you can send an open application. This means a college is allocated based on the least subscribed college at the time your application is received. However, this doesn't necessarily mean it's easier to win a place by submitting an open application. If you apply to an over-subscribed college, strong applicants at Cambridge may be 'pooled' for consideration by under-subscribed colleges. If you are applying to Oxford, you will automatically be allocated a second college, even if you stated a preference for your first choice. These mechanisms prevent strong candidates from losing out by applying to colleges of their choice.

If you dislike a particular type of college, avoid being allocated one by stating a preference. You can't change your mind once you have been allocated.

Studying medicine at Oxbridge

Wherever you study medicine, there are certain skills and certain knowledge you will be taught. Although the content of every medical school education is largely the same, information can be delivered in many different ways (p. 88). The Oxford and Cambridge courses offer a unique style of training in terms of the depth of coverage, teaching methods, and assessments.

The course The six-year course for undergraduates is divided into two stages. The first two years cover basic sciences, with a research project taking up the third year. The Oxbridge student then enters the second stage, 'clinicals', lasting three years.

- The initial three-year pre-clinical stage is when the core sciences are delivered. Students from all medical schools must learn about a vast number of subjects relevant to clinical medicine: anatomy, biochemistry, neurobiology, pathology, pharmacology, physiology, and psychology. However, whilst other courses often concentrate on the subject details directly relevant to medicine, the Oxbridge courses emphasize studying each subject in its own right and for its own sake.
- Tutorials/supervisions are incredible teaching opportunities unique to the Oxbridge medical courses.
- Very little clinical exposure (no more than a few hours a term) is provided during the pre-clinical stage. As a result, Oxbridge students are introduced to patients later than those studying elsewhere.
- Oxbridge students must submit an additional application during their third year before starting clinical medicine. Whichever institution they started at, they can choose to study at Oxford, Cambridge, or one of the medical schools in London. Although all students are guaranteed a place on a clinical course, the application process is competitive and not everyone wins their first choice.

Tutorials and supervisions In common with other medical schools, Oxbridge uses lectures to deliver core material to students. Medical students at Oxbridge also benefit from tutorials (Oxford) or supervisions (Cambridge). There are as many as four such sessions a week during the pre-clinical stage, each of which can require preparatory work (e.g. an essay or set of problems) to be completed beforehand. Such 'one-to-one' tuition is useful for solving any difficulties, as well as encouraging a deeper understanding of the course material.

It is crucial that candidates appreciate the demands that such a teaching method adds over and above a standard medical course. The time commitments are significant and not everyone is suited to the intense learning environment.

Assessment At the end of each year, most medical students sit various exams (e.g. multiple choice questions, short answer questions) to assess their competence in the subjects covered. This ensures you have met the standards required by the GMC to be awarded your degree at the end of the course (p. 278). At the end of each year in the pre-clinical stage at Oxbridge every subject is assessed by an additional exam paper that is entirely essay-based. Essays require a different set of skills from multiple choice or short answer questions.

In addition to working towards a medical degree, Oxbridge medical students work towards a 'traditional' honours degree leading to a Bachelor of Arts (BA) qualification after the first three years. This is comparable to the intercalated (BSc) degree that is available at many other medical schools (p. 87).

At the end of three years of pre-clinical training, Oxbridge medical students are awarded a 1st, 2:1, 2:2, or 3rd class degree, based entirely on performance in their third-year essay papers. The results of these papers do not otherwise count towards the medical qualification. Whilst the essays are fundamentally scientific, the pre-clinical examiners will demand a degree of literary flair. If you flinch at the mere thought of your old English literature lessons, think carefully before applying to Oxbridge.

Course differences between Oxford and Cambridge In short, there are very few. The key is to decide whether you suit the more science-oriented syllabus shared by both universities. Table 10.1 shows the main course differences.

Table 10.1 Course differences between Oxford and Cambridge

Stage	Oxford	Cambridge
Pre-clinical course	A more integrated systems-based approach (p. 88)	A more traditional core subject-based course (anatomy, physiology, etc.)
Third year BA	Most people do the 'Final Honour School' leading to a BA in medical sciences in one of five options: neuroscience; molecular medicine; myocardial, vascular, and respiratory biology; infection and immunity; or signalling in health and disease	Greater flexibility in the Cambridge Tripos exam system, which allows students to choose from a wider range of subjects in their third year with the possible option of extending their studies by another year to an additional subject, e.g. law
MBPhD programme	A PhD programme can be pursued after the pre-clinical years, although a formal MBPhD programme, like the one at Cambridge, does not exist	An additional three years of laboratory research can lead to a PhD in any science subject; often an extension of the third year research project
Clinical course	Modular assessments throughout the year; the ten-week elective is performed in the sixth year	Predominantly end-of-year exams; the seven-week elective is performed at the end of the fifth year

The Oxbridge interview

The infamous Oxbridge interview is surrounded by colourful myths, almost all of which you can disregard. After submitting your application form and completing the BMAT (p. 82), you may be invited for interview, typically in December. There are usually two interviews. Sometimes one will focus on science and the other on non-science questions. Other times they might both include an element of science and non-science.

What makes the Oxbridge interview different? Of course, almost all medical schools interview applicants (p. 264). This is to ensure that only those with the attitude and interpersonal skills required by a doctor are accepted. However, because of the unique Oxbridge course style, interviewers also want to determine whether you will thrive in their environment.

Unlike interviews at other medical schools, which use the same broad questions for each candidate, Oxbridge interviews are rarely scripted. Instead, interviewers are free to allow a conversation to develop. Although some candidates view this as an obstacle, it is better seen as an opportunity. The discursive style permits interviewers to see how you think, how you cope when faced with unfamiliar topics, and how you interact with adults in a relatively pressured environment. It also replicates the style of a typical tutorial/supervision (p. 210) so it can help you determine your suitability for this style of teaching.

Why did you apply to Oxbridge? Carefully consider your reasons for applying to Oxbridge. The last thing you need is to fumble on questions you knew would be asked. There are no 'right' answers, but you should bear in mind a few key points:

- Whilst there are plenty of attractive features (p. 204), you should focus on your interest in the academically oriented medical course, which is unique to Oxbridge. The buildings may be stunning but you are applying to study medicine, not architecture.
- In highlighting the benefits, avoid denigrating any other university and/or its course. Firstly, you do not know where your interviewers qualified from. Secondly, you are unlikely to demonstrate your best thinking by criticizing individual medical schools. It is far better to describe how the style of Oxbridge suits your own learning style and abilities.

Why would you be successful at Oxbridge? Think about skills you will need to cope with the unique style of the course. For example, four tutorials/supervisions a week, on top of five full days of timetabled work, demands effective time management.

If you're thinking about Oxbridge because you're not a 'people person', think again. Although there is little clinical training in the first three years, the Oxbridge medical courses do not exist solely to produce academic doctors. In fact, less than 5% of Oxbridge medics go on to pursue an entirely academic medical career. In common with others, Oxford and Cambridge medical schools aim to produce competent and professional clinicians.

Oxford or Cambridge? This is a topic of conversation that is worth avoiding. There are far more similarities than differences between Cambridge and Oxford.

- Usually students decide which to choose based on the type of town that would suit them best. You can only appreciate this by visiting them both.
- There are very few differences in the courses (p. 211) and to decide based on these differences would require you to have unrealistic certainty about your future career intentions. Decisions concerning third-year projects or MBPhDs are made later on in your pre-clinical education. Avoid bringing up these topics unless you are unusually well informed.

Science questions at interview A medical school interview is not designed to check your knowledge of A-level science. This should be implicit in your exam grades. However, science questions may still be asked for a variety of reasons. They could arise because your UCAS form claims an interest in a particular area of medicine. If this is the case, you need to be particularly careful that what you have mentioned truly is an interest. Doctors on the panel will not take long to discover whether or not you really know about a subject for which you claim a particular enthusiasm.

Alternatively, science knowledge may be used to see how you think around a problem. Oxbridge interviews, in keeping with their general teaching style (p. 210), aim to push students beyond material they have covered as part of a set syllabus. This means you need a solid appreciation of A-level material so you can approach science questions sensibly using first principles.

A-level science relevant to medicine Medicine is essentially the use of science to understand, diagnose, and treat disease. Biology, chemistry, and physics are all used to varying degrees. Sometimes the link is obvious: the study of cardiac physiology is directly applicable to medicine. Other areas are more subtly relevant. Your understanding of organic chemistry and the stereochemistry of inorganic molecules could be important in appreciating drug design and how compounds specifically interact with their target receptors. Physics may be tested when answering questions on the auditory system; this requires an understanding of the nature of sound waves, pressure calculations, and moments.

The style of such questions is to make you think outside of your comfort zone. Clearly, the questions you will be asked are determined by the areas studied at A-level. Having said that, do not be quick to dismiss a question because you 'haven't covered it at school'. You may need to take logical steps from A-level knowledge to reach a sensible answer. Stay flexible and remember to vocalize all of your steps and assumptions, once you've clearly thought about them (p. 214). Interviewers are interested in how you think at least as much as what you know.

Key points Keep your eyes open to topics relevant to medicine during your A-level studies. It is not possible to prepare for every potential question but fostering an interest in clinical topics might help. A rote-learned approach to answering interview questions, including science ones, will be spotted by the panel. Instead, concentrate on making sure that you have a confident grasp of all of your A-level material (p. 19).

An insider's view...

For one journalist's insights, behind the scenes of the selection process at Cambridge University, read the *Guardian* article 'So who is good enough to get into Cambridge?'.

www.guardian.co.uk/education/2012/jan/10/how-cambridge-admissions-really-work

Inside the Oxbridge interview

It is difficult to describe an Oxbridge interview, simply because every one is so different. Some colleges employ a list of questions but these only help start a general discussion. The key to answering any question is thoughtfulness, clarity, and detail. Don't be afraid to ask for a little more time to think about your responses. When you think you have an answer, vocalize all the steps you made to get you there. You do not have to always be 'right'—there is often no right answer as such—but they do want to see you are comfortable with new ideas.

The following are examples of questions that could be asked in an Oxbridge interview. Don't forget, you will still be asked common (p. 268), ethical (p. 272), and/or clinical science questions (p. 276).

> Key points When you read the science examples below, remember they are specific to a particular candidate. If you don't know the answers, don't panic, as it is unlikely your interview would have developed in this direction. Interviewers tend to follow the candidate's lead. When you answer a question correctly, they will pursue that answer to see how much you know. The result is a challenging interview that might seem impossible to another candidate. You should also remember that interviewers will coach candidates who don't know the answer but are on the right path. Bear this in mind when talking to other candidates about their interview questions.

Example I—Science questions

The following is a transcript of an interview with a student who described an interest in studying nerve conduction and action potentials at school:

Interviewer What is the refractory period for our nerves and what does this mean in terms of their frequency range?

Student The refractory period is around 1 ms. This puts an upper limit on the frequency of impulses along a nerve of around 1 kHz, since frequency is the inverse of this time period.

Interviewer So, for light entering your eye, what information about the energy is transferred by the impulse frequency along the nerve?

Student The wave-particle duality theory of light would describe the intensity of light as varying with photon frequency.

Interviewer The result of our nerves having a limit of 1 kHz to interpret light is that our eyes are relatively poor at discriminating between light intensities. Is there any way you think the eye compensates for this, to gain additional information about the intensity of light?

Student Perhaps, by possessing light receptors which react to different ranges of light intensity. Or using the iris to constrict the pupils and diminish the fraction of light reaching the retina.

Example II—Science questions

Here's an interview transcript from a student who mentioned studying oxygen–haemoglobin dissociation curves in biology:

Interviewer   How does a foetus obtain oxygen from its mother?

Student   Foetal haemoglobin has a higher affinity for oxygen than adult haemoglobin.

Interviewer   Can you think of any other circumstances in which this principle of higher haemoglobin affinity is exploited?

Student   At low oxygen pressures, such as high altitudes.

Interviewer   Take a guess at what you think the maximum altitude is that we can live for a sustained period of time, without life support?

Student   5,000 m?

Interviewer   Around that. The effect of altitude on haemoglobin is why the people of the Andes who first colonized the region were unable to have babies. What else happens to the human body with altitude?

Student   The low oxygen saturation of the blood may increase your respiratory drive, causing you to hyperventilate.

Interviewer   What is the effect on the pH of the blood?

Student   Loss of acidic carbon dioxide leads to alkalosis.

Interviewer   What is the other problem from hyperventilating?

Student   Loss of water vapour which can cause dehydration.

Example III—Problem solving

If you were put in an irregularly shaped room and asked to measure the volume, how would you do it?

When an ice cube in a glass full of water melts, what happens to the level of the water in the glass? Why? What would happen to the level if the ice cube melted in a glass of cooking oil?

Example IV—Theoretical discussion

What is science?

What has the biggest advance in medicine been and why?

If you had the power to eradicate one disease, which would it be and why?

An insider's view...

A common mistake made by students at interview is to think that the answer to a science question is our most important focus. As interviewers we are far more interested in how applicants think and how they approach scientific problems. Sometimes we don't even know the answer ourselves.

Graduate entry medicine

Chapter 11

Graduate entry medicine

Introducing graduate medicine

Graduate entry courses are accelerated, typically lasting four years instead of five. Although medical degrees in the UK usually take at least five years, this is different from other countries. In the USA, for example, school leavers enrol on a four-year undergraduate degree. Only when they graduate can they compete for the opportunity to spend another four years at medical school.

This model has now reached the UK. A number of established medical schools, and some new ones, have launched courses designed for graduate applicants. These are shorter because the course designers assume that a graduate's first degree gives them knowledge or experience that overlaps with early medical school teaching. Graduate entry medical courses vary in the types of degree they will consider for admission (p. 220).

A student's experience...

Studying medicine as a graduate is very different from my previous degree. The days are full and I am expected to sign a register at the start of almost every teaching session. But studying medicine is a lot more fun because it is immediately obvious why each fact is important. It's finally an opportunity to apply my previous study of science to problems that impact on the lives of real people.

To apply or not to apply

Just because you are a graduate does not mean you *have* to apply to graduate entry courses. You can also apply to traditional five- or six-year courses instead. In fact there are good reasons why you might want to avoid graduate entry programmes:

- Limited choice of medical schools Not all medical schools offer graduate entry courses (p. 226). If you want to study in a particular place, you might be unable to choose a graduate course.
- Workload Graduate entry courses really are accelerated. The days are full, holidays are reduced, and there is an emphasis on 'self-directed learning'. Some students call this 'do-it-yourself' medicine.
- Environment Some courses are very small (fewer than 25 students) and can feel claustrophobic.
- Competition There are lots of graduates wanting to study medicine but relatively few places. This means that accelerated courses are *much* more competitive. Applicant/place ratios vary from about 8:1 to 47:1 (p. 227).

Of course there are advantages to applying to these courses:

- Money Graduate entry courses are much cheaper. One less year of being a student can save you between £17,000 and £25,000/£20,000 (p. 15), while the extra year on a standard course means one less year in your final employment, which may mean you lose out on about £100,000 (see p. 32). Under the current system, those on traditional courses receive the NHS bursary (p. 17) in their final year but graduate-entry students are supported through years two, three, and four.
- Environment Students on graduate entry courses are (usually) older, which creates a different environment from those dominated by school leavers. You will meet people with a range of life experiences (and former careers) as well as many in your own age group.

- **Selection processes** Most graduate entry courses place less emphasis on GCSEs and A-levels. They are more interested in your degree. This can be an advantage if your earlier grades would score well in a game of Scrabble.
- **Time** Graduate entry courses save a year of studying. If you already have a degree, you might be eager to start work and enter (or re-enter) the 'real world' as soon as possible.

A student's experience...

I took the path of most graduate applicants and applied for a five-year course as a back-up choice. I was rejected by the graduate schools but offered a place on the traditional course. After doing the arithmetic, I realized I just couldn't afford five years of being a student on top of my existing student loans. It was a very sad day that I declined my offer to start medical school. If I'd thought harder at the beginning, I would have used that space for a fourth graduate course. Who knows what might have happened then?

Making a decision

Should you apply for graduate entry courses? If you are a graduate, the answer is 'probably'. The financial and time advantages, particularly having already worked through one degree, should not be underestimated. However, graduate courses can be very competitive. For this reason, many applicants include one standard course as a 'back-up'. This is a legitimate strategy but only worth considering if you can afford to pursue a five-year course. As well as an extra year of tuition and living expenses (p. 15), you will be entitled to less financial support from the Department of Health and the Student Loans Company (p. 16).

If you apply to accelerated courses, you should bear in mind the applicant/place ratio. You should also remember that other applicants, your competitors, have had more time to build strong applications too. Course selectors will expect to see a good range of work experience and extracurricular achievements. Your competitors at interview will be more confident and mature, and have a greater range of life experience to rely upon. For these reasons, you should pay even more attention to the contents of this book than school leavers.

Key points The Department of Health pays a bursary to medical students (p. 17). This covers tuition fees and, for many students, mileage, car parking, and a modest subsistence grant. Graduates on full-length courses are only entitled to this help in their final year. However, students on graduate entry courses benefit from support for the last three years. This considerably alleviates the financial burden of studying medicine as a graduate.

The academic requirements

In general, staff on graduate entry courses are more interested in your degree than your previous qualifications. GCSEs and A-levels pale in significance.

However, graduate courses have widely varying course entry requirements compared with undergraduate courses. They fall into three broad camps:

- **Strict courses** These have very clear criteria regarding the subjects they will accept and those they will not. In most cases they require a strong bioscience background. This is true of Barts (p. 239), Birmingham (p. 234), Bristol (p. 235), Imperial (p. 240), Liverpool (p. 238), and Oxford (p. 245). Others, such as Leicester (p. 237), require previous full-time paid healthcare experience.
- **Intermediate courses** These have broadly prescriptive admissions policies (e.g. Warwick, p. 248). If your degree is not explicitly listed, write and check before applying to these courses. The last thing you want is to waste a place on a course for which you are ineligible.
- **Open courses** These will consider any recognized degree. They include Cambridge (p. 236), King's (p. 241), Newcastle (p. 243), Nottingham (p. 244), Southampton (p. 246), St George's (p. 242), and Swansea (p. 252). One justification is that graduates will have developed transferable skills to help them meet the challenges of an accelerated course. In many cases, but not all, these schools require candidates to sit an entrance exam (e.g. GAMSAT, p. 221) that tests basic bioscience aptitude or knowledge. Others may require experience of science at A-level.

A student's experience...

I was very careful to find out the admissions requirements of each school I was interested in attending. One replied to say I needed a first class degree to win an interview. Having been predicted a first, I was encouraged and promptly applied. I was not shortlisted. When I asked for feedback, it turned out I had misunderstood their email. They required a *first class degree*—simply being *predicted* a first was not sufficient. It was heartbreaking to have thrown away one of my four choices on a misunderstanding.

What about grades?

Almost all graduate entry courses require an upper second class (2:1) degree. A small number will consider 2:2 degrees but such candidates may be at a disadvantage. These courses often require an entrance test (e.g. GAMSAT, p. 221), which provides another opportunity for candidates to demonstrate their ability.

- Nottingham (p. 244) and St George's (p. 242) consider 2:2 degrees. Both use the GAMSAT.
- The only graduate course that strongly prefers a first class honours degree is Birmingham (p. 234).

Although a 2:1 is usually the minimum standard, it is sometimes an advantage to hold a first class degree. At the very least it will come in handy when building a career as a doctor. However, bear in mind that not all schools award 'points' for a first during the application process. If you scored highly in your undergraduate degree, think about which medical schools are likely to value your hard work. For example, Birmingham prefers to shortlist graduate candidates with first class degrees. Alternatively, if you hold a 2:1, it might be worth avoiding these medical schools as you will be at a relative disadvantage.

Do A-levels matter?

Medical schools vary in attitudes towards pre-university qualifications. In general they are less important, although some have requirements for biology and/or chemistry at AS- or A-level. In most cases this is true of courses that do not require a bioscience subject studied at university. Graduate entry courses typically requiring chemistry at A- or AS-level include Barts (p. 239), Cambridge (p. 236), Liverpool (p. 238), Oxford (p. 245), and Southampton (p. 246). Some medical schools will accept a substantial component as part of your undergraduate degree if not offered at A-level, e.g. BSc(Hons) in biochemistry without A-level chemistry. Others have a biology requirement, e.g. Barts (p. 239) requires this to AS-level and Liverpool (p. 238) to A-level. A small number of graduate courses have science requirements without explicitly requiring specific subjects, e.g. Bristol (p. 235) requires two 'laboratory based sciences' offered at A-level. Check specific entry requirements *carefully* to avoid wasting a valuable UCAS application.

What about postgraduate qualifications?

As with degree class, admissions policies vary. Some medical schools award points for an MSc/MPhil or PhD. Others do not. Some schools (e.g. King's, p. 241) will overlook a 2:2 degree for candidates holding a postgraduate qualification. As a rule, PhDs carry more weight than Master's degrees. If you are an 'unusual' candidate in this respect, shop around to make your qualifications count. Do not be disheartened if your chosen schools do not explicitly reward your qualifications during the selection process. They may still be useful. You may well find yourself talking about your PhD thesis when asked about a 'challenging time' in interviews. In any event, your qualifications will carry plenty of weight throughout the rest of your career.

GAMSAT

Graduate courses use a number of different admission tests. Most of these are the same as those used for selection to undergraduate courses (p. 69). However, one exception is the Graduate Australian Medical Admission test (GAMSAT), which is used by a handful of courses. The following should be noted:

- A knowledge exam Unlike the UKCAT (p. 78), the GAMSAT requires academic knowledge. This includes biology and chemistry (to first year undergraduate level) and physics (AS-level).
- Three parts The exam is divided into three sections: reasoning in humanities and social sciences (75 questions in 100 minutes), written communication (2 questions in 60 minutes), and reasoning in biological and physical sciences (110 questions in 170 minutes).
- A marathon test The GAMSAT takes five and a half hours to complete with a one-hour break part way through.
- Preparation As with other admission tests, preparation is key. Sample questions and a practice GAMSAT exam are available online and from good academic bookstores.

Key points The GAMSAT is only used by a handful of graduate courses: Nottingham (p. 244), St George's (p. 242), and Swansea (p. 252). Non-direct school leavers (including graduate entrants) applying to the traditional five-year courses at Plymouth (p. 154) and Exeter (p. 122) may also have to sit the GAMSAT.

Making the most of your time

If you have spent any time in the job market, you will be familiar with the idea that a degree is not enough. Your degree (p. 220) has earned you the right to apply to a graduate entry course. That's the good news. The bad news is that, by definition, everyone else you are up against must have a degree as well. As one commentator has written: 'a degree is no longer a meal ticket to your future: it is only a licence to hunt'. Extracurricular activities mark candidates who are well-rounded, interesting, and able to balance multiple commitments (p. 41). They also give course selectors a good insight into your personality. You do not want to fall into the trap at interview of answering every question with 'During my degree...'.

One of the great advantages of being within a university environment is that your opportunities are infinite. You are only really limited by your own motivation. There are many sources of inspiration within or associated with your university:

- **Student representation groups** These usually take the form of committees within your department. They are forums for communicating student ideas to faculty members. Consider them an opportunity to improve your course and a means of interacting with academic staff. Great for winning that perfect UCAS reference (p. 190).
- **Student media** Most universities run a student newspaper, magazine, radio station, and/or television service. Learning to write well is useful for medicine—as well as anything else you choose to do. Write about topics relevant to healthcare and kill two birds with one stone.
- **Uniformed organizations** The Armed Forces have specific reserve units for students. Although students cannot be sent to war, they can be offered trips abroad and training courses, often leading to civilian qualifications. There are also opportunities to gain leadership experience. Organizations include the Officers Training Corps (Army), University Air Squadrons (Royal Air Force), and University Royal Naval Units (Royal Navy). The Police also run a system of Special Constables which could provide a unique set of experiences.
- **Volunteering groups** Most universities run a volunteering organization of some description. If not, there will be plenty of opportunities within the local community. Opportunities could include subject tutoring, helping with day trips for disabled people, or working as a refugee caseworker. They are only really limited by the time you can commit.
- **Student societies and sports clubs** Students' Unions often have hundreds of clubs and societies spanning every possible activity from knitting to paragliding. These are a great opportunity to relax and expand your range of extracurricular activities (p. 41).
- **Part-time work** Paid employment is often the best way to gain real responsibility. There are lots of 'student jobs' (e.g. bar work) but don't feel confined to these. Consider registering with a local employment agency just to keep abreast of work in the local area. Try to develop transferable skills you can talk about later on at interview. Think about communication, teamwork, and leadership. You may need to demonstrate one or all of these at some point during the selection process.
- **Additional study** Most universities run short evening/weekend courses for adult learners. You could study something outside of your core subject (e.g. archaeology) or pick up a language over the duration of your degree. Look up local colleges if your institution can't help.

- **Research** Approach your lecturers if you are interested in research. This can also serve as useful work experience. Do not be afraid to approach academics in other departments; fortune favours the brave.
- **Travel** Try to make the most of your holidays. If finances allow, or you can save enough throughout the year, there are incredible experiences to be had. Think carefully about where to go and what to do. Travel can be a great way to broaden your mind whilst having fun along the way. With tickets to/from European cities starting at £1, even cash-strapped students can find themselves exploring Prague or Vienna at the weekend. See p. 34 for more ideas in a similar vein.

A student's experience...

In two years of being in the Officers Training Corps, I launched helicopter raids on Jersey, sailed around the Canary Islands, dived in the Red Sea, and undertook Arctic survival training with Commandos in Norway. I also commanded a platoon of twenty cadets under what were sometimes very difficult conditions. But these were easy compared to the massive task of articulating so many experiences within the confines of a UCAS form.

Branching out

You might be a student but you are also part of a wider local community. There is no reason why you should not stand for election as a parish, district, or even county councillor. Likewise you could be eligible to serve as a school governor or local magistrate. Don't feel you always have to tread ground that is already well trodden by other students. If you want to stand out, branch out.

A student's experience...

Having developed an interest in my local community, I explored the possibility of becoming a magistrate. I spent a few days in the visitors' gallery at my local magistrates' court before applying. I now volunteer one day every week deciding cases alongside two other magistrates. We are advised by a legally qualified clerk but I am learning all the time. I believe (and hope) our decisions have a positive impact on the lives of victims of crime and, in many cases, on the perpetrators as well. It has certainly provided insight into what the world is like outside the university campus!

Work experience

Just like applicants to traditional courses, you will almost certainly need to undertake some work experience. Don't skip the main work experience chapter in this book (p. 49). In fact, graduate applicants should demonstrate more experience. This is for three reasons:

- **Admissions tutors expect more** You have had more time to gain work experience than students who are 16 and still at school. You also have a greater need to demonstrate a commitment to medicine—you are changing careers after all.
- **There is more competition** As emphasized ad nauseum in this chapter, winning a graduate place is particularly difficult. Your application really needs to shine to succeed.
- **The competition has more experience** On the whole, graduates tend to have very rounded application forms. They have had time to find experience and may have been collecting opportunities for years. Graduates also come from a huge range of backgrounds—some of which are naturally well-suited to the medical school selection process. It's hard to gain a better insight into healthcare than someone who worked as a nurse for 20 years, but that shouldn't stop you trying.

The good news

Fortunately there is some good news. It is, usually, much easier for graduates to arrange work experience. On the whole, this is simplest when you are still at university. You will have long vacations and support in various forms from your institution.

- Most Students' Unions have volunteering societies. Get involved.
- If your institution has a medical school, don't be afraid of it. Look at the website for clinical staff who teach on the course. They might be worth contacting. Medical students in later years will also know senior doctors who might let you shadow them or at least ask questions.
- If you live away from home, spread your net of contacts wider. Write to GPs, hospitals, hospices, etc. in your home area and around the university. Ask academics in your department and medical students as and when you come across them. Campus GPs are unlikely to permit shadowing for confidentiality reasons.
- Long university vacations are ideal for exploiting meaningful work experience. A long summer could permit work as a healthcare assistant, phlebotomist, or hospital porter.
- Careers services in higher education are much larger and better organized than at school. Book an appointment and seek advice. There might also be bursaries available to cover work experience costs.
- Watch out for St John Ambulance LINKS (voluntary groups of university students). These are student units based at most universities that offer an opportunity to learn new skills and provide first aid at major public events.

More good news

Even if you have graduated and entered the 'real world', you still have trump cards left to play.

- **Use your degree** Your degree does carry weight in the job market. Graduates could find temporary work as a doctor's secretary or research assistant. A good science education could help in securing biomedical research experience (p. 64). Many GPs need graduates familiar with scientific/biomedical vocabulary to summarize patient notes.
- **You are older** This can work in your favour. Many jobs good for work experience (e.g. phlebotomy) have a minimum age. Graduate applicants should be eligible for some roles that are inaccessible for school leavers.
- **Transport** If you are able to beg, borrow, or steal (p. 261) a car, look for opportunities further afield.

A student's experience...

I studied biomedical science and one of my favourite lecturers was a medically qualified epidemiologist. I asked his advice after a seminar and he offered to call friends of his from medical school who worked locally. This resulted in four very different hospital placements over two years. A great start to my application!

A warning

As a graduate, you may feel as if you are in a very strong position to apply to medical school. You might be bright, confident, and successful in an established career. You might have a first class degree, a PhD, and a string of research publications. Or you might have worked with patients in the NHS for years.

Whatever your position, you can *never* have enough work experience. A senior physiotherapist applying to medical school might learn more about the doctor's role (and perspective) by shadowing (p. 50). A new graduate or PhD student should aim to gain insight into the NHS as well as patient contact. Whatever your experiences as a graduate, there is *always* something you can do to improve your chances. Do not fall into complacency.

Key points Don't ever become demoralized or complacent about your application. There will always be candidates with better and worse applications than yours. The important thing is to keep working hard and learning about medicine through work experience. Persistence and diligence pay dividends eventually.

Choosing a graduate entry course

Graduate courses are similar to those designed for school leavers. The core knowledge and attitudes required to be a doctor will be covered wherever you study. In addition, most graduate courses channel graduates and school leavers into a single group for the clinical parts of the course. For example, you could receive one year of basic science teaching, then enter 'year three' alongside those who entered directly from school. However, like traditional courses, each institution has its own set of peculiarities. There are a huge range of factors, from location to course structure, which you need to consider (p. 85), including:

- **Eligibility** Graduate courses vary in their academic and work experience requirements. If this is not clear, ask. The last thing you want to do is throw away one of your four choices. See Table 11.1.
- **Year size** Graduate courses vary enormously by size. They range from Birmingham with 40 places to Warwick with 180. Some applicants prefer a small, intimate year group, others a larger, thriving cohort.
- **Composition** Some medical schools (e.g. Warwick and Swansea) only accept graduates. This creates a different environment from schools in which school leavers predominate.
- **Organization** Many graduate courses are new and still evolving and this can impact on how much you enjoy and gain from the next few years. Try to gain an overall impression from current students and staff at open days.
- **Competition** See Table 11.2; consider choosing at least one 'safe(r) bet'.

Table 11.1 Academic entry requirements for graduate entry courses

Course	Degree	Subject	AS-/A-level	Admission test
Barts	2:1	Science or health subject	Chemistry, biology	UKCAT
Birmingham	1st[1]	Life science subject	None	None
Bristol	2:1	Life science subject	None	None
Cambridge	2:1	Any	Chemistry	BMAT (optional)
Imperial College	2:1[2]	Bioscience subject	None	UKCAT
King's College	2:1[2]	Any	None	UKCAT
Leicester	2:1	Any	None	UKCAT
Liverpool	2:1	Biomedical or health subject	Chemistry, biology	None
Newcastle	2:1	Any	None	UKCAT
Nottingham	2:2	Any	None	GAMSAT
Oxford	2:1	Natural science subject	Chemistry	BMAT
Southampton	2:1	Any	Chemistry	UKCAT
St George's	2:2	Any	None	GAMSAT
Swansea	2:1[2]	Any	None	GAMSAT
Warwick	2:1	Any	None	UKCAT

[1] Although the entrance requirement is a 2:1, 'strong preference' is given to candidates with first class degrees.

[2] May accept a 2:2 together with a higher degree, e.g. MSc or PhD.

Table 11.2   Competitiveness of graduate medical schools in the UK, 2013

Medical school	Competition (applicants per offer)	Chance of interview (applicants per interview)	Success after interview (offers per interview)	Prestige (offers per place)	Competitiveness score
King's College	46.9	9.4	5.0	1.1	5
Imperial College	15.4	5.2	2.9	1.1	5
Oxford	12.7	4.3	2.9	1.1	5
Cambridge	9.2	3.5	2.6	1.3	5
Swansea	8.8	3.5	2.5	1.1	4
Barts	17.7	5.4	3.3	1.2	4
Nottingham	10.9	4.5	2.4	1.2	4
St George's	9.2	4.0	2.3	1.2	4
Newcastle	27.9	7.7	3.6	1.3	4
Birmingham	10.1	6.8	1.5	1.3	4
Leicester	8.3	5.1	1.6	1.3	3
Bristol	22.2	4.4	5.0	1.4	3
Warwick	8.9	5.2	1.7	1.4	3
Southampton	20.8	N/A	N/A	1.5	3
Liverpool	10.0	6.3	1.6	1.7	3

How to choose

The same basic rules apply as for choosing any course. Leave no website or prospectus page unread. Call if you have questions and visit on open days. Try to make contact with current students; even those on other courses will have a view on the university itself.

Make a list of all courses, then eliminate them one by one. First, strike out those for which you are not eligible to apply, then those you would not consider for geographical reasons. Continue in this way until you are left with only four.

Eligibility criteria

Table 11.1 summarizes the academic requirements of each graduate course in the UK; for the complete profiles see the next chapter (p. 228). Courses with narrow selection requirements typically advertise a list of acceptable degrees on their websites. These lists are rarely exhaustive and, if there is any doubt, you must confirm the acceptability of your degree before applying.

Selection requirements for graduate courses vary widely. As they are so competitive, you *must* shop around to find which institutions best match your application. For example, a candidate with a first class degree in biomedical science might rank Birmingham (p. 234) over King's (p. 241). This is because the pool of candidates with a 2:1 in any discipline will be larger than those with a first in a science or health subject. Similarly, an applicant with a 2:1 in history should not waste an application by applying to Birmingham.

Key points   Don't simply pick four courses on the basis of familiarity or reputation. You may need to be strategic to guarantee your ambition of graduating as a doctor.

Graduate entry medical schools

Understanding the profiles

England

Wales

Chapter 12

Graduate entry medical schools

Understanding the profiles

Many of the graduate entry medical schools have different facilities and buildings from the undergraduate courses and they all have different curriculums (at least for the first one or two years). The following pages give descriptions of every graduate entry medical course in the UK. They are designed to complement the longer profiles written for the undergraduate courses (p. 107). Two medical schools are entirely devoted to graduate applicants (Warwick on p. 248 and Swansea on p. 252) so these medical schools have full two-page profiles.

The writers To ensure the most accurate information the profiles were written in collaboration with medical student representatives from each graduate medical school (see p. ix).

Warning!

While every possible step has been taken to ensure the accuracy of this information (including multiple reviews by the admissions teams at each medical school) it is possible that there are mistakes. Furthermore medical schools are continually striving to improve their courses and methods of selecting the best students so the details may change from year to year. Before you make an important decision based on the information shown, check the medical school website or contact its admissions team.

Key to the profiles

To make it simple to compare medical schools, the profiles have been written in a consistent format, starting with a description of each medical school followed by a table (as shown on p. 231).

Graduate students join their colleagues on the undergraduate course for the clinical years at the majority of medical schools. This phase of the course is described in the profiles written for the undergraduate courses and the page reference for the relevant medical school is shown for each profile.

Entrance requirements

The entrance requirements for graduate entry courses are extremely complicated, with some taking into account GCSE, A-level, and degree results and full-time healthcare work post-qualification. Graduate schools are relatively new and many of these requirements are in a state of flux. Since there is no point in applying to a medical school when you do not meet the basic requirements, it is essential that you check the admissions website to be certain that you meet all the requirements before submitting your UCAS form.

Table 12.1 This sample profile explains the criteria we have collated for each school

Best aspects	Why studying there is better than sliced bread		
Worst aspects	Why studying there can make your blood boil		
Requirements	Degree, A-level, and GCSE requirements (please take into account the warning on p. 230)		
Type of course	Stone, Red brick, Plate glass, or Carbon fibre (p. 94)	**Year size**	Medical students per year group
Course length	Total length of course	**Admission test**	UKCAT, BMAT, or GAMSAT (p. 69 & p. 221)
Applicants	Number of applicants	**Student mix: %** **International**	Proportion of international students in a year group
Interviews	Number interviewed		
Offers	Number of offers given (p. 227)		
Competition	All medical courses are highly competitive; this subjective scale aims to highlight how they compare to other medical schools		
Work	All medical courses have packed timetables and intense workloads (expect at least 40 hours/week); this subjective scale highlights how much free time you might get compared to other medical schools		

England

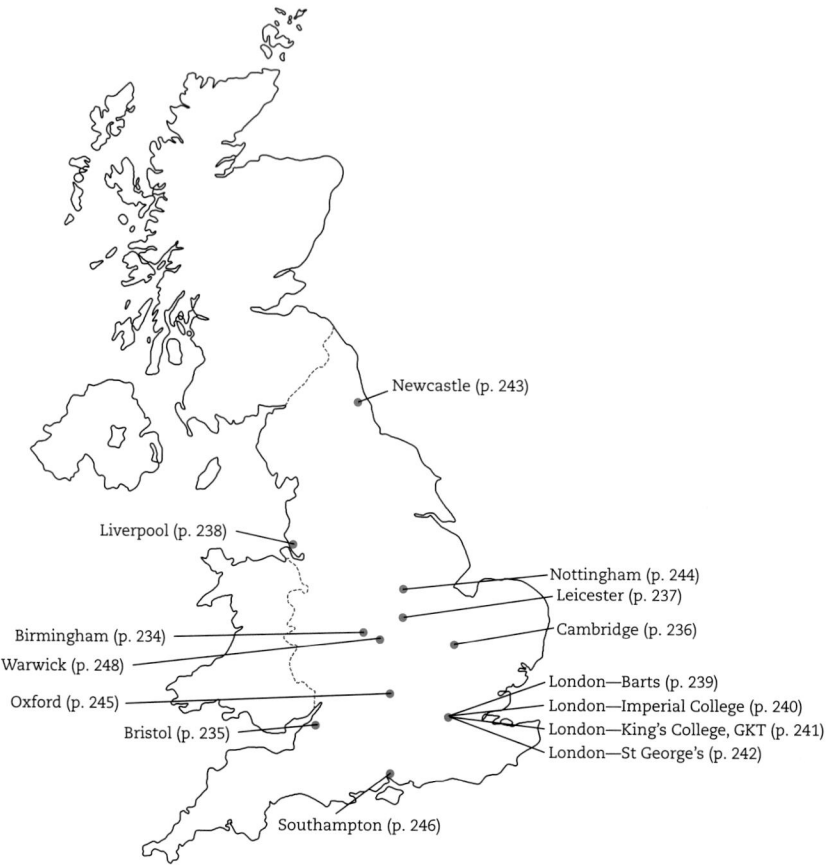

Figure 12.1   Graduate medical schools in England

Birmingham

The graduate entry course at Birmingham consists of one year of problem-based learning (PBL) and case studies followed by three clinically focused years integrated with the standard undergraduate course. You will work as part of a tutor-supervised group of about eight students in dedicated rooms. The cases are grouped into six four-week themed modules covering basic science, anatomy (including prosection), ethics, medicine in society, and behavioural science, with all these aspects integrated into each of the case studies. PBL teaching is supported by weekly anatomy sessions and tutorials with experts in the field being studied.

The first year also includes a weekly visit to a GP practice, which is always keenly anticipated and offers the opportunity to try out your clinical skills, observe clinics, and meet patients. There are also a limited number of lectures and tutorials, with the rest of the week free for self study and social activities. Two in-course assessments and feedback from the module facilitators help determine whether you are getting the right balance and are on track for the end-of-year exams. After each assessment the groups are changed, giving you the chance to work with different people. One of the best aspects of the Birmingham course is that, for the first year, each group has their own room to use at all hours as a base that is supplied with IT facilities, textbooks, anatomy models, and the all-important kettle! The small group work helps foster strong, supportive friendships that last the length of the course and beyond.

The pressure eases during the three remaining clinical years. The second year consists of clinical science lectures, pharmacology teaching, and special study modules in public health and epidemiology alongside case-based learning. The third and fourth years concentrate on exposure to the medical and surgical specialities. Integration with the standard undergraduate course during the clinical years provides an opportunity to widen your social group, whilst enjoying the challenge and excitement that the clinical setting has to offer. See p. 112 for details of the clinical course. See Table 12.2.

Table 12.2 Birmingham

Best aspects	Self-directed learning and the dedicated teaching rooms		
Worst aspects	Working with the same small group for so long leads to cabin fever at exam time		
Requirements	**Degree** preference for 1st class honours degree in life sciences. Degree should be completed prior to application; **A-level** BBB with good results in science, English, and maths		
Type of course	Red brick (p. 94)	Year size	40
Course length	4 years	Admission test	None
Applicants	535	Student mix:	
Interviews	79	% International	0% (EU only)
Offers	53		

Uncompetitive						Competitive

Working really hard						Not working/ chilling out

Bristol

Bristol's graduate entry course is a 'fast-track' programme, whereby the first two years of the standard undergraduate course are condensed and examined during your first year of study. In this context, 'condensed' means exemption from the 'Molecular and Cellular Basis of Medicine Unit' of the year one standard schedule and the student-selected component of the year two standard schedule. Graduate entry students (so-called 2 in 1s) also miss out on first-year anatomy teaching but undergo an intensive anatomy week later on to compensate. All other remaining units from years one and two are completed.

Although the needs of graduate entry students are taken into careful consideration in the design of timetables, attendance at all examined components of the year one and two schedules is impossible. It is therefore unsurprising that the challenging nature of this course requires graduate students to be proactive in prioritizing and balancing the two independently designed teaching schedules. This also inevitably demands a strong commitment to 'out-of-hours' studying.

Bristol's graduate students benefit from integration with first and second year students during their 'fast-track' year, since graduate students are taught alongside those on the standard course. After their first year, graduate students begin their clinical years along with the third year students from the five-year course.

With around 20 graduate entry students in each year, there is a fantastic sense of camaraderie. Although the first year is tough, students experience a lot of support from each other and from university staff who are always keen to accommodate the needs of students as best they can. See p. 116 for details of the clinical aspects of the course. See Table 12.3.

Table 12.3 Bristol

Best aspects	The combination of traditional systems-based teaching with early clinical contact		
Worst aspects	The frustration of not being able to attend every timetabled teaching session during the first year		
Requirements	**Degree** upper 2nd class honours degree in a human science (e.g. anatomy, physiology); **A-level** at least 'BBB', including two sciences		
Type of course	Red brick (p. 94)	**Year size**	19
Course length	4 years	**Admission test**	None
Applicants	600	**Student mix:**	
Interviews	135	**% International**	5%
Offers	27		
Uncompetitive			Competitive
Working really hard			Not working/ chilling out

Cambridge

The graduate entry course at Cambridge was established in 2001 and takes four years to complete (compared to the usual six years). You are offered a choice of three Cambridge colleges: Wolfson, Hughes Hall, or Lucy Cavendish (women only). The college provides accommodation and small group teaching (p. 210). All pre-clinical and clinical teaching is bolstered by small group supervisions, which provide a forum for detailed discussion and prevent students from falling behind unnoticed.

In their pre-clinical years, graduates are mixed with the standard course students and are taught in a mixture of lectures, practical sessions, and supervisions. In parallel graduate students receive 'level one' clinical training during the university holidays at West Suffolk Hospital (WSH) in Bury St Edmunds, 30 miles from Cambridge. The unique parallel structure provides an opportunity to immediately apply their pre-clinical knowledge to clinical scenarios at the WSH. At the start of Year 3, having completed two pre-clinical years and level one training, graduate students join the Year 5 standard course students for 'level two'. This entails specialty placements at Addenbrooke's Hospital (Cambridge) and regional hospitals throughout East Anglia. Final year 'level three training', is spent exclusively back at WSH where accommodation is provided free of charge (as it is during level one too).

The graduate programme offers the same style and high standard of teaching as the standard course (p. 118). The workload is extraordinarily tough in level one as you must keep up with the standard course students without the advantage of 26 weeks' holiday a year, but it eases as soon as level two begins and there is no longer a split focus. However, the advantage of being a graduate medic is that for the pre-clinical exams you only sit the multiple choice papers (not the essays), making the subject matter very 'crammable'. See Table 12.4.

Table 12.4 Cambridge

Best aspects	With only 22 students, the teaching and clinical exposure is very good throughout
Worst aspects	A very competitive, anxious atmosphere with fellow students very good at creating mass panic in the lead-up to exams.
Requirements	**Degree** upper 2nd class honours degree in any subject; **A-level** chemistry (in the previous seven years) plus A2/AS in at least two of physics, biology, and maths

Type of course	Stone (p. 94)	**Year size**	22
Course length	4 years	**Admission test**	BMAT (optional)
Applicants	258	**Student mix:**	
Interviews	73	**% International**	0%
Offers	28		

Uncompetitive Competitive

Working really hard Not working/ chilling out

Leicester

The graduate entry programme at Leicester was initially reserved for students with a degree in the health sciences, but entry has been extended to include graduates from any discipline who have worked in a full-time paid caring role. This means that graduate students get to train alongside graduates with a wealth of different skills, knowledge, and experiences. You can learn as much from your colleagues as from the curriculum. Leicester has a friendly learning environment, with approachable staff and a supportive 'student-parent' mentoring scheme.

Graduate students undertake an accelerated version of the pre-clinical phase of medical school, condensing two and a half years of teaching into one and a half years. This is achieved by taking more units per semester and omitting the numerous student-selected components of the undergraduate course. The workload is very intense and both evening and weekend study is essential to keep up. With good time management there is, however, still time for social activities and paid employment, although less so than for the standard course students.

The units are taught by several methods: lectures take place with the undergraduates, whilst seminars, group work, and anatomy (with cadaver dissection) are solely with other graduates, usually in a group of eight. Early patient contact begins in the second semester. The course features regular formative assessments (where the grade is for your own feedback only) and formal assessments specifically for the graduate students after each semester.

Graduate students join the undergraduate course for phase two, which is described on p. 132. See Table 12.5.

Table 12.5   Leicester

Best aspects	The diversity of graduates who are from a variety of non-science backgrounds but all of whom share a caring personality		
Worst aspects	'9 to 5' days with fewer holidays than the undergraduate course		
Requirements	**Degree** upper 2nd class honours degree in any discipline; at least 12 months' full-time postgraduate paid employment in a caring role		
Type of course	Plate glass (p. 94)	**Year size**	60
Course length	4 years	**Admission test**	UKCAT
Applicants	570	**Student mix:**	
Interviews	130	**% International**	0%
Offers	80		
Uncompetitive	🏆 🏆 🏆 **🏆** 🏆		**Competitive**
Working really hard			**Not working/ chilling out**

Liverpool

The Liverpool graduate entry course is as clinical as you can get: there is no pre-clinical year. Instead, students go straight into clinical teaching. While this might sound daunting, bear in mind that Liverpool insists on its graduate students holding a degree in biological, biomedical, or health sciences. You also needn't worry about being ill-prepared for the immediate clinical exposure—there is an intense course in essential clinical and communication skills before you are thrown in at the deep end!

The clinical teaching includes extensive problem-based learning, which forms the core of the curriculum. This allows students familiar with self-directed learning to rapidly augment their prior knowledge with just the information that they need. All of the resources of the undergraduate course are at the disposal of graduate students, including prosections from the human anatomy resource centre (HARC). During year one of the graduate course there is regular contact with second year students from the undergraduate course.

Clinical experience in the first year is based at one of the two large local university teaching hospitals (Royal and Aintree); this is complemented by community-based experience in local GP practices and visiting patients in their own homes.

At the end of their first year, graduate students sit the same examinations as the second year students on the undergraduate course. After these exams students on the graduate course merge with studends on the undergraduate course to continue their clinical studies. The rest of the clinical course is described on p. 134. See Table 12.6.

Table 12.6 Liverpool

Best aspects	Self-directed learning allows you to concentrate only on the material new to you		
Worst aspects	PBL can always be a shock to those who have previously studied on lecture-based courses		
Requirements	**Degree** upper 2nd class honours degree in a biomedical or health sciences subject; **A-level** at least 'BBB', including chemistry and biology, and an additional 'B' at AS-level and GCSEs as outlined on www.liv.ac.uk/medicine		
Type of course	Carbon fibre (p. 94)	Year size	29
Course length	4 years	Admission test	None
Applicants	500	Student mix:	
Interviews	80	% International	0%
Offers	50		

Uncompetitive						Competitive

Working really hard						Not working/ chilling out

London—Barts and The London

Graduate entry students are separated from undergraduates for the first year. During this year teaching is system-focused, considering the healthy and diseased state through a combination of lectures and practical sessions. Informal and self-directed problem-based learning sessions encourage students to work in small groups to apply their theoretical knowledge to a clinical scenario. Each system is complemented by scheduled anatomy teaching, including dissection.

Barts also benefits from an inter-professional learning module, giving graduate students the opportunity to work closely with graduate nursing students of City University, reinforcing multi-disciplinary teamworking within the medical profession.

The most popular first year module is 'Medicine in Society'. This offers early clinical exposure in community and hospital settings including home visits. The small-sized cohort gives graduate entry students an advantage in developing their clinical skills. Most teaching takes place in the smaller lecture theatres of the recently renovated Whitechapel campus, which has a warm and friendly environment amongst students and staff alike.

Exams at the end of each module include a spotter (computer-based exam consisting of images, e.g. X-rays) and a written paper with 'short answer questions' (SAQs), 'extended matching questions' (EMQs), and 'single best answer' (SBA) questions. At the end of the year, there are four exams, one SAQ, one SBA/EMQ, one spotter, and one objective structured clinical examination (OSCE).

In their second year, graduate students join the third year of the undergraduate course and begin their clinical training at some of the best teaching hospitals in London. See p. 136 for more details of the clinical training. See Table 12.7.

Table 12.7 London—Barts and The London

Best aspects	Early clinical exposure to both patients and other medical professionals via the inter-professional learning module
Worst aspects	Summative course assessments approximately every six weeks
Requirements	**Degree** upper 2nd class honours degree in a science or health-related subject (only your first degree will be considered); **A-level** at least 'BB' in AS-level biology and chemistry if these subjects are not a significant component of your degree

Type of course	Carbon fibre (p. 94)	Year size	50
Course length	4 years	Admission test	UKCAT
Applicants	1212	Student mix:	
Interviews	181	% International	10%
Offers	~100		

Uncompetitive						Competitive

Working really hard						Not working/ chilling out

London—Imperial College

Imperial's graduate entry programme provides some of the best clinical attachments that London has to offer with many affiliated hospitals being of international prominence. If you can keep up Imperial's 'work hard, play hard' ethos, you'll see why doctors at all levels compete for training in North West Thames.

Standing between you and your MBBS are four demanding years. The first year covers the whole syllabus of the first two years of the standard course. It's a 9 to 5 schedule, with a couple of hours of homework thrown in, but this is the time that you'll form close friendships with the ~47 other graduates. Students are highly motivated, each enthusiastically contributing their own unique experiences and scientific background to their group. The learning environment is challenging but good teamworking makes things easier.

Teaching is split between lectures, tutorials, PBL sessions, and lab work. The first year is organized into themes. The 'Cellular and Molecular Science' module is still evolving and remains largely self-taught whilst the 'Regional Systems and Anatomy' (including cadaveric dissection) is very popular amongst students. A clinical attachment also runs alongside with tutorial groups lead by clinicians. Imperial's international research ensures teaching by leading researchers which provides great insight into cutting-edge medicine.

On completion of the first year, you will join the undergraduates as they undertake their third year. The transition to clinical study is fairly painless and is regarded as the reward for a tough, textbook-filled first year. Following their third year, graduates join the finalist undergraduates and stay with them until graduation. See p. 138 for details of the clinical aspects of the course. See Table 12.8.

Table 12.8 London—Imperial College

Best aspects	Strong group ethic; quick progression to clinical years; famous hospitals with top clinicians and access to world-leading research		
Worst aspects	Being a young course, Imperial is still modifying the delivery of the curriculum; some flexibility is often required from students		
Requirements	**Degree** upper 2nd class honours degree or PhD across a range of biological sciences and a 'good' UKCAT score (usually scoring 640–650 across all sections) (p. 71)		
Type of course	Stone (p. 94)	**Year size**	47
Course length	4 years	**Admission test**	UKCAT
Applicants	783	**Student mix:**	
Interviews	150	**% International**	20%
Offers	51		
Uncompetitive			Competitive
Working really hard			Not working/ chilling out

London—King's College

As one of the few courses in the UK that doesn't require a science background, the King's graduate course offers the chance for a medical qualification to those who don't know their sphincter ani externus from their olecranon when it comes to basic medical science.

While the regular course takes two years to cover the 'Introduction to Medical Science' curriculum, the graduate course whisks you through in the first 'transition' year. This is intense, often involving a mind-boggling seven hours of lectures per day. Lectures are organized into weekly scenarios which demonstrate the clinical relevance of the medical science that you're learning.

Anatomy is held in particularly high regard at King's. Teaching occurs throughout the transition year, and is delivered through dissection in one of the best anatomy facilities in the country.

The reward for surviving the epic first year is joining year three of the regular MBBS, and the remainder of the course is completed in a standard (non-accelerated!) fashion, with abundant opportunities for learning languages, conducting small research projects (in the form of student-selected components), or for study abroad (in the form of peripheral attachments) along the way.

The 'fifth' year (your fourth) kicks off with the elective period, which is an enjoyably long eight weeks (plus two weeks of summer holiday).

The graduate route is tough but certainly not impossible for total science novices, as demonstrated by an encouraging flow of arts and social sciences graduates through the course. See p. 140 for further details of the clinical course. See Table 12.9.

Table 12.9 London—King's College

Best aspects	Well established course; dissection; being taught at the internationally renowned hospitals of Guy's, King's, and St Thomas'; diverse patient mix; long elective period		
Worst aspects	Relatively tough, lecture-heavy first year; frequent exams		
Requirements	**Degree** upper 2nd class honours degree in arts or sciences, or lower 2nd class honours degree plus a master's degree with merit, or a PhD; A-/AS-levels no longer matter!		
Type of course	Red brick (p. 94)	**Year size**	28
Course length	4 years	**Admission test**	UKCAT
Applicants	1500	**Student mix:**	
Interviews	160	**% International**	5%
Offers	32		
Uncompetitive			Competitive
Working really hard			Not working/ chilling out

London—St George's

The graduate entry programme at St George's University of London (SGUL) is the first of its kind in the UK and is based on a scheme developed at Flinder's University in South Australia. The success of the SGUL model is reflected by its recent export to SGUL Nicosia in Cyprus.

The SGUL graduate course is founded upon problem-based learning (PBL), requiring self-motivation and a lot of small group work in the first two years. Instead of a systems-based course (e.g. Respiratory) the course is based on cases. There are lectures but learning is largely self-directed with students reading around subjects, and in between tutorials. Areas of focus are outlined in Learning Objective lists (known as LOBS) which are released on a weekly basis. The style of learning can be tough for students arriving from non-scientific disciplines, but experience has shown that they perform just as well. The teaching style is varied: a typical week includes two days of PBL, two days of lectures, and a day of clinical skills. Exams are frequent, meaning everyone stays on top of their work and no one falls behind.

After the first year, students in the graduate programme join those on the traditional five-year course at the beginning of their third year. This year alternates between six-week blocks of PBL and clinical placements. Students are sent to numerous hospitals including Tooting, Kingston, Croydon, St Helier, and Epsom. Subsequent years are made up entirely of clinical attachments. Final year students go even further afield and accommodation is usually provided for placements that cannot be feasibly commuted from St George's.

What really sets St George's apart is the friendly and supportive atmosphere. The course is geared towards making you a good FY1 doctor and former students often remark that they feel better prepared than their new colleagues. See p. 142 for more details of the clinical course. See Table 12.10.

Table 12.10 London—St George's

Best aspects	Friendly, modern course in a truly multi-disciplinary environment
Worst aspects	GAMSAT; over-reliance on students' own resourcefulness; the administration can feel disorganized
Requirements	**Degree** lower 2nd class honours degree in any subject, or a higher degree such as MSc, MA, MPhil, or PhD

Type of course	Plate glass (p. 94)	**Year size**	116
Course length	4 years	**Admission test**	GAMSAT
Applicants	1291	**Student mix:**	
Interviews	324	**% International**	0%
Offers	140		

Uncompetitive					Competitive

Working really hard					Not working/ chilling out

Newcastle

Newcastle welcomes a wide range of graduates and health professionals onto its accelerated course. Its students have come from backgrounds as diverse as computer science, forensics, palaeontology, and psychology. Graduate students cover two years of undergraduate medicine in a single year before joining the undergraduate course in its third year. The course attracts highly motivated students who are able to organize their time effectively.

A large component of the learning is self-directed and utilizes a hybrid of problem-based learning, whereby cases are tackled in small groups chaired by extremely knowledgeable tutors with medical backgrounds but learning outcomes are provided to focus your self-directed study. The university also provides lectures tailored towards the graduate students, with a faster pace of content. There is always plenty of interaction between the highly experienced lecturers and the smaller audience.

There are three exam periods in the first year, which assess knowledge, clinical reasoning, and practical skills. Students also formatively assess each other throughout the year, so there are always opportunities to identify one's strengths and weaknesses. A small amount of time is spent on hospital visits, meeting patients, and putting into practice some of the skills you have been learning about.

The small year makes for a tight-knit group; many students appreciate studying alongside highly motivated colleagues from different backgrounds. There is great support from personal tutors who guide students throughout the year, ensuring adequate progress and a healthy work–life balance.

After the first year, graduates join the third year of the undergraduate course to develop their clinical and knowledge skills further; see p. 148 for more details. See Table 12.11.

Table 12.11 Newcastle

Best aspects	Great support from all your tutors and colleagues
Worst aspects	The pure intensity of the course; you don't know what self-directed study is until you have a go at the accelerated programme!
Requirements	**Degree** upper 2nd class honours degree in any discipline or a practising healthcare professional with a post-registration qualification

Type of course	Carbon fibre (p. 94)	Year size	25
Course length	4 years	Admission test	UKCAT
Applicants	920	Student mix:	
Interviews	120	% International	0%
Offers	33		

Uncompetitive — Competitive

Working really hard — Not working/chilling out

Nottingham

The broad entry requirements ensure a massive variety of students both in terms of age and background, with biomedical science graduates alongside 30–40% from non-traditional including the odd musician and Army Officer!

The first 18 months take place at the Royal Derby Hospital site, distinct from the undergraduate course (p. 150). It utilizes problem-based learning with students arranged into groups of eight. Four and a half hours every week are dedicated to working on a case from initial presentation to diagnosis and definitive management. PBL sessions are supported by lectures, workshops, and clinical skills learning. There is a strong emphasis on clinical relevance; parrot-fashion rote learning is discouraged. Although some students find PBL doesn't match their learning style, there are enough lectures and workshops to ensure all personalities are catered for. There are also opportunities to work with graduate nurses on a shared family study to learn how to work in multi-disciplinary teams early on in the course.

Teaching is well adapted to the mature intake and is relaxed and friendly. Although the course becomes intense at times, learning feels like a collaborative effort between staff and students, with very approachable teaching staff.

After the first 18 months, graduate students join the undergraduate course halfway through their third year to complete a seven-week clinical practice course before entering the final two years together. All medical students then complete the intensive clinical training phase together at hospitals around the Trent region (Derby, Nottingham, Mansfield, and Lincoln). After completing the initial 18-month pre-clinical phase, some students move to Nottingham, as it is more convenient for teaching, campus facilities, and the nightlife. See p. 150 for more details of the clinical phase. See Table 12.12.

Table 12.12 Nottingham

Best aspects	Clinical placements from the start; learning in a friendly environment
Worst aspects	Formative assessments every six weeks; learning at a brisk pace!
Requirements	**Degree:** lower 2nd class honours degree in any subject, a minimum of 55 in section II of the GAMSAT, 55 in section I or III, and at least 50 in the remaining section in order to gain an interview, significant healthcare work experience

Type of course	Red brick (p. 94)	**Year size**	91
Course length	4 years	**Admission test**	GAMSAT
Applicants	1197	**Student mix:**	
Interviews	265	**% International**	2%
Offers	110		

Uncompetitive	🏆	🏆	🏆🏆🏆	🏆🏆	🏆🏆	Competitive

Working really hard						Not working/ chilling out

Oxford

The graduate course is for those who don't need spoon-feeding. With fewer than 30 in each cohort, the graduates are a close-knit group and soon develop a Blitz-spirit as they proceed through the course together. Year one is tough. There is no escaping this, as the syllabus is broad and the pace demanding. Essentially it means students need to work out for themselves what's important, then go and find the necessary material.

The syllabus is largely systems-based and teaching is organized accordingly. Seminars focus on 'extension' topics (further reading around each system), leaving most core knowledge to be gleaned from private study. Alongside seminars, most of which are voluntary, clinical 'problem' sessions are scattered throughout the year to cement independent science study in a clinical context. Colleges also provide tutorials for their own students, typically in groups of two or three, although the quality and number of tutorials varies widely. The course organizers are keen to respond to student needs which led to the recent addition of dedicated time in the anatomy dissection room.

Throughout the first year, one day each week is spent in primary or secondary care learning practical medicine. Early clinical exposure helps contextualize library work and reminds students why they applied to medical school in the first place. This is different to the traditional Oxford course (p. 152), in which students have more limited clinical exposure during the first three years.

After first year exams, students can relax slightly as they are integrated with the traditional course for laboratory sessions and medical and surgical attachments. Specific graduate-course seminars and tutorials continue throughout the second year until full integration with the traditional course in year three onwards. Graduates traditionally perform well in the final exams—practical evidence that the first couple of years are worth so much hard work! See p. 152 for more details of the clinical course. See Table 12.13.

Table 12.13 Oxford

Best aspects	Tutorials and lots of clinical contact		
Worst aspects	High expectations; teaching yourself medicine		
Requirements	**Degree** upper 2nd class honours degree in applied and experimental sciences; **A-level** two sciences, including chemistry; 'evidence of scholastic excellence in the broadest sense'		
Type of course	Stone (p. 94)	Year size	28
Course length	4 years	Admission test	BMAT
Applicants	380	Student mix:	
Interviews	88	% International	10%
Offers	28		

Uncompetitive ▢▢▢▢**▢** Competitive

Working really hard ••••••• Not working/ chilling out

Southampton

Students on the graduate course are treated as adults from the outset; there's a dedicated staff team and a strong emphasis on self-directed learning. The graduate programme is closely modelled on the undergraduate medicine course (p. 158). During the first two (largely pre-clinical) years, teaching is based around systems. Although lectures make an appearance, problem-based learning predominates and groups focus on weekly topics from the system under study. Case material helps identify key learning points for the group. During the week there is a combination of basic science lectures in Southampton, and clinical teaching at the Royal Hampshire County Hospital and in GP practices. In total, one and a half days a week are spent in clinical environments during the first two years.

In year three, the graduates join fourth years on the traditional course for clinical rotations through medicine, surgery, paediatrics, obstetrics and gynaecology, general practice, and psychiatry. The final year comprises attachments in specialities across Dorset, Hampshire, Wiltshire, Surrey, and the Channel Islands. Assessment is ongoing throughout the final year with mini-clinical examinations building up to a grand finale of three written papers and an objective structured clinical examination (OSCE). Finals are now in February and the following few months used to prepare for practice by taking part in a student assistantship, spending time in a speciality of your choosing, and an elective period. See p. 158 for more details of the parts of the course shared with the undergraduates. See Table 12.14.

Table 12.14 Southampton

Best aspects	No interviews; a dedicated graduate-entry medicine staff team for the first two years; good pastoral support; long summer holidays	
Worst aspects	Self-directed learning: opportunity for some, or nightmare for others	
Requirements	**Degree** upper 2nd class honours degree in any subject; **A-level** chemistry or AS-level chemistry *and* biology/human biology.; **GCSE** minimum grade C in maths, English, and double award science (or equivalent)	
Type of course	Plate glass (p. 94)	**Year size** 40
Course length	4 years	**Admission test** UKCAT
Applicants	1250	**Student mix:**
Interviews	No interviews	**% International** 7.5%
Offers	60	

Uncompetitive 🏆　🏆　🏆🏆　🏆🏆　🏆🏆🏆 Competitive

Working really hard ～～～～～ Not working/ chilling out

Warwick

Warwick is unusual in only accepting applications from graduates (of any subject); there are no school leavers. This means there is an adult atmosphere about the whole course, which is designed with the graduate learner firmly in mind.

University The medical school was purpose-built in 2000, including a lecture theatre, common room, clinic facilities, seminar rooms, and a computer suite. These facilities are available 24 hours a day; which is great for night owls, and everyone else at exam time! There is also a Bio Med Grid, which incorporates technology, leather couches, and a biomedical reference library, for those who prefer to spend as little time as possible in the physical library. Local hospitals are up to 15 miles away but most students work at the new £500 million University Hospital in Coventry. The hospital includes a Clinical Sciences Building for members of the university, including students, to gain respite from patient areas. Car parking is a problem but few are brave enough to rely on public transport in the clinical years.

Course All medical students study for four years. In the first year, students are taught basic science arranged by physiological system (e.g. locomotion, brain, and behaviour) using lectures, small group work, and clinical encounters. The second year begins with a period of largely case-based learning with students gradually spending more time in the clinical environment until they are spending all their time on core rotations, including general practice, orthopaedics, medicine, surgery, and psychiatry. Year three also combines case-based learning with clinical placements, including medicine and surgery but also more specialized fields, e.g. emergency medicine, paediatrics, and obstetrics/gynaecology. In the final year, students rotate through any clinical placements not yet completed as well as arranging an elective of their choice. The final exams happen in March and are followed by an 'assistantship' in which students are attached to a clinical team, given real responsibilities (under appropriate supervision), and can set about the task of learning to be FY1 doctor. This aims to smooth the (otherwise disorienting) leap from student to doctor.

Warwick Medical School has bought £1 million-worth of plastinated cadavers from controversial anatomist Gunther von Hagens, to assist in the teaching of anatomy. These real anatomical specimens are a unique opportunity to really 'get to grips' with the human anatomy.

Unlike most medical schools, Warwick insists on a 1:1 consultant/student ratio in the clinical years. This means plenty of opportunities to get involved and ask questions but does make it harder to slip away early on sunny afternoons!

Lifestyle Medical students join in with all the activities on central campus but also run their own clubs and societies, co-ordinated by Warwick Medical Society (MedSoc). These include medic rugby, football, cricket, hockey, and netball clubs, and a range of academic and arts societies exclusively for medical students. There are also volunteering opportunities both locally and further afield in Sri Lanka and Ghana. When the medics aren't studying, playing sports, or saving the world, there are plenty of MedSoc socials and formal balls. Recreational facilities on central campus include 60 acres of outdoor playing fields, a running track, tennis centre, aerobics studio, gym, squash courts, indoor climbing centre, and a 25m swimming pool. Most of these are available to medical students for a bargain price of £49 a year!

Factoid Warwick goes out of its way to help students undertake work experience, research, and travel. Past bursary recipients have kayaked through Tibet, surveyed different cuisines in Mexico, and studied body image on the beaches of California. See Table 12.15.

Table 12.15 Warwick

Myth	A new medical school full of old students producing 'nice' doctors who don't know very much
Reality	A contemporary school with state-of-the-art facilities and a modern approach to clinical education
Personality	Very diverse; new medical students range from 23-year-old graduates to those who finished their PhDs more than 30 years ago
Best aspects	One consultant per student in the clinical years; learning in an adult environment; exposure to patients from the second week
Worst aspects	9–5 teaching on most days; only two weeks' summer holiday after the first year
Requirements	**Degree** upper 2nd class honours degree in any subject

Course length	4 years	Structure	Campus
Type of course	Plate glass (p. 94)	Year size	178
Typical offer	2:1	Admission test	UKCAT
Applicants	2187	Student mix:	
Interviews	420	% International	7%
Offers	246		

Uncompetitive ▢▢▢▢▢ Competitive

Low living costs ▢▢▢▢▢ High living costs

Working really hard ▢▢▢▢▢ Not working/chilling out

Contact details	The Education and Development Team, University of Warwick, Coventry, CV4 7AL
Tel: +44 (0) 24 7657 4880, Web: www2.warwick.ac.uk/fac/med/study/ugr

An insider's view...

At Warwick there is a 1:1 ratio of students to consultant doctors in the clinical years. This means students often receive one-on-one teaching and are assigned a different specialist to oversee their progress throughout each clinical rotation. Each consultant has a team of junior doctors so there are always plenty of clinical teachers available. This model is ideal for graduate students, who develop strong professional relationships with their senior colleagues and make the most of time on the wards.

Dr Jane Kidd, Director of Undergraduate Medical Education

Wales

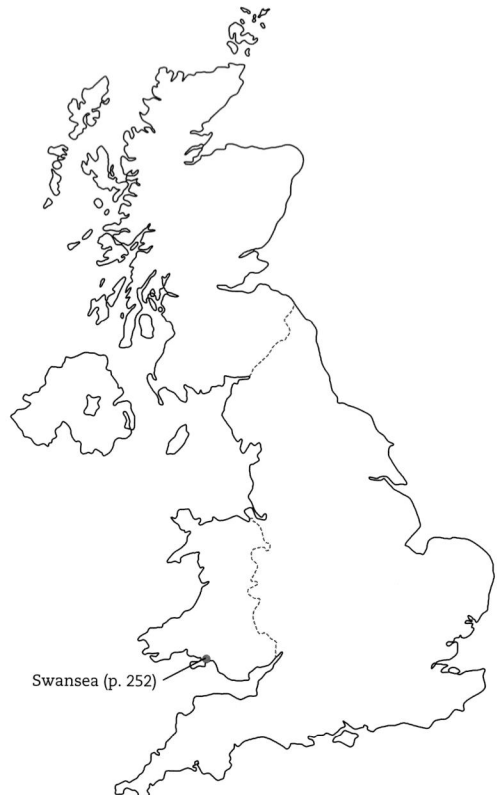

Swansea (p. 252)

Figure 12.2 Graduate medical schools in Wales

Swansea

Swansea and Warwick (p. 248) are the only two graduate-only medical schools in the UK. The course at Swansea is relatively new (established 2004) and aims to reduce the acute shortage of doctors in Wales. It is specially designed to help graduates of any discipline achieve the core knowledge required for work as a doctor.

University The university is the third largest in Wales and has its foundations in the early 20th century. It became an independent degree-awarding institution in 2007 when it devolved from the University of Wales. All the facilities at Swansea are centred on the beach-front campus and so everything a student could ever want is never more than a short walk away.

Swansea's medical school is located on the main campus and contains everything needed to study effectively, including lecture theatres, an anatomy suite, clinical skills laboratories, and a medical student common room. Singleton Hospital, a 550-bed district general hospital, is right on the edge of campus and, as well as providing a very convenient place to see patients, it contains a clinical skills lab and a 24-hour library.

Course The first two years are predominantly university based but there is still significant clinical exposure. Teaching is organized around a case-based 'learning week' format. At the start of each week a clinician or scientist introduces a patient case and, throughout the week, clinical sciences (anatomy, physiology, pharmacology, etc.) are taught in a way that is clinically relevant and linked back to the case. On Fridays there is a clinical forum, run by the week leader, to consolidate the knowledge learned throughout the week.

During the first two years, students have three five-week clinical apprenticeships based in hospitals around Wales. Alongside this, students also participate in Swansea's unique and innovative Learning Opportunities in a Clinical Setting (LOCS) programme, in which students are able to choose half-day experiences from a huge range of different clinical settings. Popular examples include observing autopsies, psychiatry in HM Prison, cardiothoracic surgery, and shadowing a midwife.

The final two years are spent working in hospitals and GP practices throughout south and west Wales. Commuting to some placements is very difficult with limited public transport. Although not essential, a car is a major asset to students on this course. Assessment is structured along three educational 'domains' mapping directly to the GMC's *Tomorrow's Doctors* standards and outcomes. Assignments and exams require hard work, but there is the opportunity for one re-sit.

Students especially interested in research can find ways to make the most of the new state-of-the-art Institute of Life Sciences research facilities, based on campus.

Lifestyle Although halls of residence are available, most graduate medics live in affordable privately run accommodation close to the campus. The medical school is extremely outdoors- and sports-oriented. University facilities include the 50m Wales National Pool, a running track, tennis and squash courts, and a newly refurbished gymnasium. The Gower beaches are ideal for surfing, kite-boarding, and other water sports. Swansea medical students have a keen sense of social responsibility and run a number of national and international fundraising projects. The medical school itself has close links to the Gambia and China.

Factoid The Gower Peninsula was Britain's first Area of Outstanding Natural Beauty. With world-class waves and so many beaches to explore, you'll be forgiven for not going home in the summer. See Table 12.16.

Table 12.16 Swansea

Myth	Cardiff's poor younger brother
Reality	A modern perspective on the age-old tradition of teaching medicine; the result is competent, knowledgeable, and dedicated doctors
Personality	Make things happen
Best aspects	The enthusiasm of the clinical leaders; a feedback system which enables the views of students to make an impact on continually improving the course; the beaches
Worst aspects	Small cohort may breed cabin fever; little holiday due to intensity of course; prosection instead of full cadaveric dissection; lots of rain.
Requirements	**Degree** first or upper second class degree degree in any subject or lower second class degree with a higher degree (MSc or PhD); **GCSE** 'C' in maths and English or Welsh; classification as a 'home' (UK/EU) student

Course length	4 years	Structure	Campus
Type of course	Plate glass (p. 94)	Year size	70
Typical offer	2:1	Admission test	GAMSAT
Applicants	700	Student mix:	
Interviews	200	% International	0%
Offers	80		

Uncompetitive		Competitive
Low living costs		High living costs
Working really hard		Not working/ chilling out

Contact details	School of Medicine, Swansea University, Singleton Park, Swansea, SA2 8PP Tel: +44 (0) 1792 602 618, Web: www.swan.ac.uk/medicine

An insider's view...

In Swansea we welcome graduates with a first or upper second degree in any subject and at any one time we may have up to a third of the class qualified in non-science subjects—history, languages, philosophy, etc. This enriches both the staff and the student experience. Students with non-science degrees are not disadvantaged. Indeed, many of them are among our academic 'high flyers'. Part of our success is due to the individual attention that we can give students in a school that is 'small but perfectly formed' and many of our students take leadership roles across Wales and beyond, e.g. in Wilderness medicine, the Surgical Society, the Rural and Remote Health Track, and the Swansea–Gambia link.

Prof. Judy McKimm, Dean and Professor of Medical Education

Non-traditional applications

Chapter 13

Non-traditional applications

Non-traditional qualifications

It's a common complaint of admissions tutors that all medical school applications look the same. Most applicants are predicted straight 'A' grades, play sport for their school, and play a musical instrument to a high standard.

Of course, medical school applications do not always look this way; successful applicants may have a wide range of grades, qualifications, and social backgrounds. It is important to be aware of how such diversity will affect your chances and be handled by medical schools, so this chapter explores how applicants with different qualifications (p. 256), non-traditional backgrounds (p. 258), health problems, and criminal records (p. 260) should approach their applications.

Academic challenges

Neither medical students nor doctors have to be geniuses. But medical school is competitive and applications need evidence of high academic achievement and commitment to learning. Medical schools want to know that applicants are able to cope with the equivalent of three rigorous A-levels (p. 20) over two years.

Re-sitting A-level modules If you get a low mark on one of your A-level or AS-level modules you will probably have the option of re-sitting it for a small fee. So long as you do this within the standard two-year timeframe, medical schools will not be informed that you have re-sat the module. You need to balance the effects of an increased workload caused by re-sitting and the effects this might have on the modules that you are currently studying (and which you will not get a chance to re-sit as easily). In the sciences you are more likely to benefit from having learned the additional material you have covered since your exam, in order to achieve a higher score at the re-sit.

With this in mind you should avoid any mention of re-sitting modules in your personal statement (and perhaps ask your referee not to mention it in their reference). The only time it may need mentioning in the school reference is if you are being predicted less than their standard offer.

Re-sitting entire A-levels Unlike re-sitting modules, medical schools take an extremely dim view of re-sitting A-levels or taking longer than two years to complete them. Attitudes vary between different medical schools (see p. 285 for more details); some simply refuse to take applicants with re-sits while others will only consider them when there were extreme and well-documented mitigating circumstances (and typically straight 'A's on the re-sits).

Missing your offer This is dealt with on p. 282.

> **Key points** While re-taking A-level modules during the usual two years is well tolerated, re-sitting entire A-levels or taking longer than two years to complete them means your chances of getting into medical school are low. If you are in this situation you can either apply to the more lenient medical schools using the school reference (p. 190) to document the mitigating circumstances (which need to be extreme) or study another degree and apply as a graduate (p. 216).

Non-traditional qualifications Most British applicants to UK medical schools will base their applications around A-levels or Scottish Highers. One common alternative is the International Baccalaureate (IB). Medical schools often have a standard offer for IB students, just as they do for those sitting A-levels, and this can usually be found on the medical school website. Many schools also require chemistry (and sometimes biology) to be taken at a higher level.

Medical schools accept many other equivalent qualifications. Admissions teams are advised by their university international office as to what grade or score is required from such applicants. You must contact universities in advance of applying through UCAS to confirm this information and get their response in writing. Although your school, government, or exam board advise that a given score is equivalent to 'A*AA' at A-level, British universities might not share this view. Do not waste a UCAS space on an institution that does not recognize your qualifications.

Breaks from education There are many reasons why applicants might have taken time away from education. Although there is nothing wrong with taking time out, e.g. for employment or through illness, medical schools will often require evidence of recent academic success and an explanation of breaks in education.

- **Graduates** Graduates in employment will usually apply to graduate entry courses (p. 216). These courses expect applicants to have breaks from education, although evidence of recent study benefits applicants too.
- **Mature non-graduates** Although mature candidates bring additional life experience, they need to demonstrate that they are as academically capable as students fresh out of A-levels. Evidence of achievement in recent study is very important for these applicants.
- **Illness** If illness has meant time away from education, this must be documented carefully. Your circumstances should also be supported by strong references. Illness can mean additional insight into healthcare and be turned to your advantage (p. 196). But medical schools may want to establish whether health problems will prevent you from completing the course. Evidence of recent good health and recent study may allay such concerns.

There are many ways to provide evidence of recent academic success.

- **Local colleges** These institutions offer a range of courses, from NVQs to A-levels. They are a good place to start if you do not meet the necessary grade requirements. If you already have strong A-levels, consider taking another one (maybe chemistry) to re-establish former studying habits.
- **Short university courses** Most universities run short courses aimed at the public. These sometimes lead to qualifications (e.g. certificates and diplomas).
- **Distance learning** If you want to delay sitting in classes until after receiving a medical school offer, you might consider distance learning. The Open University (www.open.ac.uk) runs lots of courses in natural sciences and healthcare (among others), leading to certificates, diplomas, and degrees. As these are formally accredited, they serve as strong evidence of current academic ability. Constituent colleges of the University of London similarly run accredited and respectable distance learning programmes: www.londoninternational.ac.uk.
- **Access courses** These are aimed primarily at applicants without the right qualifications to get a medical school offer. They offer good evidence of recent study (p. 258) but do not guarantee you a place at medical school.

Non-traditional backgrounds

Medicine attracts a huge range of different people. There is a growing understanding that patients are best served by a diverse medical profession. This means diverse strengths, backgrounds, and experiences.

EU students Students from European Union (EU) countries outside of the UK can apply for UK medical school places on an equal footing with UK students. They need to demonstrate proficiency in English (the specifics of this vary between medical schools) and check that their qualifications are suitable (p. 107). Students from the EU can apply to UK medical schools through UCAS with the same form and deadline as UK students.

International students Medical schools may only permit a quota of international applicants each year. Most medical schools consider all international students equally, while some, including Cardiff and Manchester, give priority to applicants from countries unable to train enough doctors for their own population.

International students are charged higher fees than applicants within the EU. These fees increase during the clinical years. It is not unusual for tuition fees (excluding transport, accommodation, etc.) to be around £17,000/year, rising to £30,000/year during the clinical course.

As the number of international students is limited, these applications are often dealt with differently and they may be even more competitive than applications from UK/EU candidates.

Mature students The term 'mature students' refers to three different groups.

- **Graduates** See p. 216 for guidance on graduate applications.
- **Non-graduates with suitable qualifications/grades** If you fall into this group, see p. 257 before approaching your application.
- **Mature applicants without suitable qualifications** These applicants will either need to sit A-levels through a further education college or complete an access course.

Access courses These are courses run by institutions that do not have a medical school (e.g. further education colleges) and aim to help mature students applying for medicine to demonstrate recent academic study. The courses usually involve one year of full-time study. It is very important to do your research before embarking on an access course. Many medical schools do not recognize courses in place of formal qualifications and some only accept applications from students at specific institutions. In all cases, medical schools require an access course pass at a pre-determined level, usually 'distinction' or above 70%. Access courses may also have specific admission requirements, e.g. some only accept candidates from their local area. Table 13.1 introduces some of the major access courses available in the UK; some courses have already had students accepted to certain medical schools, while others have not been tested. It is best to check with medical schools before starting the course.

> **Key points** Medical schools rarely accept access courses as compensation for poor A-level or degree performance. This is not their purpose. Ask individual schools if there is doubt about whether you will be eligible after an access course.

Table 13.1 A selection of access courses available in the UK

Institution	Location	Partnerships
City and Islington College	London	Students have been accepted by at least five medical schools
College of West Anglia	King's Lynn, Norfolk	Former students accepted by 20 medical schools, including some graduate entry courses
Lambeth College	London	Explicitly accepted by St Andrews, Leicester, and St George's University of London
The Manchester College	Manchester, Lancashire	Explicitly accepted by Manchester and Leicester
Sussex Downs College	Lewes, East Sussex	All students guaranteed an interview at Brighton and Sussex Medical School; also recognized by Leeds, Leicester, Manchester, and St George's University of London.

Foundation courses These are usually run by a medical school or its partner institution. Like access courses, they require one year of full-time study and are aimed at applicants without the qualifications necessary for medical school; however, students are guaranteed a place at a specific medical school afterwards. Medical schools offering foundation years include Bristol (p. 116), Cardiff (p. 180), Dundee (p. 170), Durham (p. 120), Keele (p. 126), King's (p. 140), Leeds (p. 130) run through the University of Bradford, Liverpool (p. 134), Manchester (p. 146), Sheffield (p. 156), Southampton (p. 158), and St George's (p. 142).

> Key points Although the terms 'access courses' and 'foundation courses' are sometimes used interchangeably, only foundation courses guarantee you a place at medical school.

Transferring between courses It is not usually possible to transfer into medical school from a non-medicine university course. Transfers between medical schools are only permitted in exceptional circumstances. In general, transferring is not a viable route into medical school.

A student's experience...

I left school at 16 with average GCSEs and worked with my uncle as a bricklayer. When work dried up, I took a job in a nursing home. I must have mentioned to someone that I'd have liked to study medicine because one of the staff nurses gave me a college prospectus advertising access to medicine. I had no idea this was an option for someone with my skills and qualifications. The college provided huge amounts of support (including advice and mock interviews) and a year later I embarked on a new career at a London medical school.

Fitness to practise

There is no shortage of hurdles to jump over before winning a place at medical school. For some applicants the biggest of these is determining whether they are 'fit' to work as a doctor.

What is fitness to practise? Fitness to practise refers to the suitability of students and doctors to work within the medical profession. Each medical school has its own Fitness to Practise Committee whose job it is to ensure all students meet minimum professional standards. Committees are independent but act under guidance from the General Medical Council. They convene whenever concerns are raised about an applicant's fitness to practise. Common areas of concern include:

- Criminal activity Particularly those relating to fraud, offences against property (e.g. theft), violence, and sex offences.
- Drug or alcohol abuse Including driving under the influence of alcohol/drugs, supplying drugs, and drunkenness affecting daily life.
- Dishonesty Concerns may be raised about cheating in school exams, plagiarizing coursework or UCAS personal statement, or lying on the UCAS form.
- Health concerns Any student with long-term disability or chronic illness will need to declare this.

You must contact medical schools in advance of applying if any of these apply. Withholding information will be interpreted as further dishonesty and is likely to attract severe sanctions, e.g. expulsion. The fitness to practise procedure at a typical medical school is as follows:

- Applicant enquiry Applicants make a confidential enquiry to the admissions office stating their personal circumstances. Although a decision cannot be made at this stage, the admissions tutor may know from experience how certain problems are dealt with by the Fitness to Practise Committee. Details in writing may be required before an application is submitted.
- Application The UCAS application process proceeds independently.
- Fitness to practise process If your application has been successful, the Fitness to Practise Committee convenes to consider your particular case. You may be allowed to proceed, subject to certain conditions, or have your offer withdrawn if you are not considered fit to practise.

As fitness to practise is usually considered after the admissions process, declarations made beforehand should not influence whether you receive an offer. However, this may vary between institutions, so ask if uncertain.

Physical disabilities Disability is not a bar to studying medicine. Its definition (under the Disability Discrimination Act 1995) includes any substantial, adverse impairment lasting 12 months or longer. This includes mobility problems, hearing and visual impairments, epilepsy, and chronic disease (e.g. diabetes). Almost 13% of UK medical students have a disability falling under this definition.

Medical schools need to establish that candidates are likely to complete the course and be fit to practise medicine afterwards. This does not mean students can be turned away simply because they would be difficult to support. The Disability Discrimination Act 1995 requires employers (and academic institutions) to make 'reasonable adjustments' to accommodate disabilities. An applicant's fitness to practise should only be in doubt where there is a high risk that the applicant could not finish the course, or work as a doctor, despite reasonable adjustments.

Mental health problems As with physical impairments, mental health problems should be declared through UCAS. These issues are dealt with separately from your general suitability to study medicine. Although a history of mental health problems is not itself incompatible with medicine, it raises two key questions that the Fitness to Practise Committees will consider as part of their duty of care both to you, the potential student, and to the general public:

- **Risk to patients** Some uncontrolled mental illnesses could pose a risk to vulnerable patients.
- **Risk to mental health** Medicine is a physically and mentally demanding discipline—there is lots of pressure and a heavy exam load during and after medical school. This could aggravate some mental health problems.

Medical school policies on mental health vary. Decisions will depend on the condition, severity, response to treatment, insight, and interference with day-to-day professional life.

Learning impairments Although all medical students have achieved good grades, learning impairments such as dyslexia still feature for many. Fitness to Practise Committees must establish whether an applicant with dyslexia will be safe to practise as a doctor. In most cases, applicants performing highly in previous academic work have learned to compensate for their impairment. But medical schools may be interested in whether affected applicants have insight into problems they could potentially face in the future (e.g. safe prescribing).

> **Key points** Applicants must raise potential fitness to practise issues in advance (or at the time of) applying. Fitness to Practise Committees will not be sympathetic to applicants hiding health problems or criminal records.

Serious communicable diseases All medical students (and doctors) perform procedures that carry a risk of exposing the patient to blood (e.g. blood tests). For this reason, successful applicants are subject to blood tests for blood-borne viral infections (HIV, hepatitis B, and hepatitis C). If you are found to have one of these infections you may lose your place on the medical course or have the course modified so that you avoid risk-prone procedures. New medical students are also screened for other infections (e.g. tuberculosis) and immunity to rubella and chicken pox.

Criminal records New medical students must apply for an enhanced Criminal Records Bureau (CRB) disclosure. Regular CRB checks include all convictions, cautions, reprimands, and final warnings regardless of how long has passed since they were incurred. Enhanced disclosure includes checking with local police forces that can add any additional information, e.g. about ongoing investigations or cases not leading to conviction. Fitness to Practise Committees will consider the nature and time of offences before deciding whether fitness is impaired. They will also consider whether allowing a candidate with a criminal past to work as a doctor could pose a risk to patients or bring the profession into disrepute.

> **Key points** Minor traffic offences (e.g. speeding) do not have to be declared unless they resulted in a court summons or criminal proceedings.

How to succeed at interview

Chapter 14

How to succeed at interview

The medical school interview

The vast majority of medical schools choose to interview potential medical students and the interview is a common source of anxiety. This chapter takes you through how to prepare (p. 266), questions to expect (p. 268), and answering ethical questions (p. 270). It also has some useful background information on medicine (p. 276) and healthcare (p. 278).

Importance of the interview

Medical schools choose to interview for three reasons:

- **To select the best students** With as many as 20 applicants for each place, medical schools do not have an easy time choosing who to accept. Furthermore most applicants have at least 'AAB' predictions, work experience, and a range of extracurricular activities. The interview helps selectors make this difficult decision.
- **To select the best doctors** All medical graduates are guaranteed a job as a doctor. You are not just applying for a course, you are being considered for a whole career. Few jobs with such responsibility and a training budget of £250,000 have such short interviews.
- **To assess communication** Medicine is all about people so doctors need to communicate well. This is easier to assess at interview than on a form.

Who is the ideal candidate?

There is no such thing as a 'typical' medical student; medicine welcomes all genders, races, religions, and sexualities. Instead, interviewers are looking for evidence of your potential to become a good doctor. This can include everything from commitment to medicine to your attitudes, values, and personal qualities. However, medical school selectors cannot see into the future, so judgements are based solely on your UCAS application, admission test results, and behaviour within the interview room.

How does the interview usually work?

Interviews vary enormously between different medical schools. Often there are two interviewers and sometimes a small panel. The interviewers may be doctors and/or other people teaching at the medical school, such as scientists and social scientists. Some medical schools also invite senior medical students and lay representatives (i.e. people not involved with the medical school) to join selection panels.

If you are faced with a panel, don't panic. In most cases, one or two people will ask questions while the others watch and make notes. Don't be thrown by this: all applicants will have the same experience. Remember, the panel interview aims to gain a more balanced view of your suitability.

Interviewers usually score your performance against set criteria. These are the same for all applicants to ensure fairness and consistency. To get an idea of what the criteria are likely to be, you should read *Good Medical Practice* and *Tomorrow's Doctors* (p. 278). These lay out the qualities necessary for a successful doctor. The exact criteria used will, however, vary between medical schools. Interviewers may use a mark scheme that incorporates these qualities and helps provide consistency throughout the process. An example score sheet is included on p. 265.

In many cases, applicants are each given a score during the interview and ranked against each other, with the top interviewees receiving an offer. When ranking applicants, some schools include other factors such as UCAS form score and performance on admission tests. Others go solely on performance at interview. Some schools are open about these details and provide an admissions statement on their website. If they do not, it cannot hurt to call and ask.

Example interview mark scheme

- Clear reasons for wanting to study medicine (10 points).
- Understanding of what doctors do (20 points).
- Learned about teamworking during work experience (10 points).
- Displays appropriate attitudes: can describe suitable examples, e.g. of empathy and integrity (30 points).
- Confidence and clarity of answers: demonstrates appropriate communication skills (30 points).
- Overall impression of candidate suitability: including academic ability, intellectual curiosity, and common sense (20 points).

How to find out more

Once you are invited to interview, do lots of research to avoid surprises on the day.

- Read the interview letter very carefully. This should provide most of the information you need, including a time, date, and interview location.
- Check the medical school website (p. 107).
- Telephone or email the medical school admissions office (p. 107). Ask about the status of the interviewers (e.g. doctors, lay people) and the length and format of the interview. Consider asking for the interviewers' names too.
- If you do manage to get the names of your interviewers then do some internet research. Where do they work? What department are they based in? Do they have a special interest in teaching or research? All this information can help gain an idea of each interviewer's perspective.
- Use open days or personal contacts (including those made at open days) to ask about interview questions.
- Use medical school entrance forums (p. 338) to find out what other candidates were asked. Use this information with caution as questions and interviewers frequently change. However, it can give a good idea of the types of question you are likely to be asked.

Key points The key to succeeding at interview is preparation. This includes everything from undertaking extracurricular activities (p. 41) and work experience (p. 49) to practising potential questions the week before. Remember the five Ps: proper preparation prevents poor performance.

Preparing for the interview

Acing interviews requires long-term and short-term preparation. You have been preparing for this moment ever since you decided to apply. The harder you have worked to build a strong application, the easier it will be to sell yourself at interview. However, the next couple of pages are about short-term preparation. This means going into the interview with a good idea of what you are going to say and how you will conduct yourself.

Gaining medical knowledge There is an assumption that really interested candidates will know something about medicine. This doesn't mean you have to understand the pathophysiology of pseudopseudohypoparathyroidism (in fact most final year medical students won't), but you should know some basic details about common medical conditions (see p. 276 for examples). This can simply mean reading about conditions you hear about during A-levels and work experience or reading useful publications (e.g. *Student BMJ* and *New Scientist*, p. 337).

Keeping up to date If there has been a widely publicized medical news story in the last few weeks or months, you must know about it. This should not require much effort; for example, just looking at the BBC News website's 'Health' section every few days should do it. There are many other sources of useful information including websites, RSS feeds, podcasts, newspapers, and magazines. Make sure you pick a respected and reliable source rather than just the most readable. Candidates who are up-to-date on interesting or controversial medical news really stand out.

Content of a medical interview After greeting you, interviewers will often start with one or two predictable questions (p. 268), followed by discussion about your application form, and then ethics (p. 270) and/or science (p. 276) questions. Most schools employ stand-alone questioning techniques. This means questions will not always flow from one another and are unlikely to change regardless of how you answered earlier questions. Put any 'bad' answers behind you and move on.

Practising for interview Even the most confident applicant can be unnerved by an interview panel. For this reason, practice is the best way to avoid wasting your efforts so far. The ideal scenario for mock interviews is to have an older person with some knowledge about the course interview you; school teachers can be very useful here. If you know a doctor (or even a senior medical student) use them too. Your aim should be to try to recreate as much of the experience of a real interview as possible. That includes the introduction, types of questions, the duration, and formal closures. Your 'interviewer' will help put you on the spot, challenge your responses, and, hopefully, provide feedback afterwards.

Keep up to date with current medical issues

- Check the health pages on the BBC News website regularly.
- Most newspapers run a health supplement during the week; find one you like and follow a few topics.
- Don't forget to keep abreast of non-medical current affairs as well; there are health implications of almost every news story. *The Economist* provides a good weekly summary of the world's news in a single magazine.
- Most publications have RSS feeds or regularly updated podcasts available on iTunes to help you keep up to date with a certain newspaper or publication. You may need to subscribe to (and occasionally pay for) some RSS feeds or podcasts.
- Radio 4 runs informative medical programmes—use BBC iPlayer to find these.

Before the interview As soon as you are invited to interview, find out as much as you can about the process (p. 264). Make sure you have clothes suitable for interview in advance. Whatever you choose to wear, you should look smart to make the best possible impression. Remember, you are applying to join the medical *profession* and should look professional.

- Men should ideally wear a suit, but at least a shirt and tie. Shirts should be tucked in and ties kept an appropriate length.
- Women should wear a skirt/trouser suit or blouse with trousers/skirt. Clothes should not be too revealing.
- Both sexes should consider removing any piercings (besides simple ear piercings for women).

Interviewers are not assessing your appearance but they do have to gauge each candidate's personality in just 30 minutes. Medicine is a conservative profession and your interview is not the time to push boundaries.

The day of the interview Arriving in good time is vital. This gives you plenty of time to overcome unexpected obstacles *en route* and prevents you feeling rushed or flustered. Plan well ahead and have maps ready to locate the interview room when you reach the university. If possible, get someone to drive you as this will reduce stress associated with public transport and connecting journeys. Read any notes you have prepared to jog your memory of responses to predictable questions (and your BMAT essay, see p. 82) and flick through a newspaper for any important medical stories that the interviewers simply could not ignore. You should arrive for the interview at least 15 minutes before it is due to start, but avoid arriving three hours before and camping in reception.

The interview Interviewers' decisions are not finalized within the first 30 seconds, but first impressions really do matter. Follow the interviewers' lead; usually you will be introduced and offered the chance to greet and shake hands with each of the interviewers. Avoid vice-like or weak handshakes and try to appear confident. After a greeting you will probably be offered a seat, which is likely to be across a table from the interviewers. Sit in a comfortable position, but ideally upright or leaning slightly forward. Avoid slouching or leaning back (and definitely don't put your feet on the table!). Try to make eye contact with the person talking to you (without staring) and smile when appropriate.

If you have tics, or know you respond in a particular way when nervous, try to overcome the temptation. Interviewers expect a degree of nervousness but they will become impatient after 30 minutes of spinning a pen or tapping your leg. Keeping still makes you seem more confident.

Always make sure you answer the specific question asked and do not be afraid to take the time you need to consider a response. Applicants often grow anxious about sitting in silence but, contrary to popular belief, you do not have to fill every quiet moment with sound. Take a glass of water if it is offered. Not only will it prevent you drying out but also it can offer you a suitable pause to think a little longer about questions. Preparation is important but the panel do not want to hear you acting out a carefully rehearsed script. Ideas should be fresh in your mind.

Predictable questions

Whilst it is impossible to anticipate all the questions you will be asked at interview, there are some you should expect. This is because the interview panel are looking for specific knowledge or qualities (p. 192), some of which can only be elicited in a limited number of ways. Use the following examples as a guide but be prepared to answer questions on similar topics that are worded differently. Remember, every answer you give is an opportunity to highlight important values that might be on the mark scheme.

Tell us about yourself This question is supposed to 'break the ice' but can fluster any candidate. Very often the idea is simply to help you relax—the interviewers are not expecting a biographical account of your entire life up to the present day. Briefly describe the subjects you study, the school you attend, and what you do with your spare time. Include an interesting (but not outrageous) fact if possible. Try to keep your answer relatively brief. Don't be afraid to repeat information on your UCAS form—there is a good chance the interviewers have not read it thoroughly. There is no excuse for not answering this question well as it is an early opportunity to make a strong first impression.

Why do you want to be a doctor? Think very carefully about this question, as it *will* come up. There is no 'correct' answer and you should be honest when articulating your own motivations for studying medicine (p. 4 and p. 194). However, do not under any circumstances go to interview thinking the answer is 'obvious' and one you can articulate on the spot. Most applicants find it very difficult to articulate their reasons and those without a confident and fluent response to this question risk disaster at interview.

It is worth remembering that interviewers may not always accept your answer and move on. They may challenge your reasons. If your greatest desire is to help people, why not become a nurse? If you like science so much, surely a chemistry degree would be more appropriate? Think carefully about these questions beforehand. Use this book and your work experience (p. 49) to prepare appropriate responses.

How do you relax? This is another question that almost always appears in some form. It is asking how you unwind, but do not let your guard down. This is a serious question and the panel are not interested in how you like to lie-in at the weekends or take long bubble baths. Medicine can be a stressful career and interviewers want to see that you have durable coping mechanisms. Use this as an opportunity to demonstrate your extracurricular achievements (p. 41) and transferable skills (e.g. teamwork and time management skills). Like all interview questions, this one offers the opportunity to make a good impression, if you are well prepared.

An insider's view...

I began the interview like every other, by asking the candidate why he wanted to become a doctor. He replied—whilst ticking off three fingers—'money, status, power'. Quite taken aback, I asked him to explain his reasoning. He started to talk about when his grandma was ill and how he had a lot of contact with her GP. Thinking he might yet redeem himself, I encouraged him to continue. He had met her GP on a number of occasions and was particularly impressed by...his car.

Even the most predictable interview question can be answered badly!

What was the most challenging thing you faced during your work experience? Your answer will clearly depend on your personal experiences but this should not stop you brainstorming answers in advance. Related questions could ask about the most 'interesting' experience, whether anything concerned you, and whether there was anything you thought could have been dealt with differently. Ideally you should have noted important events in a reflective diary during (or shortly after) each placement (p. 58). This is an opportunity to talk about your work experience, show you learned something, and demonstrate that you can reflect on experiences.

'According to your personal statement...' Questions from your UCAS form (p. 186) may be asked for several reasons. It could raise a topic of particular interest to the interviewer or there might be a discrepancy with something you said at interview that they want to clarify. Alternatively, the interviewer may just be filling time. Regardless of the motive, try to anticipate these questions before you get to the interview. If you've written that you read every issue of *New Scientist*, be prepared to discuss articles that you have read recently. You should be able to talk around topics described in your personal statement without simply repeating what you've written.

Do you have any questions for us? Most interviews will end with the selectors asking if you have any questions for them. There are two ways to approach this. If you genuinely have a sensible question, then ask. Perhaps it is unclear from the website and prospectus how many students can pursue an intercalated degree (p. 87). If the course is split between pre-clinical and clinical phases, you might want to know how much clinical exposure there is in the first couple of years. Such questions can show you have thought hard about how the course is structured. However, be careful not to ask questions that are answered elsewhere: you will come across as wasting time and having not prepared adequately. For the same reason, do not make up questions just to appear interested. It is perfectly acceptable to say all your questions were answered by the prospectus/website/open day.

Once you have dealt with this final question, you are usually free to thank the interviewers and say goodbye before heading for the door.

An insider's view...

Perhaps the most important advice for the interview day is to be yourself. If you have thoroughly prepared, then your enthusiasm and suitability for medicine will come through.

Key points There is no excuse for answering predictable questions poorly. Every applicant who prepares properly should answer these questions well. However, many candidates become flustered as the obvious questions are often difficult to answer convincingly on the spot. Don't throw away a medical school offer because you didn't prepare.

Ethical principles

It is useful to think through some ethical dilemmas before arriving at your interview; a number of these are found on p. 272. While you are unlikely to guess what questions you will be asked, these pages will allow you to practise the thought process necessary to answer them. These two pages describe the principles that medical students and doctors are taught to apply to such issues.

The principles

Ethical thinking in medicine is governed by a number of fundamental principles. Think about each of these when answering ethical questions.

Autonomy This principle recognizes that individuals have a right to control their own lives. In medicine this means that, where possible, patients should be helped to make decisions about their *own* care. Instead of deciding on a course of treatment, doctors should try to discuss the pros and cons of each available option, allowing the patient to give informed consent (p. 273). This approach can increase patient satisfaction and ensure they comply with the agreed course of treatment.

Beneficence This really just means 'do good'. Of course, if ethical dilemmas could be resolved by simply doing 'good', there wouldn't be a need for these pages. Beneficence usually means doing what is in the interests of the patient. However, as you will see from the scenarios on p. 272, this can be difficult to determine when doctors and patients have different ideas about what is in the patient's 'best interests'.

Non-maleficence Similar to the principle of beneficence, non-maleficence simply means avoiding harm. In fact, 'first, do no harm' has been a principle of medicine since ancient times. For example, doctors should take care not to use treatments that inadvertently cause harm to patients, even if the aim is to cure disease.

Justice This principle means treating all patients fairly and equally, for example without prejudice in relation to factors such as ethnicity and religion. It can also refer to fair distribution of healthcare resources. For example, in the UK, it is generally accepted that patients in one area should have access to the same treatments as those living elsewhere.

Dignity All patients have the right to respect from healthcare professionals. For example, doctors should avoid judging individual patients and should be courteous at all times. The duty of confidentiality is closely related to protecting patients' dignity.

Integrity and honesty Integrity means acting according to a consistent set of values and principles and acting with a sense of 'honesty'. In most cases, doctors should be honest to protect the trust patients have in the medical profession. Honesty is also important to allow autonomy—without honest information, patients cannot make decisions about their illness and treatment.

> **Key points** Some people argue that each consultation should be seen as a meeting of two experts. The doctor is an expert on disease and the patient an expert on their experience of the illness and their own priorities when seeking treatment.

Practical use of ethical principles

These principles guide daily medical decisions. For example, most people accept that doctors should keep their patients' personal details confidential. You could just accept confidentiality, but it can also be justified according to the core principles described in **The principles**:

- Autonomy Patients have a right to choose who knows about their medical problems.
- Beneficence Failing to preserve confidentiality rarely results in a benefit, although there are exceptions to this, for example the patient with HIV who has not told their partner.
- Non-maleficence Sharing personal information can cause great harm to patients (e.g. embarrassment or discrimination).
- Justice All patients have an equal right to confidentiality.
- Dignity Disclosure of sensitive medical details could cause a loss of patient dignity.
- Integrity Doctors are expected to maintain patient confidentiality at all times even when talking to friends or publishing research.

Although ethical dilemmas posed in interviews are often about 'big issues' (p. 272), doctors have a duty to act ethically in their day-to-day work as well. Interviewers could well ask, 'Why should patient records be kept confidential?' or, 'Should doctors always tell patients what is wrong with them?' In all cases try to keep these core values in the back of your mind.

Conflicting values

It is also important to recognize that ethical principles often conflict with one another. Should patients be allowed to make decisions (autonomy) that will cause them harm (non-maleficence)? Should the NHS provide fertility treatment (autonomy and beneficence) if this means there is less money available for cancer treatments (justice)? It is when these principles conflict that an ethical 'dilemma' arises. Although you will be expected to have an opinion, you should recognize that there is rarely a single correct answer. Try to understand all sides of the argument and reach a balanced answer. The interviewers are trying to understand how you think, not expecting you to solve an age-old ethical problem in five minutes.

An insider's view...

Ethical questions are phenomenally helpful to interviewers. They help us assess candidates' intellectual agility, core values, and insight into medicine as a profession. However a candidate chooses to answer our question, we will always take the contrary viewpoint. This isn't because we are unfriendly or generally disagree—it is simply a way of expanding the discussion and encouraging the candidate to think about the issue from different perspectives.

A few ethical dilemmas

Although dilemmas rarely have clear, definite answers, a logical approach should always be employed when considering them. Consider each option available in terms of the core ethical principles (p. 270). Try to retain a degree of impartiality and consider both sides of the argument. If you have strong personal beliefs, carefully consider how you might present them in an interview situation. As there is no 'right' answer, you are unlikely to impress course selectors by dogmatically clinging to one point of view at the expense of others. Doctors often have to tread through difficult ethical territory and interviewers will want to assess your ability to develop a balanced understanding of complicated issues. This is not to say that you should not have (or even express) a view. Doctors have to make decisions as well so, after considering all sides, do not be afraid of suggesting your preferred solution.

Abortion

This debate typically occurs between 'pro-life' and 'pro-choice' groups. Pro-life groups claim that a foetus is a human being who should not be killed whereas pro-choice groups emphasize a woman's right to choose what happens to her body.

The debate is often said to hinge on when life begins. Is it at the moment of conception, when the nervous system forms, when the heart first beats, or at birth? There are also other issues at stake: whether terminations are justifiable when the child would be born with profound disabilities and where the line is drawn between 'abortion' and 'murder'.

In the UK, legal abortions occur up to the 24th week of pregnancy, or later if there is serious medical risk to the mother's health or gross foetal abnormality. Abortion requires the signed agreement of two doctors that there is a greater risk to the woman's physical or mental health (or to that of her current children) if the pregnancy is allowed to continue. However, this is true of all pregnancies (the risk of childbirth is higher than that of abortion) so the Abortion Act 1967 effectively allows any woman to have an abortion before the 24-week limit.

Stem cells

Before cells differentiate into skin, bone, liver, or another tissue type in the body, they are known as undifferentiated precursor cells. At this stage they have the potential to become some (or even all) of these 'differentiated' cell types. Embryos are a rich source of stem cells that, once recovered, can be used to grow tissues in laboratories to create accurate disease models, improve understanding, and, potentially, find cures for disease. Stem cells can also be transplanted into patients and have been tested in conditions such as Parkinson's disease; in theory whole new organs can be grown from them without the risk of transplant rejection. The cells are taken from surplus embryos created during *in vitro* fertilization treatments. Again, those who believe life starts at conception sometimes consider the process of obtaining stem cells to be 'murder'. In the future it might be possible to use stem cells induced from adult cells (induced pluripotent stem cells) or collect the sparse population of stem cells still present in adults.

A similar topic involves putting a human cell nucleus into an animal cell to form a chimera or hybrid for research. Some groups describe such techniques as 'playing God' and worry about fully grown human hybrids. In UK law hybrids are not allowed to grow beyond a small cluster of cells before they are destroyed.

Euthanasia

This describes deliberately ending a person's life for their 'benefit'. Some argue that this need arises when a person's quality of life has deteriorated to such an extent that dying 'with dignity' is a better option than continuing to live an unbearable life. This issue may arise in patients suffering severe pain or those who have lost all motor functions and so are unable to speak or move (e.g. advanced motor neurone disease).

Opponents often fall into two camps: those who believe in the sanctity of human life and the immorality of taking life in this way, and those who argue that euthanasia might be misused by relatives or devalue populations (e.g. the elderly) who feel pressured to relieve their burden on friends and family. Euthanasia currently amounts to murder in the UK, although assisted suicide is lawful in nearby countries such as the Netherlands and Switzerland (such as through the organization Dignitas, which has attracted much media interest). Supporters of euthanasia describe its illegality as a violation of personal freedoms and human rights. Opponents argue that, although everyone has a 'right to life', there is no 'right to death'.

Key points Note the important difference between euthanasia and assisted suicide. In the former, the patient's life is ended by another person. For example, some criminals in the USA are executed by lethal injection. Euthanasia can be voluntary or involuntary. Assisted suicide is different. In this case the patient ends their own life, but with help from a third party. For example, a doctor might prescribe drugs that the patient chooses to take themselves. Both euthanasia and assisted suicide are illegal under UK law as it currently stands.

Consent and capacity

In order to carry out a test, operate, or examine a patient, it is necessary to obtain consent. Touching a patient without consent may amount to battery. For consent to be valid, it must be informed (i.e. the patient must know the potential benefits and risks), given voluntarily, and given by a patient with *capacity* to consent. Capacity is the ability to understand, retain, and use information relevant to the decision. It may be lacking due to, for example, mental illness, brain damage, or intoxication.

When a patient lacks capacity, the medical team must make any decisions in their best interests. The team should take into account many factors, such as the patient's previously expressed wishes (when they had capacity), their personal beliefs, and the thoughts of their family. Ethical dilemmas often arise when the various contributors disagree but, ultimately, doctors (or a court) make the final decision.

The question of capacity is more complicated when dealing with children. This area of law is informed by an important case from 1985: *Gillick v West Norfolk Health Authority*. Mrs Gillick sought a declaration that GPs should not prescribe contraception to her daughters, who were aged under 16. She argued that this encouraged minors to have sex. However, the court found that children can have capacity to request contraception if they possess sufficient intelligence, comprehension, and maturity. A similar principle is applied to other dilemmas involving children.

Ethics in modern healthcare

You probably encountered ethical dilemmas during your work experience, perhaps without even realizing it. If you haven't yet finished your work experience, keep an eye out for ethical issues—they are pervasive. Some commonly encountered dilemmas are introduced below. Try to think about these, identify the issues raised, and develop a personal view where possible. Again, this is not a complete list so keep abreast of the news, read articles online, and discuss what you read with other people.

Access to resources

The National Health Service is a massive organization paid for by the taxpayer. It costs over £100 billion every year. Although taxation can be increased, most people appreciate that the NHS has a limited budget. One inevitable consequence of limited resources is that the NHS cannot pay for all treatments all the time.

- Luxury treatments Should the NHS pay for potentially 'non-health-related' issues such as *in vitro* fertilization (IVF) and gender reassignment? In a budget-limited system, some people believe funds should be allocated to patients with diseases instead. Others argue that psychological wellbeing is an NHS responsibility because it is an important part of health.
- Expensive drugs Should the NHS pay for very expensive drugs? One drug used for breast cancer (Herceptin) costs around £22,000 per patient every year. What about expensive drugs that only work occasionally or increase life expectancy by only a few weeks?
- The 'postcode lottery' One aspect of the NHS is that it is broken into individual NHS trusts. This is so that healthcare resources can be tailored to the needs of particular populations living within each area. However, one consequence of allowing local trusts a degree of independence is that resources may be available to people living in one area and not those living elsewhere. This is called the 'postcode lottery'. For example, some NHS trusts refuse to pay for Herceptin. Some allow three cycles of IVF on the NHS whereas others only permit one. This has important implications for principles of fairness and equal treatment (see 'Justice', p. 270).

Private healthcare

Although most patients are treated by the NHS, some pay for treatment through private hospitals. These often employ doctors who also work for the NHS. Those supporting private healthcare argue that patients should have choice about where they are treated. If patients want to pay extra, why should anyone stop them? They also argue that by seeing a private doctor, patients do not clog up NHS appointment times and waiting lists. It is also worth remembering that private patients essentially pay twice for healthcare since they still pay for the NHS through taxes.

However, others argue that NHS doctors should not support private healthcare. This is for two reasons. The first is fairness—why should people with money receive 'better' treatment and in less time than those in the NHS? The second argument claims that private healthcare undermines the NHS. Because NHS waiting lists are often long, it is claimed that doctors should be spending more time in the NHS rather than in private practice. However, doctors working privately could argue that work done in their free time is no-one else's business.

Nurse practitioners (NPs)

These are Registered Nurses who see new patients with undiagnosed conditions. They are responsible for ordering appropriate investigations, reaching a diagnosis, and treating patients. Some people believe this is a natural extension of the nursing role. It also allows individual nurses to take on more responsibility as they develop their careers. However, others fear NPs are encroaching on the perceived role of doctors. This is followed by concerns over whether NPs are adequately trained to diagnose and treat patients safely.

Screening

This is the process of looking at a great number of people to identify those with disease who do not yet have symptoms. The idea is that early diagnoses will improve health outcomes. One of the best known screening programmes in the UK is for breast cancer. Women between the ages of 50 and 70 are invited for a breast X-ray ('mammogram') every three years.

Although it sounds like a great idea, there are a number of downsides. Screening can lead to over-diagnosis, misdiagnosis, worry, and a false sense of security when screening suggests there is no disease. It is expensive and some screening tests also carry risks of their own. For example, mammography is used to screen for breast cancer but carries a risk of causing cancer by exposing women to radiation. These reasons explain why there are only screening programmes for a small number of diseases.

Medical students

As a medical student you will be expected to spend a lot of time with patients. In many cases, you will learn personal details about patients, examine them, and see them in a state of undress. Of course, doctors do these things, but only when necessary to help diagnosis and/or treat patients. Medical students do not contribute to patient care directly and so it is harder to justify why they should risk causing discomfort or embarrassment to patients.

However, on the other hand, medical students must see patients if they are to become competent, safe doctors. Do you think patients have a moral obligation to help with this process even if it causes them discomfort?

Key points Keep a diary of everything you see during your work experience that makes you think. These issues will almost always have an ethical dimension. Consider each aspect of the situation in the light of the ethical principles on p. 270. Wherever possible, follow up the case and find out what decisions were actually made. Try to understand the perspectives of everyone involved (e.g. doctor, patient, and relatives). Talk through everyday ethical dilemmas with the staff you are working with. This will help you understand the system of ethics that is (or should be) applied within the NHS.

Science in the medical interview

As a doctor, you will diagnose and treat patients with many diseases. Medical schools ideally want to select applicants with more than a passing interest in health and illness. Some diseases are of particular importance (or public interest) and it is a good idea to be prepared to discuss these at interview.

Diabetes

This is caused by a deficiency or failure of the hormone 'insulin', which normally instructs cells to absorb and convert sugar (glucose) into its stored form, glycogen. Diabetes is characterized by weight loss and excessive volumes of urine because glucose goes into the urine and causes large amounts of water to be retained in the urine by osmosis. There are two types of diabetes: type 1 in which insulin is not produced and type 2 in which it has a reduced effect. For this reason, insulin must be injected to treat type 1 but may not be needed to treat type 2. High levels of glucose in the blood can cause complications over time, including damage to the blood vessels (heart attack, stroke), eyes (retinopathy), and nerves (neuropathy, altered sensation or movement). Type 2 diabetes is more common with obesity and so, as the average waistline expands, it is becoming an increasingly common problem.

> **Key points** Some medical schools will expect a greater degree of scientific/healthcare knowledge than others. For example, Oxbridge interviews are likely to travel in this direction (p. 212). Ask each individual medical school, or people who have previously been interviewed there, whether there is a scientific element to the interview.

Myocardial infarction

This is more commonly known as a 'heart attack'. Cholesterol is deposited in the walls of arteries, producing a plaque that can impair the flow of blood to cells. Like all organs, the heart needs a blood supply and this comes from the coronary arteries that bring oxygen to the muscle (myo-) of the heart (cardio-). When these arteries become blocked the myocardium can die, potentially resulting in death of the patient.

A similar process also causes strokes. If a fatty plaque/clot in an artery in the neck breaks off, it can travel through the circulation and block an artery in the brain. This may cause infarction of brain tissue. Other strokes are caused by bleeding into the brain.

Cancer

Most cells in the body divide to replace themselves. Very few individual cells survive from birth to old age without becoming replaced. This process is tightly controlled by signals within and between cells, which ensure that they divide appropriately. However, like any process, it can go wrong. When cells begin dividing uncontrollably, they can start invading adjacent tissues and even spread to distant sites in the body (for example via the blood), and this is called cancer.

Cancer can affect any cell in the body at any age. However, a number of factors can make it more likely. For example, chemicals in tobacco smoke can lead to lung cancer, some inherited genes can increase the likelihood of developing bowel cancer, and ultraviolet light can cause genetic defects that lead to skin cancers.

Age is also an important factor. For a cell to become cancerous it must accumulate a number of genetic 'errors'. With increasing age there is more time for these errors to occur and this is why cancers are more common in the elderly. This is important as people now live to an older age and so many cancers are becoming more frequent.

HIV/AIDS

Human immunodeficiency virus (HIV) is spread horizontally (through sexual intercourse or blood-to-blood exchange) or vertically (from mother to child). The virus replicates in white blood cells, which are part of the normal immune system. The infection can have a long incubation phase in which the patient can infect others but lacks any symptoms.

When the white cells are depleted, the patient begins to contract unusual infections. This is known as acquired immunodeficiency syndrome (AIDS). Although anti-retroviral drugs are very effective at treating the disease, they are expensive and not always available in the developing world.

Pandemics

This describes an infectious disease that spreads across continents or even worldwide. Recent pandemic scares include severe acute respiratory syndrome (SARS), avian influenza, and swine flu.

Every disease has a certain level at which it is expected in a certain population. This is usually quite low, because the population possesses collective immunity, i.e. most people are immune and so the infection is unable to spread quickly. However, such immunity may not exist when a completely new infection is introduced. New infections have the potential to infect an entire population before individuals become immune.

Viruses are particularly adept at changing as a result of antigenic shift. Every year, changes in the surface proteins (antigens) of the influenza virus mean that a new 'flu' jab has to be designed. Occasionally an antigen on one virus is swapped (or recombined) with those from a completely different virus. The result is a dramatic shift in virus surface proteins and an entire population whose immune systems can no longer react quickly to the novel virus. If these infections are not identified and quarantined early, they can spread throughout the whole world.

Although the entire population is susceptible, the new infection does not have to be particularly severe. The mortality rate might even be similar to the virus from which the newly recombined one was derived but, because such a large population is affected, pandemics can result in many deaths.

Key points Your goal should not be to learn all about health and disease. There will be plenty of time for that later once you are at medical school. Instead, take opportunities to pay attention when anything is mentioned about health. This will show interviewers that you are interested in healthcare and understand issues from outside your A-level syllabus, and will stop you making naïve mistakes at interview.

Also, you never know when something learned now will win you valuable marks during an exam in a couple of years' time!

Useful things to look up

This is not an exhaustive list of things you must know before interview. However, knowing about important issues and institutions in medicine could demonstrate insight to the course selectors. Don't be caught out though. If you use one of the phrases below, an interviewer is likely to ask you what it means. Whether you consider this a risk or an opportunity depends on how well prepared you are.

General Medical Council (GMC) The GMC is the organization responsible for registering and regulating doctors within the UK. It also ensures that medical schools meet a minimum standard. Any doctor in the UK can be 'referred' to the GMC if their 'fitness to practise' is in doubt. This could be because of poor health or concerns about their ability and/or behaviour. The GMC is often criticized by the public for protecting doctors, and by doctors for being too harsh.

Good Medical Practice This is a document published by the GMC that sets out the values and standards expected of registered medical practitioners. It is very short and worth reading before your interview. Search the GMC website (www.gmc-uk.org) for *Good Medical Practice*.

Tomorrow's Doctors Another document from the GMC that describes the knowledge, skills, and attitudes that must be learned at medical school. This document and *Good Medical Practice* help inform mark schemes for UCAS forms and interviews; use the GMC website (www.gmc-uk.org) to find *Tomorrow's Doctors*.

British Medical Association (BMA) Unlike the GMC, which regulates doctors, the BMA represents them. It is the registered trade union for all doctors and medical students in the UK. The BMA provides a number of services but a key role is negotiating with the government over issues such as doctors' pay and working conditions. It also speaks for the medical profession, often providing opinions on important health issues.

Royal Colleges Most specialities within medicine are organized into specific professional bodies, known collectively as the Royal Colleges. These aim to improve the standards and training of each group of doctors. There are many Royal Colleges, including the Royal College of Surgeons and the Royal College of General Practitioners. These organizations also set postgraduate exams, which must be passed before a doctor can become a GP or specialist trainee (p. 8).

Evidence-based medicine (EBM) This is an important move in medicine towards applying science to clinical practice. It requires treatments to be supported by evidence, not simply by 'expert' opinion. This requires every treatment to be thoroughly evaluated by clinical trials before it is recommended for use by doctors.

National Institute for Health and Clinical Excellence (NICE) An organization set up to standardize the treatments available in different parts of the country. NICE publishes reports considering the evidence of each new treatment, then makes a recommendation based on its cost effectiveness. As a result, NICE decisions are often controversial as national priorities that consider cost do not always please doctors, patients, or the public. The NICE website is at www.nice.org.uk.

Modernising Medical Careers (MMC) The programme for postgraduate medical training was introduced in 2005. It changed the structure of how doctors are trained up to the level of consultant or GP. See p. 8 for the career structure following MMC. This programme was very unpopular with doctors, in part because the number of speciality training posts available only covered about half the number of applicants. You can read more about MMC at www.mmc.nhs.uk.

Multi-Disciplinary Team (MDT) Modern healthcare is a team effort and the team is growing! You will already be familiar with doctors and nurses. But there are also physiotherapists, speech and language therapists, clinical psychologists, physician assistants, and operating department practitioners, to name only a few. Even experienced doctors struggle with the number of different uniforms seen in a single hospital. During work experience, you may have attended an MDT meeting in which different healthcare professionals come together to discuss patients. A good understanding of how the MDT works can show that you have the right attitude to become a doctor.

Patient-centred care This is all about putting the patient first in healthcare. For example, patient welfare should be placed above other considerations when deciding upon a course of investigation or treatment. One aspect of patient-centred care is involving patients, wherever possible, in their own care.

Clinical governance A system by which NHS organizations are expected to foster an environment of clinical excellence to ensure patients receive the best possible standard of care. This includes teaching, research, audit, and handling complaints.

Professionalism Although difficult to define, this word is used frequently to describe how doctors should act. It can refer to many different things, often at the same time, including maintaining skills and knowledge, keeping an appropriate relationship with patients, teamworking, taking responsibility, and honesty.

Key points Health is important to people. This means there is a lot written about it—far more than you could ever hope to read in a lifetime. But the more you read, the more insight you will have into the NHS and the medical profession.

An insider's view...

Candidates with genuine insight into the NHS really stand out. Most candidates will know something about medicine and/or the NHS. This might be because of family connections or because they keep abreast of the news. Just occasionally, you come across a candidate who has a fundamental grasp of what it is like to be a doctor and to work within a state-funded healthcare system. There is no 'one thing' these candidates say to identify themselves—the panel can just sense that they really understand.

If things don't work out

Chapter 15

If things don't work out

If you don't win an offer

The number of applicants to British medical schools far exceeds the number of places. This means that many applicants (even those with a string of A/A* grades and work experience) will not be successful on their first attempt. The next couple of pages take you through how to react if you are faced with four rejections through UCAS. If you did receive an offer but didn't achieve your grades, jump ahead to p. 284.

Everyone responds differently to a final UCAS rejection. Anything from numbness to earth-shattering disappointment is completely normal. Some applicants view this as a personal rejection; however, many who would have made great doctors are rejected every year—there are simply not enough places to train everyone.

- **Take a break** For many applicants this is their first ever taste of failure. It is normal to feel disappointed, lost, and even angry. Don't do anything rash; take a few days to come to terms with the situation. Consider catching up with any friends or hobbies that were neglected during the application process.
- **Speak to other people** Most unsuccessful applicants find it helps to talk about their experience. Friends, family, and teachers are often good sources of support. For a more anonymous sounding board consider online forums (p. 338)—these also offer information and support from other applicants.
- **Reflect** Talking to others is therapeutic but also helps with reflection and future planning. Once you feel ready you need to address some big questions. Do you still want to study medicine? Why were you unsuccessful? What are you going to do now? These are discussed in more detail below.

A student's experience...

I was rejected without interview by all four medical schools. When I sat down with the careers advisor she pointed out that I'd applied to four of the most competitive institutions. I didn't even meet the minimum GCSE requirement for one of them. I spent so much time studying and organizing work experience that I hadn't researched the courses well enough.

Do you still want to study medicine?

A rejection at this stage does *not* mean you cannot win a place at medical school and become an excellent doctor. Many current medical students (and senior doctors) got in on their second, third, or even fourth attempt. However, it is also true that not everyone is suited, or even wants, to be a doctor. This can come across to admissions staff when they read an application and result in four rejections. Other applicants become disillusioned with medicine, talk themselves out of applying, or become interested in something else during the UCAS process. There are a number of questions you should ask yourself at this stage:

- **Why do you want to study medicine?** Your reasons for studying medicine need re-visiting (p. 4). Are they still relevant to you? Would other careers (p. 287) satisfy your requirements at least as well, if not better?
- **Are you being realistic?** Although many applicants win a place on the second attempt, you don't want to spend years fruitlessly applying to medical school. You must undertake an honest appraisal of your application and abilities. Most people are bad at doing

this—they either *under*estimate or *over*estimate their position. Try to recruit someone else to the process, ideally someone whom you trust to be completely honest. A teacher or school careers advisor could help identify whether you are willing to invest the time needed to make a successful re-application. Although you should take advice, remember that the final decision is yours alone.

Why were you unsuccessful this time?

Understanding why you were unsuccessful is vital if you intend to re-apply. Some factors (e.g. A-level grades) are difficult to change whereas others (e.g. work experience) are more amenable to improvement. Things to consider include:

- Invitations to interview A strong indication comes from whether you were invited to interviews. If four medical schools sent rejections without interview, there is a problem with your UCAS application or admission test result. Review your grades, school reference, and personal statement. If your reference is glowing and grades all read 'A/A*', there is probably something wrong with your statement. Similarly, if you were invited to interview four times but didn't win a place, you need to work on this aspect of your application. Or you could apply to an institution that does not routinely interview candidates, i.e. Southampton (p. 158) and Edinburgh (p. 172)
- Admissions requirements Did you meet all the necessary admissions requirements? This includes apparently 'unimportant' things such as a minimum grade in GCSE English.
- Feedback from medical schools Institutions vary in willingness to provide feedback. Although most send a standard reply with advice for unsuccessful applicants, others provide specific feedback if approached. Don't come across as challenging or in disagreement with their decision. Instead, emphasize that you want to learn from the experience of applying. If necessary, wait a week to cool down after receiving their decision.

Your options

If you didn't receive an offer, you have four broad options. Think carefully and talk to other people about where you are going to go from here.

- Keep trying this year It's very unusual for medical schools to enter clearing but they do occasionally. Check the clearing lists on the UCAS website as soon as you get your A-level results. Alternatively, it's sometimes worth a telephone call a few days after A-level grades are released and before the start of term. Medical schools have been known to re-consider borderline applications if they have spaces unfilled. This is only really an option if you were rejected after interview; candidates who weren't shortlisted are unlikely to be considered borderline.
- Re-apply Learn as much as you can from this experience, take a gap year (p. 30), and start planning your re-application. This *could* be the best thing that ever happened to you, although you won't know it yet.
- Graduate entry Take up one of your non-medicine options and consider applying to medical school as a graduate. This needs careful thought so read p. 218 before choosing this option.
- Make other plans Think about alternative science or healthcare careers (p. 287).

Key points You are making important career decisions. Although you should listen to other people and seek advice where possible, the final decision is yours alone.

If you miss your offer

Most successful applicants are made a conditional offer based on exam grades. The medical school will set a threshold (e.g. 'AAAb') that guarantees the applicant a place if they achieve the necessary results. Some medical schools stipulate additional requirements (e.g. grade 'A*' in chemistry). This means another hurdle for applicants to trip over and many do not achieve the required grades.

Trying your luck

Medical school offers are not set in stone. If you just missed your offer, call and explain your situation. Admissions teams tread a fine line between making too many and too few offers for the number of places they have available. It is only on results day that they find out whether they under- or oversold their course. If they have places left, you might just call at the right time.

> Key points Keep a list of telephone numbers for the admissions staff at medical schools at which you hold offers. If you miss your grades, call straight away for advice. There might still be a chance if you are proactive and don't give up at the first obstacle.

Extenuating circumstances

If your exam performance was adversely affected (e.g. by illness or bereavement) this should ideally have been recorded at the time of the exam. If not:

- Evidence Collect all available evidence attesting to the circumstances and their potential impact on your exam performance. A death certificate, doctor's note, or letter from another appropriate professional is a good place to start.
- Support To ensure your claim sounds plausible you will need support from your school. Ideally your referee will write an additional letter and/or contact medical schools on your behalf. Talk to them early if this is a possibility.

This route is only for those genuinely affected during their exams. Medical schools are unlikely to be impressed by a complaint based on minor circumstances. Similarly, while extenuating circumstances could result in sympathy for a narrowly missed 'A' grade, they are unlikely to account for a string of 'D's.

Challenging your grades

Every year around 20,000 exam candidates (GCSE and A-level) have their grades changed after re-marking. If your results were considerably less than expected or you were very close to meeting your offer, there is little to lose from querying your results. Candidates cannot usually liaise directly with exam boards so you must contact your school in the first instance. Do this quickly as there are deadlines to meet for re-marking and medical schools need to know as soon as possible. It normally takes about 18 days for a priority re-mark (i.e. if a university place depends on the result) or 30 days otherwise.

The process varies between exam boards but costs range from £15 (for a clerical check) to £45 for a full re-mark. Your school can also request to see your marked exam script. The full process for appealing A-level grades is as follows:

- School submits an enquiry to the exam board, which re-marks or re-moderates the necessary papers.
- If you (and your school) are dissatisfied with the result, you can appeal. The result will be considered under the exam board appeals procedure.
- The final stage is an external appeal to the Office of Qualifications and Examinations Regulations (Ofqual).

At every stage, keep medical schools for which you hold an offer informed so they don't prematurely give away your place.

A student's experience...

I was devastated on results day when I scored 'ABB' instead of the 'AAB' needed to meet my offer. On calling the medical school I learned that they did not have any last minute vacancies. I appealed both 'B' grades and my history mark was revised to push me into an 'A' grade. Fortunately the medical school was sympathetic and took me as an 'extra' onto their course. Exam boards are not infallible after all.

Re-sitting

One option is to re-sit A-level modules. Although AS module re-sits are well tolerated, medical schools are suspicious about A-levels taking longer than two years (p. 256). Medical schools permitting re-sits usually require extensively documented mitigating circumstances and 'A' grades in all subjects re-taken.

- Medical schools that strongly discourage re-sit candidates include: Aberdeen (p. 168), Barts (p. 136), Bristol (p. 116), Glasgow (p. 174), Manchester (p. 146), Newcastle (p. 148), Oxford (p. 152), St George's (p. 142), and UCL (p. 144).
- Brighton and Sussex (p. 114), East Anglia (p. 160), Exeter (p. 122), Keele (p. 126), Liverpool (p. 134), Plymouth (p. 154), and Sheffield (p. 156) do not take an overly negative view of re-sat A-levels, although they may require straight 'A' grades from re-sit candidates.
- Others will only consider A-level re-sits from candidates with mitigating circumstances who previously applied to their course. These include Cardiff (p. 180), Imperial (p. 138), Nottingham (p. 150), and Queen's University Belfast (p. 164).

Key points Be realistic about your grades. If you worked hard but scored 'CCC', take advice about whether you could achieve the 'AAA' necessary for most re-sit applicants.

Dealing with poor grades

If re-sitting is not an option, your poor grades will make it much harder to win a place. Access courses (p. 258) are not substitutes for poor A-level grades. If you do still want to pursue medicine, your best option is to do so as a graduate. This means starting a degree in another subject (e.g. anatomy or biomedical science) then applying to graduate entry courses (p. 216). An upper second class honours degree may be considered in lieu of strong A-levels. However, this is a long (and potentially expensive) option that requires careful thought (p. 218).

If things still aren't working out

Commitment and persistence are important qualities. But there is a point at which every unsuccessful applicant should re-consider their career options. Applicants falling into this category include those with:

- Surprisingly poor results without mitigating circumstances.
- Four rejections who are unwilling to take a year out.
- Unsuccessful UCAS applications for a second or third time.

Most UCAS applications to medical school include two other (often bioscience-related) courses. Applicants not receiving offers to study medicine may be tempted to pursue one of these instead. The ultimate aim might be to find a career outside medicine or to apply for graduate entry courses three years later.

Graduate entry medicine

These courses are accelerated (i.e. four years' duration) and aimed at graduates. Although most require a degree in a related field (e.g. biomedical science), others consider graduates in any subject. Most require an upper second class honours (2:1) degree, which is achieved by over 55% of UK graduates. More details about graduate entry courses can be found on p210.

> Key points Don't panic if you're unsuccessful first time. Avoid studying another course just for the sake of going to university. If you are considering a non-medicine degree, make this a deliberate choice after carefully considering your options.

Many unsuccessful applicants begin another degree with the intention of studying medicine later on. This is a legitimate route but requires careful thought.

- Time An honours degree followed by four years at medical school is a total of seven years. This is two years longer than a regular medical course.
- Money Home (and EU) students pay over £9,000/year tuition for degrees at British universities (p. 15). This is without considering accommodation, food, and other expenses for two years. Two years' lost earning power can amount to more than £200,000 (p. 32).
- Competition Graduate courses attract between 10 and 55 applications for every place. This compares to between four and ten applicants for traditional courses. Many graduate applicants will have first class degrees, PhDs, and many years of work experience. This means accelerated courses can be much less accessible than their traditional counterparts. Sometimes it's worth taking a year out (p. 30) and re-applying for a five-year course instead.

That's not to say you shouldn't pursue the graduate route. There are many advantages to completing another degree first.

- Better qualified The graduate route means another degree on your CV. This can score additional points when choosing a speciality and applying for work as a doctor in years to come. However, many traditional courses permit medical students to complete an intercalated degree in just one year.
- More experience A first degree means three additional years to arrange work experience. It will also mean you are more experienced, more confident, and more mature when applying to medical school again.
- Alternative careers Many students find new interests at university. You may develop an interest outside of clinical medicine, perhaps in research.

Thinking outside of medicine

The future is bright for any university applicant with strong A-levels. If you are thinking about alternatives to medical school, consider again what it was that made you want to be a doctor. If you lean towards knowledge and discovery, there are options within science you should explore further. If your motivations were based on helping or working with people, look at other careers within healthcare. Of course science A-levels do not confine you to these fields. The UCAS website (www.ucas.ac.uk) lists courses from aerospace engineering to zoology.

It's important to remember that, however fixated you have become on medicine, there are many careers in the world. Take time to think about them properly.

Careers in science Table 15.1 gives an idea of what science (specifically bioscience) graduates do after graduating. Almost half spend three or four years working towards a research degree (e.g. PhD). The latter is usually funded by a stipend (~£14,000/year). Depending on the field of interest, researchers work in a laboratory on graduation. They are responsible for many of the discoveries that change the diagnosis and treatment of disease in medicine.

Other relevant careers include research in the pharmaceutical industry, teaching, patent law (e.g. protecting intellectual property rights), marketing of new products (e.g. to doctors), and public understanding of science.

Table 15.1 Destination of bioscience graduates

Employment	42%	
Further study	44%	Usually taught MSc or research degrees (e.g. MRes or PhD)
Unemployed	9%	Including those travelling post-graduation
Unknown	5%	

Careers in healthcare You will have come across many different healthcare professionals during your work experience. Most healthcare professions are accessible through degree courses, some of which are extremely competitive. Graduate healthcare careers include nursing, physiotherapy, radiography, and occupational therapy; use a similar strategy to get relevant work experience for these professions (p. 49).

Making the most of medical school

Chapter 16

Making the most of medical school

So you're going to be a doctor...

Congratulations—you've made it! Having achieved the difficult task of getting in, you can now look forward to spending the next few years living, studying, and socializing at university. University can, and should, be one of the greatest experiences of your life, provided you get off to a good start. Unfortunately many new undergraduates are ill-prepared for the realities of university life and enter with a mindset that is uninformed and unsustainable. There can also be practical hurdles to catch out unsuspecting 'freshers', from mix-ups with the Student Loans Company to sitting degree-level exams for the first time.

The following chapter offers an insight into university life, as well as advice on how best to settle in (p. 292). There are some tips for learning (p. 294) and living (p. 298) as a university student, which can be different from even the most independent A-level student experience. These pages will also be relevant to medical school applicants who have not yet secured a place, as they paint a picture of life as a medical student. Finally, the importance of early career decisions will be covered—taking a step towards your possible future medical career as a doctor (p. 302).

What will university be like?

Everyone has a different opinion about what university is like and you will hear various descriptions of students, from being lazy and hung-over to studious and nerdy. The accounts will depend on the story-teller's own personal experiences and prejudices. Of course, the truth is somewhere in between.

University life will probably be different from your student experiences so far. Not only is the material delivered in a different format (p. 88), but you are likely to be one of the many students who are living away from their parents for the first time (p. 298). It is worth remembering that you will not only be a university student studying for their degree, but also are a doctor-in-training. This adds an additional dimension to your learning experience and one that is different from students in other disciplines. With all this change happening at once, starting university can be a daunting time. The key to success is finding your feet early on (p. 292) and knowing what to look out for and what to avoid.

What can I look forward to?

- **Making friends** If you look past the horrible cliché, you may begin to appreciate the fantastic opportunity that starting university offers. This is the largest and most diverse group of people you will ever meet. Starting university is a great opportunity to expand your horizons and form a new group of interesting friends, some of whom you will stay close to for the rest of your life.
- **Joining the profession** You're not only a medical student, you are a student *doctor*. This is reflected in your course content, which includes both professional and academic content (p. 294). With the status of joining the medical profession comes significant responsibility for you as a student doctor, even at this early stage (p. 297).

- **Life skills** Although this is likely to be your first experience of living away from home for a long period of time, you should seize the opportunity to gain independence. University is a time for maturity and developing a sense of personal identity.
- **New beginnings** One of the best things about university is the genuine opportunity to *be yourself*. The cohort of students are less likely to be judgemental than your school colleagues—so if you've held back in your academic, social, or personal life, this is your chance to show your true colours.

What should I avoid?

- **Solitude** Homesickness is common when starting university, as is the fear of not fitting in or finding any close friends. Often this is something you can get through together with the friends you make during Freshers' Week (who will inevitably feel the same).
- **Excessive debt** With the amount of financial support in place for university students, you shouldn't struggle to live comfortably, provided you are sensible with your finances (p. 298). Debt is inevitable after completing a medical degree, but careful spending can limit the final bill (p. 15).
- **Alcohol** Students are not exempt from the excessive drinking culture of 'Binge Britain'. It is worth remembering that doctors suffer one of the highest rates of alcoholism of all the professions. Medical school is a time to form a *healthy* relationship with alcohol. At best, a heavy night risks wasting the next day through the haze of a hangover. At worst it can result in death or severe injury (spend any Friday night in A&E to witness this first-hand). Drunken misdemeanours can also bring students to the attention of their institution's Fitness to Practise Committee (p. 260). You do not want a written warning on record for the rest of your professional career. So, if you are partial to an alcoholic beverage, learn self-restraint early.
- **Sex** Freshers' Week is all too often the source of regretful one-night stands, fuelled by the excitement of independence and cheap alcohol. It is worth bearing this in mind when you start university.
- **Recreational drugs** The GMC (not to mention the law) looks very dimly on drug abuse and you risk ending your career before you've even qualified. Being a student does not absolve you from your responsibilities as a citizen or as a professional-in-training.
- **Re-sits** Exams are an inevitable part of any university course and provide an opportunity to assess how well you are learning the subject. They represent another milestone and a step closer to becoming a doctor. However, you do need to prepare early to avoid re-sits. There is a limit to the number of times you can repeat medical school exams, usually once unless there are exceptional circumstances, after which you may be asked to repeat the year or leave the course.

Starting university

There are often mixed emotions when starting university. Parents may be upset about releasing their 'child' alone into the world for the first time. Students themselves may experience a mixture of excitement at the prospect of new experiences and anxiety that it will fail to 'work out'.

In fact, you will probably find yourself looking back fondly on the emotional rollercoaster of starting university only weeks after arriving, having happily settled in and dispelled any misconceptions that you had formed. The following will hopefully help you to reach this sense of nostalgia more quickly.

Arriving at university

You should receive specific instructions by post, telling you where to go and what to do on your first day. Most first year students arrive a week before academic term begins, which provides an opportunity to participate in a week of activities organized solely for them (see the box **Freshers' Week**).

You will probably need to exchange paperwork with the university authorities when you first arrive. Successful completion of these administrative challenges is rewarded by a room key, map, and timetable. The timetable will be useful for finding out when and where you need to be for various academic introductions and social gatherings. You can then begin the arduous task of unloading a car full of belongings into your new room (if you have been successful in persuading your parents to offer their services—highly recommended!).

Settling in

You will find it a lot easier to settle in if you are well prepared with all of your everyday necessities.

- Bedding It's best to check what will be included with your accommodation before you arrive but most students prefer to bring their own pillows and duvet covers.
- Home decor Student rooms aren't renowned for their palatial furnishings, so it is worth bringing a few home comforts: pictures, cushions, throws, and beanbags. There are often poster sales that run during Freshers' Week too.
- Entertainment Remember that you will be spending a fair amount of time in your halls of residence, so it's worth bringing along something to keep yourself entertained when you have a moment to relax. Books, an iPod, DVDs, speakers, musical instruments, sport accessories, and games consoles can be fantastic respite material (if used wisely).
- Documents Remember to bring important documents that the university/medical school will need to see prior to you starting the course. This may include student finance/Local Education Authority letters, criminal record (CRB) checks, and vaccination forms. Photo ID (driving licence/passport) is often necessary for banking matters and has a role in proceeding past doormen at local bars and clubs.

- Computers All universities have significant computing resources for their students, but it is helpful to have access to a computer in your own room. A laptop has the added benefit of portability, which will be useful for clinical attachments. You won't need anything too advanced—most medical students use their computers for creating documents and slide presentations, checking their email, and browsing the internet. Don't forget to look for student deals on computers and software and university grants can help to contribute towards the cost (p. 16).
- Clothes As a medical student you will need a smart wardrobe for working on the wards and in general practice, as well as day-to-day clothes. The NHS has a 'bare below the elbow' dress code, meaning that sleeves must be rolled up (or short-sleeved shirts worn). If you choose to wear a tie, it needs to be tucked into the shirt or worn with a tie-clip so as not to hang loose. Also bear in mind that your wardrobe needs to (ideally) see you through the entire term at university, so be prepared for formal occasions that might require a lounge suit/cocktail dress or black-tie outfit/ball gown.
- Bike At some universities, cycling is a common mode of transport. Visiting on an open day will have helped to determine whether a bike would be useful. If you do take one, remember to bring a heavy-duty bike lock, helmet, and lights.
- Don't forget... Towels, coat hangers, lamps, extension cables, kettle, crockery, cutlery, and cookware, washing-up cloth, tea towels, Blu-Tack®/drawing pins, stationery, and tea/coffee. A 16–25 Railcard is an immensely valuable investment, offering one-third off rail journeys for £30/year, and all students are eligible. You may also want to bring along your chequebook together with bank cards as this is handy for joining clubs and societies that have an initial fee. If you have to wait for your bank account to be activated, bring enough cash to last a couple of weeks.
- Storage space Storage can be limited so you should avoid bringing too many needless extras before you know how much space is available. Find out whether you have to move the contents out of your room between terms.

Freshers' Week

Every year around the middle of September, freshers (another word for first year university students) across the UK begin a week of activities, organized by the university and student committees (e.g. JCR and MedSoc). Whilst most of it is voluntary, the activities organized are often great ways to get to know your colleagues as well as your surroundings and are definitely worth attending. You will also gain a better idea of the services and facilities that are available. Look out for the societies fair, where you can join one of the hundreds of societies covering every conceivable interest. You may also get university 'parents', students in the years above who will be able to dispense their advice (of variable quality). Rumours about medic initiations can often run rife during Freshers' Week and it is common for students to feel anxious about what they may be asked to do. Suffice to say, you should only take part in what you feel comfortable with, whilst not forgetting your professional responsibilities (p. 291).

Learning at university

There are fundamental differences between the teaching at sixth form and in higher education. The uniqueness of higher education requires a new approach to learning.

How is university education different from A-levels?

- **Content** It goes without saying that the material you will cover at university will be different. In fact, it's not just the details of each subject that will be new to you but the way in which subjects are pursued. Lectures offer a starting point to help you read around the subject so the learning is more *self-directed*. You will develop a deep understanding across a wide range of topics relevant to medicine. Such breadth and depth can seem daunting at first.
- **Resources** Unlike your sixth-form education, you will spend a great deal of time reading material from textbooks, journals, and websites.
- **Teachers** There will be 'teachers' at university but their role is less obvious than at sixth form. They may deliver lectures, lead practical classes, or oversee PBL presentations but, unlike high school, they will have other commitments in their area of expertise. This might include leading a research team or working full-time as a doctor. As a result, they are better seen as a resource for clarifying uncertainties than a source of *spoon-feeding*. Textbooks and online resources are your new best friends.
- **Dynamic curriculum** Medicine is constantly changing, from the understanding of the basic sciences (e.g. how the brain works or the pathophysiology of heart failure) to clinical developments (e.g. chemotherapies in cancer treatment or the indications for a particular operation). This information comes from ongoing research, so your lecture material is only ever a snapshot of current knowledge. Students must be aware of new research findings and gaps in medical knowledge, as well as the details that are understood.
- **Professional dimension** Unique to medical students are the legal and ethical elements of your role as a future doctor. These require additional teaching to reflect the social implications of implementing biomedical knowledge.
- **Exams** The exams you will take during your pre-clinical and clinical years will depend on the university at which you study (p. 92). They are likely to include the following: multiple choice, short answer, essay, and practical questions (based on lab data, histology slides, and pathology specimens) and prosections (anatomical specimens from which you are asked questions). Clinical exams include mock interviews with actors, clinical examinations of patients with diseases, and practical clinical skills (e.g. taking blood from a plastic model). You may also be exposed to oral examinations or 'vivas'.

What will I learn?

Medicine is a broad subject, which is taught in a variety of ways (p. 88).

- **Basic clinical sciences** Traditional courses focus their pre-clinical teaching on the individual subjects upon which medicine is based. This includes everything from biochemistry to psychology.
- **Systems-based courses** These teach the important principles of each subject in a series of lectures that are linked by a common set of organs. For example, studying the renal system will involve understanding the physiology of the normal kidney, visualizing the anatomy of the urinary tract in the dissecting lab, gaining an appreciation of the congenital and acquired diseases that affect the kidney (via pathology and genetics), and learning the pharmacology of drugs that act on the kidneys. As you can see, by the end of the pre-clinical years, students from all types of course will have a similar understanding of how the body works and what can go wrong. This enables them to focus entirely on its pragmatic application on the wards in the clinical years.
- **Clinical attachments** After a few years of book learning, medical students begin their full-time clinical attachments. Up until this point your clinical exposure could have been anything from once a week to bi-annual patient contact, depending on your type of course (p. 88). In the clinical years most students are assigned to medical or surgical teams in hospital for four to eight weeks at a time.

A student's experience...

I found it quite difficult to immerse myself in the esoteric detail of my pre-clinical course, which was taught as basic clinical sciences. It is difficult to see the immediate relevance of lectures when you are learning about the intricate molecular interaction between oxygen and haemoglobin. I found this depth of study made it particularly challenging to stay focused during my revision. Fortunately I am now in the clinical stage of my medical course, studying the subject I originally signed up for. It is a lot more enjoyable when there is a clear purpose to your efforts.

Learning at university cont ...

How will I learn pre-clinical medicine?

The following teaching methods are used to different extents, depending on your course type (p. 88). However, most courses include at least some of each type.

- **Lectures** One speaker usually teaches the entire cohort of medical students for 50 minutes. The size of the audience therefore depends on the medical school but it can be over 300. The format is often a slideshow presentation and, if a handout is provided, this may be a printout of the slides or notes to accompany the lecture content. Your decision to take notes will depend on the quality of the notes you receive and how well the textbooks cover the same material. Remember, lectures are fantastic for grasping principles for the first time, but the minutiae can often be found elsewhere so don't worry about catching every word.
- **Seminar** Smaller groups, usually between 10 and 30 students, are taught by one teacher. There is usually an element of participation, either through small group exercises or direct discussion between the teacher and the group. Seminars are often used to reinforce important topics or teach discursive subjects such as law and ethics.
- **Problem-based learning cases (PBL)** The number of PBL cases you will complete will greatly depend on the type of course (p. 88). PBL cases usually take place over a week in which a small group (eight to ten students) are given a problem/clinical scenario to learn about independently over the week. The group reconvenes at the end of the week to share their findings.

> **Key points** If you are presenting a slideshow, always have a clear set of objectives at the beginning and key messages at the end. You should also remember to restrict the amount of text on each slide to just a few short bullet points.

- **Dissection** Human cadaveric dissection is increasingly being replaced with the use of pre-prepared prosections (professionally dissected specimens) to teach anatomy to medical students. However, full cadaveric dissection is still found at many medical schools. Others use prosections, plastinates (prosections that are solidified), plastic models, or electronic methods of teaching anatomy.
- **Practical classes** During your pre-clinical education, you are likely to encounter various practical classes in order to further understand physiology, biochemistry, pharmacology, and histology. Practical skills are often neglected by medical students, who see them as an enjoyable escape from intense lectures. Whilst they are often enjoyable, they are also examinable and offer easy marks at exam time provided the material is well understood and time is invested in producing a complete workbook.

> **Key points** Every subject has a list of aims and objectives that you are expected to complete by the end of the course. It is useful to familiarize yourself with these before beginning the relevant lectures or laboratory classes. This can help you concentrate on the material that is examinable (i.e. the aims/objectives) and focus your attention on 'high yield' information.

How will I learn clinical medicine?

In many ways, clinical attachments are like apprenticeships. Groups of medical students (usually between two and eight) are assigned a clinical firm to 'shadow'. You may follow a ward round and even write in the patient notes. Your firm's doctors will run clinics in which they assess outpatients and determine their management (e.g. considering a patient for surgery or altering their drug treatment), which you can also attend.

- **Good manners** You must always remain polite, *especially* towards patients. Your kindness towards them will often be reciprocated by their permission to allow you to examine them or perform procedures.
- **Lend a hand** Don't be afraid to get stuck in. Practical tasks on the wards always need doing and you will be actively contributing to the running of the ward. Ask if you need help, only do what you are comfortable with, and *never* expose yourself or a patient to risk.
- **Attending theatre** You should receive an introduction to surgery and theatre etiquette before beginning your first surgical attachment. There is a strict hierarchy within the operating room, with the scrub nurse placed squarely at the top! Introduce yourself to the whole team as soon as you enter an operating theatre. Ensure that everyone is happy with your attendance and not just the consultant. Ask where they would like you to stand and be careful not to touch anything within the 'sterile field'.
- **Scrubbing in** This can be a useful experience if the surgeon is willing to teach in theatre. But be warned: surgery might look exciting but soon loses its appeal after the fifth hour of holding a retractor in position. Although you must experience assisting (especially if your consultant says you should), your time could often be better spent elsewhere. Ask your consultant if you feel you could learn more from seeing patients on the ward or in clinics instead.
- **Attention to detail** Good students soon learn that there is a wealth of detail they can never hope to master if they want to pass their exams. You won't face a question on dosing regimens of anti-retrovirals in finals, so learning them is not a good use of time. Learn what interests you but remember it is a *strong* grasp of *basic* knowledge and underlying principles that will get you through the exams.
- **Books or patients?** It's difficult to achieve the right balance between clerking patients and learning theory. Clinicians will encourage you to take histories, examine patients, and consider their management. The ability to diagnose patients cannot be achieved from books alone. That said, it is easy to overlook the quantity of information you will need to know for your clinical exams, so it is important that you strike the right balance.
- **Asking for help** Don't be afraid to ask. You can do almost anything with appropriate supervision—ask someone to teach you. You are there to learn.

An insider's view...

He who studies medicine without books sails an uncharted sea, but he who studies medicine without patients does not go to sea at all.

Sir William Osler, an important doctor

Living at university

If the different style of learning at university wasn't enough for you to get used to, living as a student will definitely require pause for thought. Many students find themselves having to manage finances, maintain a work–life balance, and look after themselves for the first time. Hopefully this transition to independence hasn't come all at once but, if it has, you are certainly not alone. The following advice should make this transition easier and point you in the right direction should you come across any difficulties.

Money Page 15 covers the cost of medical school in detail. Suffice to say you will be spending in the region of £200–400 a week on tuition fees, rent, and living costs. The first two are fixed, but the estimate of living costs is very dependent upon your lifestyle as a student. The lower boundary doesn't prevent you from socializing, nor does the upper estimate guarantee you stardom within the upper echelons of the university high life. You will need to determine your weekly budget early on. It is worth checking that your 'books balance' every so often to ensure you are not overspending.

Should you run into financial difficulties, you have several options to consider after parental contributions have run dry. You could seek a larger loan through the Student Loans Company if you are not already claiming the maximum amount. If your circumstances have changed, you may be eligible for re-assessment or perhaps a grant/bursary from the university. You could consider a part-time job but beware that this does not interfere with your education. Professional trainee loans of up to £25,000 are another option but the interest rates are often high and should be avoided if possible. Credit cards should be avoided at all costs as these debts can increase dangerously due to the high interest rates.

> **Key points** Should you find yourself in excessive debt, you need to re-assess your current expenditure to avoid making the situation worse, as well as prioritizing any debts you have to pay. Do not ignore the issue. Seek advice from pastoral tutors, Students' Union services, and/or the Citizens Advice Bureau.

Health Whilst learning about the ills of others and how to treat them, it's often easy to overlook your own health. University offers a bewildering array of hazards, from fresher's flu to alcohol intoxication. Moreover, the intensity of the course makes it easy to become run down and it is important that you register with a local GP.

Make sure you inform someone if you are feeling particularly unwell and be alert to any signs of danger (in yourself and your peers). For meningitis, these may include: headache, fever, vomiting, neck stiffness, drowsiness, avoidance of bright lights, and non-blanching bruises.

Central to your health is your mental wellbeing. Whilst the overall incidence is low, doctors have one of the highest rates of depression, alcoholism, and suicide of any profession. There are various services on hand including your GP, welfare tutor, and university pastoral support services. The Samaritans can be contacted 24 hours a day on 08457 90 90 90.

Key points Beware the phenomenon of the hypochondriacal medical student. As you study disease every day, you may begin experiencing symptoms or recognize a rare syndrome in yourself. This is normal and local GPs expect a steady stream of concerned medical students throughout your course. Fortunately this wears off and you are less likely to self-diagnose Kartagener's syndrome or bubonic plague after the third year.

Work–life balance Maintaining a work–life balance is an issue that arises for every student and medics are no exception. With so much to condense into a short period of time, you quickly run the risk of being over-run with lecture handouts and an ever-growing reading list. Two extremes of students can materialize. One stays up until the early hours in a vicious state of catch-up, trying, often with limited success, to cover *everything*. The second student stacks their workload for the coming holidays, admits defeat, and concentrates on socializing. Neither is an ideal strategy for success.

It is nearly impossible to be familiar with all of your course materials at any one time during term. More importantly, it is not necessary. If you are examined regularly (via modular tests) then there is a limited amount of information you must know for each test. Otherwise, simply concentrate on having a good understanding of the principles of your subjects and addressing the difficult concepts whilst the material is fresh in your mind. It would be foolish to begin learning esoteric details for an exam that is nine months away.

Adopting such a strategy should give you enough time in the day for personal respite. How you choose to utilize this is entirely up to you, but free time need not be unproductive. It is possible even at this stage to take up enjoyable activities that can be directed towards your medical CV later on (p. 303).

Hobbies and interests Application forms for medicine are teeming with extracurricular activities and voluntary services that are often impossible to continue to the same extent at university. Medical schools look for this breadth to ensure students can cope with pressure beyond the A-level syllabus and have coping mechanisms that are adequate for the pressures of medical school.

Finding a life outside of medicine is essential to the health and wellbeing of student doctors. Whether it is a morning run, working for a student newspaper, or being a committee member for the medical society, you will find it difficult to cope without some type of outlet. You may wish to continue a hobby from your school days or pursue a completely novel interest that has caught your eye during Freshers' Week (p. 293). Just make sure you have something that you can regularly participate in, which takes your mind off the workload.

An insider's view...

It's not unheard of for a medical student to work themselves into ill health. Previously top A-level students can arrive at university with an unrealistic level of academic standards and their downfall is precipitated by a failure to establish a network of friends or develop interests outside of medicine. It is important that new medical students possess the coping mechanisms to overcome the difficulties they may face and seek assistance when necessary.

A day in the life of a student doctor

The following entries give you an idea of the day-to-day life of a pre-clinical and clinical student. Note there will be some differences between course types (p. 88) and the exact content of the lectures will obviously depend upon how far along you are during the course.

A day in the life of a pre-clinical student...

08:20 Get out of bed after hitting the snooze button for the fifth and final time. No time for breakfast. Run for the bus to the hospital. Just miss it...

09:05 Creep into the back of the first lecture, the third of six lectures on the hypothalamic–pituitary axis. Need to read about this later; as it goes completely over my head!

10:00 The next lecture is on pregnancy. The handouts are a little sparse so it's worth getting out a notepad and taking some notes.

11:05 Grab a quick coffee before attending a PBL session on genetics and development. I am assigned to a group of seven medics (four of whom I've never met before). Our presentation is on epigenetic disorders and I have to research Prader–Willi syndrome.

12:30 Chat to friends then grab a quick bite at the canteen.

13:30 Neuroanatomy teaching in the dissection laboratory: this session is on the motor system looking at prosections of the cerebellum and spinal cord. I spend the hour receiving informal teaching from demonstrators and reading posters that accompany the anatomical specimens.

15:00 Pharmacology practical, investigating the effect of drugs on the neuromuscular junction. We apply various drugs like acetylcholine to a guinea pig ileum and measure its response using an electrical transducer. The experiment is a complete failure but it's an enjoyable exercise nonetheless.

16:30 Meet up with my 'student-selected component' tutor to discuss my upcoming project in the Department of Psychiatry. I will be writing a 4,000-word dissertation on the neurodevelopment of obsessive compulsive disorder (OCD)—an area I found fascinating when it was briefly covered in our lectures last year.

17:15 Get to the sports pitches for lacrosse training—an intense session in preparation for the inter-university competition later on in the month.

18:30 Stop by the library to pick up books on genetics for the PBL presentation and endocrinology to fill in the gaps from the morning lecture.

19:00 Get home and cook myself a student special—pasta with pesto—then finish off some pharmacokinetics calculations for a seminar tomorrow.

20:45 Watch a bit of TV before getting ready to go out.

22:00 Meet up with friends at the union bar, play a few games of pool, and catch up on the latest gossip.

00:30 Check the alarm is on for 7:30 and hit the sack.

A day in the life of a clinical student...

07:45   Wake up; shower and breakfast before leaving the house.

08:15   Arrive at a friend's house who is driving four of us to our current cardiothoracic placement ten miles away.

09:00   Wait for the doctor to arrive for a cystic fibrosis clinic.

09:30   The Specialist Registrar (SpR) arrives half an hour later, after attending to emergencies on the ward. Thankfully I brought along my *Oxford Handbook of Clinical Medicine* and so managed to refresh my knowledge about the condition beforehand.

09:45   See the first patient, a 15-year-old girl recovering from pneumonia whose symptoms have worsened. The patient is given an additional course of oral antibiotics and is told to return in a fortnight for a trial of nebulized saline.

10:30   The second patient fails to turn up so the SpR uses the opportunity to teach me about cystic fibrosis; this morning's reading proves particularly useful.

11:00   The next appointment is a routine follow-up reviewing a patient's drugs. There is an interesting discussion on the risks and benefits of long-term antibiotics and the patient decides to 'watch and wait' her chest symptoms.

11:30   Final patient is particularly tearful and prefers that a student doctor is not present during his assessment. I attach myself to the physiotherapist and dietician and sit in on a few of their consultations.

12:30   Grab lunch at the hospital canteen then go to a clinical lecture on asthma and its management.

14:00   Change into scrubs and asked the scrub nurse if I can observe the scheduled lobectomy. I had previously clerked this surgical patient a few days ago on the ward. He had been diagnosed with lung cancer after smoking for 25 years.

14:20   The surgeon arrives and offers me the chance to scrub in. I spend the next two and a half hours assisting with the lobectomy—holding retractors, 'following-through' with sutures, and providing suction.

17:00   Head home, but get stuck in rush-hour traffic.

18:00   Cook dinner then head to the medical school where there is a guest speaker at the Surgical Society talking about the history of plastic surgery and offering advice for students interested in pursuing this speciality.

20:30   Return home and attempt to complete a poster presentation I am producing with an SpR. We hope to send it off to be considered for a conference.

22:45   Admin: send out an email in my capacity as vice president for the Jazz Society, arranging the next rehearsal and confirming the location for the weekend's gig.

23:30   Skim a few pages of a non-medical book before falling asleep.

The importance of early career decisions

Only ten years ago, the career path of medical students was vastly different from what it is today. The longer hours meant that junior doctors were exposed to more clinical medicine and the job application system allowed student and junior doctors to develop a wealth of experience before selecting their chosen speciality.

Medicine is becoming increasingly competitive, with doctors having to make career decisions earlier in their training. Applicants have had less time to distinguish themselves and demonstrate an interest in their career of choice. This section explains why making career decisions early is important and how to pursue them.

Why is it necessary?

With increasing competition, reduced working hours, and the new job application programmes (foundation, core training, and specialist training; see p. 8), student and junior doctors now have to demonstrate their clinical interests at an early stage. This is difficult because final year medical students and junior doctors have very similar CVs with which they need to distinguish themselves in order to win their choice of positions. The inflexibility of the new training programmes also makes it difficult to change career once you have committed to a particular speciality. So not only does your choice of speciality have to come after less clinical experience but also you need to be absolutely sure early on.

But it isn't all bad. The process of trying to identify your chosen speciality early on allows you to engage more closely with medicine and actively identify, or dismiss, future career options.

How do I decide?

- **Clinical attachments** Student doctors are in a fantastic position to determine their future careers. The apprenticeship style of teaching (p. 297) means that you have the opportunity to shadow many specialities as a student doctor. Unfortunately, most students fail to exploit their placements for this purpose and instead focus entirely on training to become junior doctors. Whilst this *is* important, it does not exclude the possibility of considering each speciality as a potential career destination.
- **Asking the right questions** There are many factors to consider when making a career decision: working hours, on-call work, salary, competition, and so on. Pick the SpR and consultant's brains and ask them as much about the lifestyle of their speciality as about the work itself.
- **Student groups** There are often student special interest groups around each speciality that are established in medical schools. These groups tend to arrange regular events/workshops and often receive lectures from guest speakers about the subject.

Key points You may find the junior doctor's teaching to be more relevant than the SpR's and consultant's when it comes to nailing down the basics for finals. But if you find yourself interested in a particular speciality, there is no substitute for shadowing the senior members of a clinical team and exploring their roles.

- **Student-selected modules** Every medical course includes components where the student themselves decides on an area to study. The student's efforts could be expressed in the form of a dissertation, poster, or presentation. They can be great ways to learn about an area of medicine in greater depth.
- **Outside the box** The majority of medical students enter a career in hospital medicine or general practice. However, a small minority choose to step outside these traditional confines to use their expertise in less common environments...military medicine, medical law, forensic psychiatry, tropical medicine, aid work, medical management consultancy, expedition medicine, and prison medicine to name but a few. Keep your eyes (and options) open!

How to direct your medical CV

Once you've made a decision about an area you want to specialize in, you need to demonstrate an interest. Consider some of the following:

- **Student-selected modules** Use this opportunity to pursue a project under supervision from a consultant within your speciality of interest.
- **Audits** An audit refers to a process of review and implementation of change to improve the quality of patient care and outcomes. You start by collecting data on whether *set standards* are being met (e.g. measuring whether pulse oximetry is being recorded for all chronic obstructive pulmonary disease (COPD) patients in a GP clinic). You may then identify *areas of change* based on your data (e.g. investing in more pulse oximeters, which you have found to be shared between consulting rooms). If a *change is implemented* (e.g. purchasing more oximeters for the practice) then you can *re-audit* after a certain time in order to see whether your results have improved.
- **Research** The importance of research in your medical career cannot be overstated—it not only offers extra CV points but also provides an experience of how science and medicine develop. Intercalated degrees offer a fantastic opportunity in your pre-clinical career for getting published (p. 87).
- **Medical press** Publications do not necessarily have to come from scientific or clinical research. Writing for the medical press, such as a student journal, can highlight your interest and enthusiasm. Note that peer-reviewed articles are of much higher status than those published in other forms (e.g. student magazines).
- **Prizes** These can be useful in demonstrating your success in clinical exams. The application process for your first job ranks students by quartiles within their universities (top 25%, second 25%, third 25%, and bottom 25% are each assigned a different number of points). Prizes can highlight additional success. The Royal Colleges (p. 278) also offer prizes for essays written by medical students. These are often under-subscribed and so worth trying for if you have a talent for writing.

Key points Medical school is the beginning of a career, so begin thinking about the direction of your career from the very first day. Invest in a medical careers guide early, such as *So you want to be a brain surgeon?* It is in the same series as this book and covers all the available careers in medicine (not just brain surgery).

Appendix

Chapter 17

Appendix

UKCAT section 1 questions

Time allowed 2 minutes

Scottish devolution

In September 1997, Scotland held a referendum on the question of devolution. Over 60 per cent of eligible voters went to the polls, and they voted in favour of both questions on the ballot-paper. On the first question, asking whether there should be a Scottish Parliament, 74.3 per cent of voters agreed, including a majority in favour in every Scottish local authority area. On the second question, asking whether that Parliament should have tax-varying powers, 63.5 per cent of voters agreed, including a majority in favour in every Scottish local authority area except Orkney and Dumfries & Galloway. In response to the results of this referendum, the UK Parliament passed the 1998 Scotland Act, which was given Royal Assent on 19 November 1998. The first members of Scottish Parliament (MSPs) were elected on 6 May 1999, and the Queen formally opened the Scottish Parliament on 1 July 1999, at which time it took up its full powers.

Under the terms of the 1998 Scotland Act, the Scottish Parliament has the authority to pass laws that affect Scotland on a range of issues. These issues are known as 'devolved matters', as power in these matters has been transferred (or 'devolved') from a national body (the UK Parliament at Westminster) to regional bodies (the Scottish Parliament, the National Assembly for Wales, and the Northern Ireland Assembly). Education, Agriculture, Justice, and Health (including NHS issues in Scotland) are among the issues devolved to the Scottish Parliament. The Scottish Parliament also has the power to set the basic rate of income tax, as high as 3 pence in the pound.

The 1998 Scotland Act also provides for 'reserved matters', which Scots must take up through their MPs at Westminster rather than through their MSPs. Such reserved matters, on which the Scottish Parliament cannot pass legislation, include Foreign Affairs, Defence, and National Security.

In Scottish parliamentary elections, each voter has two votes: one vote for the MSP for their local constituency, and one vote for the candidate or party to represent their Scottish Parliamentary Region. There are 73 local constituencies, and eight Scottish Parliamentary Regions; each local constituency is represented by one local MSP, and each region is represented by seven regional MSPs. These local and regional MSPs account for the total membership of the Scottish Parliament. Thus, every Scotsman or Scotswoman is represented by a total of eight MSPs (one local and seven regional).

UKCAT section 1: Questions

Based on the passage on p. 306, answer the following four questions.

1 In the 1997 referendum, more voters in Dumfries and Galloway were in favour of a Scottish Parliament than were in favour of the tax-varying powers for a Scottish Parliament.
   A True
   B False
   C Can't tell

2 The Scottish Parliament can raise the basic rate of income tax by 3 pence in the pound.
   A True
   B False
   C Can't tell

3 NHS issues in Wales are among the issues devolved to the National Assembly for Wales.
   A True
   B False
   C Can't tell

4 There are a total of 129 MSPs in the Scottish Parliament.
   A True
   B False
   C Can't tell

UKCAT section 2 questions

Time allowed 2 minutes

Linden Grove School is designated a Specialist Language College. All students at Linden Grove must study at least one language to GCSE level and many students take GCSEs in two languages. All students in Year 11 at Linden Grove take at least one of three languages:

61 students in Year 11 study French

35 students in Year 11 study German

47 students in Year 11 study Spanish

These numbers include students who take a single language, as shown in the first chart, as well as students taking more than one language, as shown in the second, third, and fourth charts.

No student in Year 11 studies more than two languages.

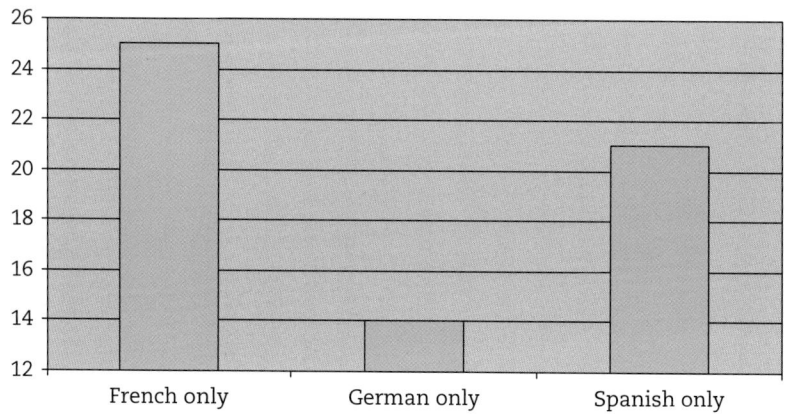

Students in Year 11 Who Study One Language Only

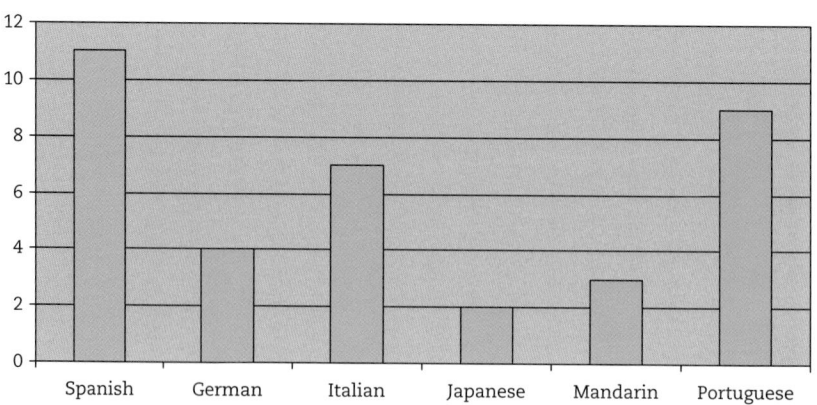

Second Languages of Students in Year 11 Who Study French

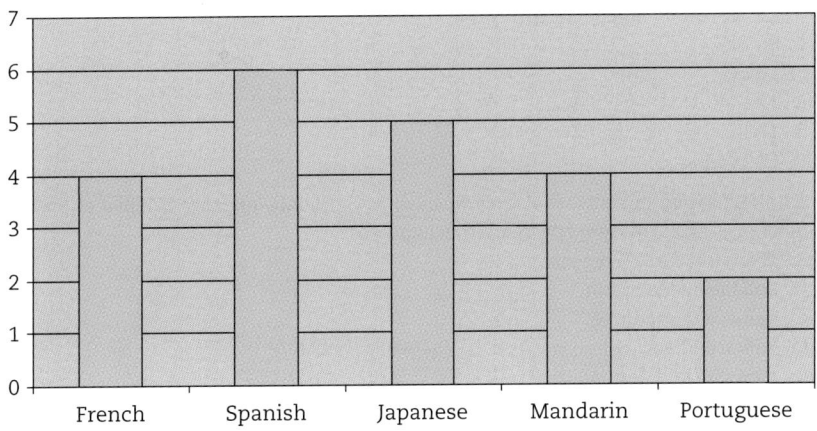

Second Languages of Students in Year 11 Who Study German

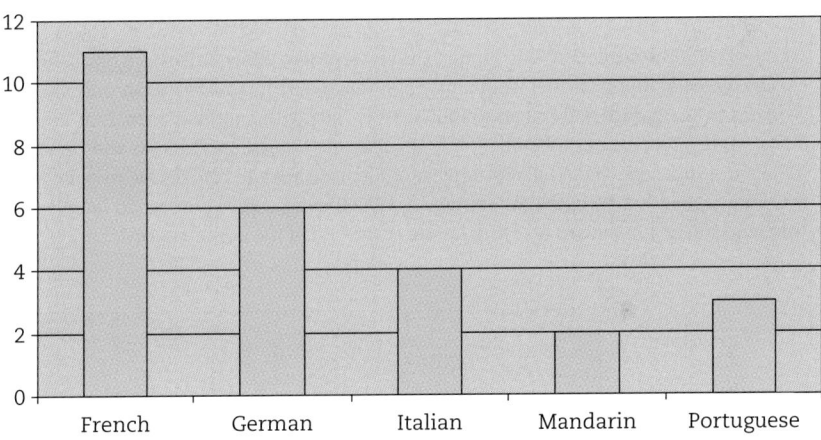

Second Languages of Students in Year 11 Who Study Spanish

UKCAT section 2: Questions

1 What is the total number of students in Year 11?
   A 80
   B 101
   C 122
   D 143
   E Can't tell

2 The number of students who study Spanish as their only language is equal to the total number of students that study which two languages?
   A Mandarin and Portuguese
   B Italian and Mandarin
   C Italian and Japanese
   D Italian and Portuguese
   E Japanese and Portuguese

3 What percentage of students who study German also study Mandarin?
   A 4%
   B 11%
   C 19%
   D 26%
   E 43%

4 At the start of the academic year, Linden Grove decides to allow Italian as a first-language choice. Three students switch from studying French and Italian to Italian only and one switches from Spanish and Italian to Italian only. During the autumn term, four new students joining Year 11 opt for Italian only; one selects French and Italian; and three take Italian and Japanese. Half of all Portuguese students in Year 11 also decide to switch their first language to Italian in the autumn term. Which chart shows the second languages of students in Year 11 who are studying Italian at the end of the autumn term?

A

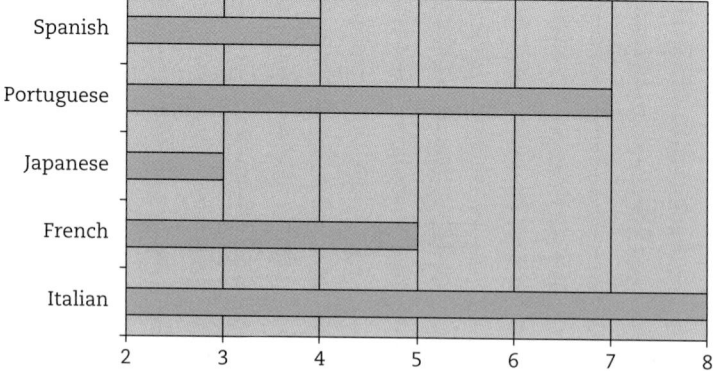

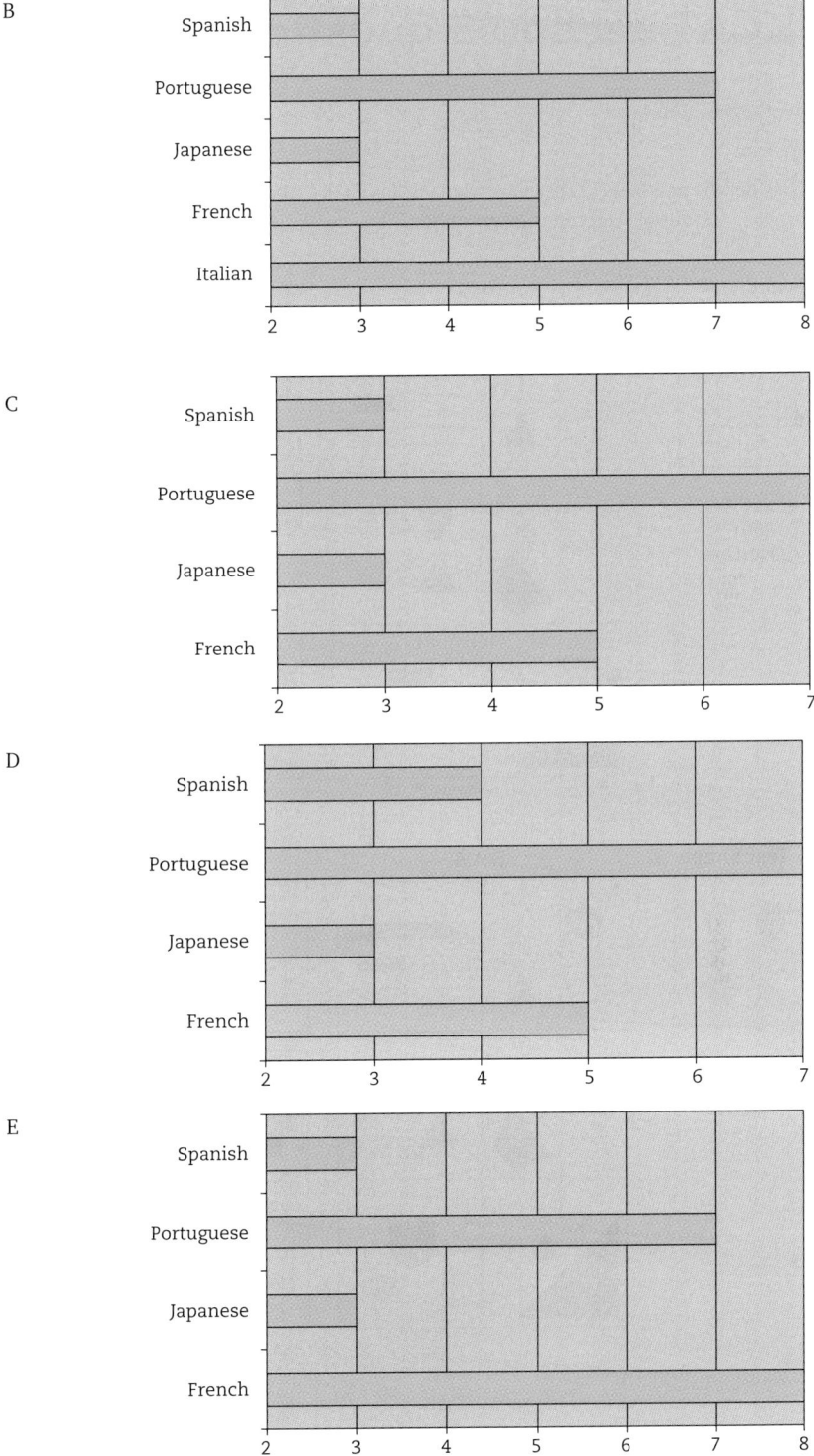

B

Spanish				
Portuguese				
Japanese				
French				
Italian				

2 3 4 5 6 7 8

C

Spanish				
Portuguese				
Japanese				
French				

2 3 4 5 6 7

D

Spanish				
Portuguese				
Japanese				
French				

2 3 4 5 6 7

E

Spanish				
Portuguese				
Japanese				
French				

2 3 4 5 6 7 8

UKCAT section 3 questions

Time allowed 1 minute

Directions:

- Consider the pair of sets (which are the same for all five test shapes).
- For each test shape select one answer only.

1. Test Shape

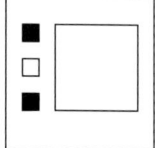

- ° A. Set A
- ° B. Set B
- ° C. Neither

Set A

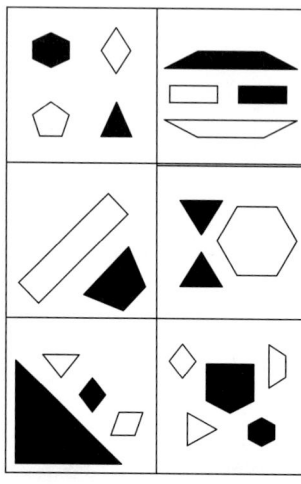

Set B

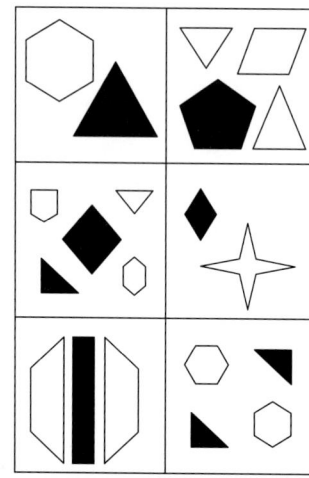

2. Test Shape

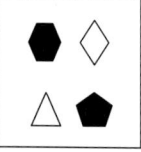

- ° A. Set A
- ° B. Set B
- ° C. Neither

Set A

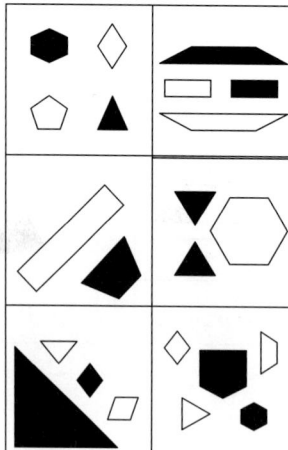

Set B

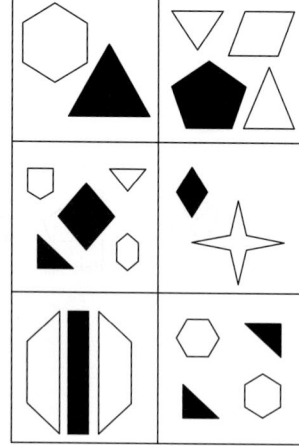

3. Test Shape

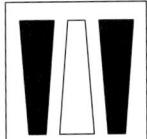

° A. Set A
° B. Set B
° C. Neither

Set A

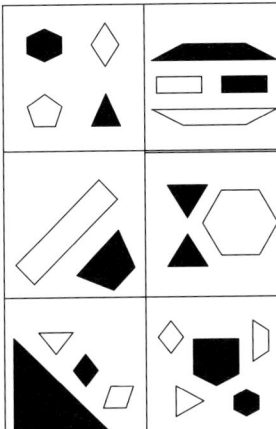

Set B

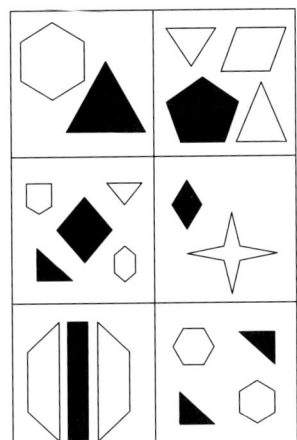

4. Test Shape

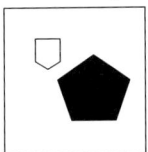

° A. Set A
° B. Set B
° C. Neither

Set A

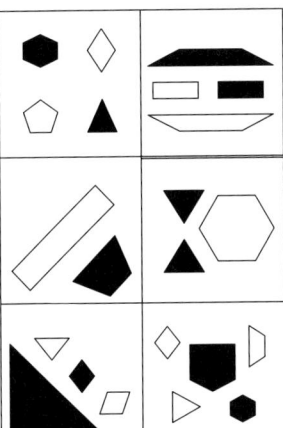

Set B

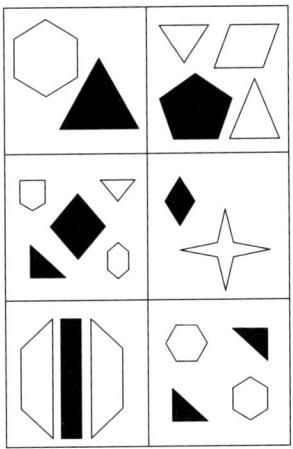

5. Test Shape

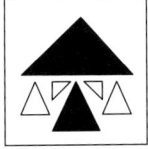

° A. Set A
° B. Set B
° C. Neither

Set A

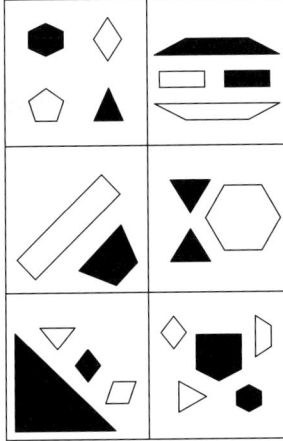

Set B

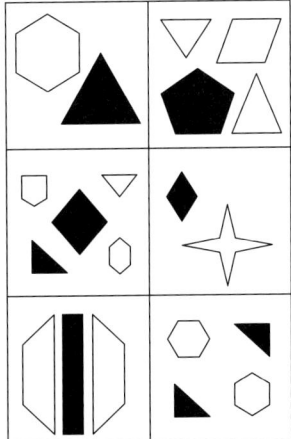

UKCAT section 4 questions

Time allowed 7 minutes

Medieval tapestry code

Whilst cleaning a 14th-century tapestry, employees at the British Museum discover a previously undetected and rather elaborate code woven into its fabric. The code appears to consist of a series of letters and numbers, grouped together in sequences as coded messages, that appear to tell a story. The employees call in an art historian, who hires you as his assistant to decipher these newfound codes.

On examining the tapestry, you determine that some of the information is strange or incomplete, but all of the messages contain some logic. Indeed, the code seems to follow certain patterns that indicate that an internal logic is built into its use. Thus you must make your assessments based on the codes rather than what seems the most predictable or literal translation. Every code has a best answer that makes the most sense based on all the information presented, but remember that this test requires you to make judgements rather than simply apply logic and rules.

Table 17.1 Table of codes

Operators and general rules	Specific information
	Basic codes
A = multiple	1 = I
B = opposite	2 = you
C = down	3 = man
D = group	4 = horse
E = danger	5 = sword
F = noble	6 = tree
G = into	7 = brave
H = special	8 = move
	9 = take
	10 = fight
	11 = creature
	12 = castle
	13 = goblet
	14 = search

UKCAT section 4: Questions

1 What is the best interpretation of the coded message: C12, 1, 9, F(B3)?

   A Down from the castle, the noblewoman takes me as her equal.

   B The countess was my downfall.

   C I am taking the duchess into the castle.

   D I took the countess down from her castle.

   E The duchess and I found our downfall at the castle.

2 What is the best interpretation of the coded message: F(7,3), E8, 5, B(G6)?

   A The brave duke pulled the dangerous sword out of the tree.

   B The brave duke risked pushing the sword into the tree.

   C The duke bravely moved away from the treacherous tree with sword in hand.

   D The knight pulled the sword out of the tree.

   E The knight risked pulling the sword out of the tree.

3 What would be the best way to encode the following message: Many armies of knights came to the castle seeking the Holy Grail?

   A AF(7, 3), 8, G12, 14, H13

   B AF(7, 3), 8, D4, G12, 14, H13

   C ADF(7, 3), 8, G12, 14, H13

   D ADF(7, 3), 8, G12, 9(14, H13)

   E ADF(7, 3), 8, D4, G12, 14, H13

4 What is the best interpretation of the coded message: B(7, 3), 8, 10, (7, 3), 14, B10?

   A On his quest for peace, a fearful man sometimes moves against a brave one in battle.

   B A coward fights on, while a fearless man seeks peace.

   C A man who is not a knight went and fought one who was on a search to end the war.

   D A serf must go fight a knight in the name of peace.

   E Peace is found when serfs and knights refuse to fight.

5 Which of the following would be the most useful and second most useful additions to the codes to convey the message accurately?

   Message: The perilous woodland creatures alarmed my horse with their vulgar sounds.

   A Peril

   B Woodland

   C Disturb

   D Vulgar

   E Noise

UKCAT section 5 questions

Time allowed 7 minutes

Read the following scenario and answer the questions that follow.

> You are shadowing a Foundation Year 1 doctor in your local hospital for work experience. After just a morning of shadowing, you have noticed that the junior doctor appears inattentive, tired, and has not completed any of the jobs tasked to him on the morning ward round. He has also not responded to the last five bleeps he has received, and asks you to go and buy him a coffee while he 'recuperates' in the doctor's mess.

How appropriate are each of these responses by the medical student in this situation?

1 Ask the junior doctor why he appears to be neglecting his duties and putting his patient's safety at risk.

   - A very appropriate thing to do
   - Appropriate, but not ideal
   - Inappropriate, but not awful
   - A very inappropriate thing to do

2 Offer to buy him a coffee providing he responds to his pager.

   - A very appropriate thing to do
   - Appropriate, but not ideal
   - Inappropriate, but not awful
   - A very inappropriate thing to do

3 Report the junior doctor to your human resources point of contact at the end of the working day.

   - A very appropriate thing to do
   - Appropriate, but not ideal
   - Inappropriate, but not awful
   - A very inappropriate thing to do

4 Volunteer to answer his pager in the hope this will encourage the junior doctor to complete his professional duties.

   - A very appropriate thing to do
   - Appropriate, but not ideal
   - Inappropriate, but not awful
   - A very inappropriate thing to do

How important are these options in response to this scenario?

5 To ascertain, with certainty, whether the junior doctor is under the influence of alcohol.

- Very important
- Important
- Of minor importance
- Not important at all

6 Share your observations with the junior doctor's superiors, if you are concerned.

- Very important
- Important
- Of minor importance
- Not important at all

7 Identify if the pager is working and whether the junior doctor is currently responsible for answering his pager, before raising your concerns with anyone else.

- Very important
- Important
- Of minor importance
- Not important at all

8 Establish the junior doctor's medical school ranking in order to gain an impression of his clinical expertise.

- Very important
- Important
- Of minor importance
- Not important at all

UKCAT answers and explanations

UKCAT section 1 answers

1. (A) True

This statement needs to be evaluated carefully. We're told in the first paragraph that Dumfries & Galloway was one of two local authority areas in which a majority of voters were not in favour of a Scottish Parliament having tax-varying powers. So the percentage of voters in favour of this question in Dumfries & Galloway must be 50 per cent or less. We're also told that a majority of voters 'in every Scottish local authority area' were in favour of having a Scottish Parliament. Dumfries & Galloway is one of these areas, so a majority of voters, or more than 50 per cent, were in favour of a Scottish Parliament. We don't know the exact number of voters in Dumfries & Galloway, but there must have been more in favour of a Scottish Parliament (at more than 50 per cent of voters) than were in favour of tax-varying powers for that parliament (a number of voters at or below 50 per cent). So the statement is True.

2. (B) False

This statement is also rather challenging and requires you to read and think very carefully. The last sentence of the second paragraph tells us that the Scottish Parliament can 'set the basic rate of income tax, as high as 3 pence in the pound.' However, this statement says that Parliament 'can raise the basic rate of income tax by 3 pence in the pound'. Thus there must already be a basic rate of income tax, unspecified here, which is to be raised. Whatever the starting basic rate, raising it by 3 pence in the pound would result in a basic rate of income tax above 3 pence in the pound, which takes the rate beyond the level the Scottish Parliament may set it at. So the statement is False.

3. (C) Can't tell

The passage tells us very little about the National Assembly for Wales; its existence is merely noted, in brackets, as one of the regional bodies to which certain powers have been 'devolved', or transferred, from the UK Parliament at Westminster. We are told in the next sentence that 'Health (including NHS issues in Scotland)' are among the issues devolved to the Scottish Parliament, but we cannot infer from the passage that similar issues in Wales are devolved to the Welsh National Assembly. We simply know nothing from the passage about this Assembly, other than that it has some powers devolved to it. So the answer is Can't tell.

4. (A) True

This statement requires you to do some maths, which shouldn't prove too difficult, so long as you don't misread the passage! We're told that Scotland is divided into 73 local constituencies, each with one local MSP, and also into eight parliamentary regions, each with seven regional MSPs. So there are $73 \times 1 = 73$ local MSPs and $8 \times 7 = 56$ regional MSPs, making a total of $73 + 56 = 129$ MSPs in the Scottish Parliament. The statement is True.

UKCAT section 2 answers

1. (C) 122

We can eliminate one answer straightaway: we seem to have enough data to calculate the total number of students in Year 11, so the answer can't be Can't tell. Eliminate (E). The calculations, however, are not quite as straightforward as you might think, particularly if you did this question quickly, as it's not simply a matter of adding the number of students in the summary: 61 + 35 + 47 = 143. These numbers include students who take a single language, as well as students who study two languages. Looking at the three charts, we see that students who study French and German, French and Spanish, or German and Spanish are counted twice. You must subtract them from the total of 143, so 143 − 11 − 4 − 6 = 122, and the correct answer is therefore (C).

2. (E) Japanese and Portuguese

For this question, we need to read our charts carefully and do some basic sums—again, nothing terribly challenging, but it's very easy to make an error in the rush of trying to get through the question. First, we need the number of students studying Spanish as their only language. The first chart shows this as 21. We can then quickly count the number of students studying the other languages:

> Italian: 7 + 0 + 4 = 11
> Japanese: 2 + 5 + 0 = 7
> Mandarin: 3 + 4 + 2 = 9
> Portuguese: 9 + 2 + 3 = 14

Of those figures, we can only equal 21 by adding 7 and 14, the numbers of students studying Japanese and Portuguese, so the correct answer is (E).

3. (B) 11%

Questions about percentages are very common on the UKCAT and the key is to read carefully and make sure you don't make an error in your maths, as the common errors will likely be listed as wrong answer choices. This question asks for the percentage of German students who also study Mandarin. We see from the initial summary that 35 students study German. From the chart of second languages of German students, we see that 4 of these students also study Mandarin. So our percentage is 4/35 × 100, or 11%. The answer is (B).

4. (C)

Occasionally the UKCAT will give you a question where the answers are new charts! These can be time-consuming. A good tip is to work backwards from the data in the answers and see if you can eliminate any of them straightaway on this basis. In this instance, charts (A) and (B) include Italian as a second language. However, the question asks for a chart showing the second languages of students studying Italian. Thus, Italian can't be a second language choice, so we can eliminate (A) and (B). We can then scan the remaining three charts for differences in the data. For instance, all three remaining charts list the number of Japanese students as 3 and Portuguese students as 7. So we cannot determine which is correct on the basis of these students. So let's try Spanish: we're told one student switches from Spanish and Italian to Italian only. There were 4 such students, so the number in our chart should be 3. That eliminates (D). Originally there were 7 students studying French and Italian; we're told that 3 switch out of this group and 1 new student joins during the autumn term. Thus the total number of French and Italian students in our chart should be 5 and the answer is (C).

UKCAT section 3 answers

1. (A)

This set is all about colours and sides. In Set A, the total number of sides on the white shapes in each item is equal to the total number of sides on the black shapes. In Set B, the total number of sides on the white shapes is twice the total number of sides on the black shapes. The size, arrangement, or type of shapes is irrelevant. Our first test shape includes white shapes with a total of 8 sides and black shapes with a total of 8 sides, so it fits into Set A.

2. (C)

This test shape includes a black hexagon and pentagon, with a total of 11 sides, and a white diamond and triangle, with a total of 7 sides. Thus it fits into neither set and the answer is **(C)**.

3. (C)

Counting the sides here, we find a total of 8 sides on the black shapes and 4 sides on the white shape. This test shape fits into neither set, so again the answer is **(C)**.

4. (A)

This test shape contains two pentagons, one white, one black. As they have the same number of sides, the answer is **(A)**.

5. (B)

The final test shape in this set is the least like the rest of the lot, presenting two black triangles and four white triangles. The black shapes have a total of 6 sides and the white shapes a total of 12 sides. Therefore this test shape fits into Set B.

UKCAT Section 4 answers

1. (D)

Literal translation: down(castle), I, take, noble(opposite(man))

The basic approach with Decision Analysis is to write down the literal translation—taking care to group the elements of the code with commas or brackets, fitting the original. Then you can eliminate any answers that omit elements, or don't combine them correctly. Starting here with C12, or down(castle)—answers **(A)** and **(D)** keep these elements clearly together. Eliminate **(B)**, which omits the castle, and also **(C)**, which swaps 'down' for 'into' (which is a different letter in the code). Be very suspicious of **(E)**, which seems to separate 'down' and 'castle' (turning 'down' into 'downfall', a more elaborate concept than the code suggests). The three remaining answers contain 'I', but answer **(E)** drops out when we come to 'take', which is not included. The final element of the code could well become 'noblewoman', as in **(A)**, or 'countess', as in **(D)**. The elements of the code have been exhausted without accounting for the concept 'as her equal', which finishes **(A)**, so this cannot be correct. The correct answer is therefore **(D)**, which includes all the elements of the code and nothing more.

2. (E)

Literal translation: noble(brave, man), danger(move), sword, opposite(into(tree))

You don't need to take the code elements in order to eliminate answers. Here, the easiest might be the last element, which must mean something like 'out of the tree'. This matches answers **(A)**, **(D)**, and **(E)** and eliminates **(B)** and **(C)**. We might next consider the element 'danger', which is linked to 'move', which eliminates **(A)**, as this choice links 'danger' with 'sword'. The difference between **(D)** and **(E)** then is the difference between 'pulled' and 'risked pulling'—only the latter accounts for both 'danger' and 'move', so **(E)** is correct.

3. (C)

This question works in reverse, so we can go straight to the answers and see what elements they have in common; we can then make our judgements and eliminate as appropriate. For instance, the answers all start with 'AF(7, 3)' or 'ADF(7, 3)'—which best matches the start of our message, 'Many armies of knights'? The correct answer for question 2 rendered 'F(7, 3)' as 'knight'. In the code, A means multiple and D means group, which would account for the 'many armies'. Eliminate answers **(A)** and **(B)**, as they omit the 'group' code (and would thus mean something like 'many knights'). All remaining answers include 8, 'move', and G12, 'into the castle'. They also include 14, 'search', and H13, 'special goblet', which would fit 'Holy Grail' in the message. These elements and nothing more are found in answer **(C)**, which appears to be correct. Checking quickly, we can see that answer **(D)** groups the search and special goblet with code 9, 'take', which does not make sense with the message, and answer **(E)** adds in D4, or 'group of horses', also not in the message. This question also points up the value of using your correct responses from previous questions to help understand the patterns in the code, as these can recur again and again.

4. (B)

Literal translation: opposite(brave, man), move, fight, (brave, man), search, opposite(fight)

This coded message includes a 'brave man' and his opposite, so eliminate answers that don't: answers **(C)**, **(D)**, and **(E)** all render 'brave man' and the opposite as 'knight' and 'serf' (or 'not a knight'), but we've seen that the code requires F, noble, to indicate that a brave man is in fact a knight. So that leaves **(A)** and **(B)**. Comparing these, it's quickly clear that answer **(B)** accounts for all the elements in the code and nothing more; answer **(A)** jumbles the order—moving the 'quest for peace' to the beginning and attributing it to the 'fearful man'; answer **(A)** also adds the element 'sometimes'. The better fit, and correct answer, is **(B)**.

5. (C) and (E)

This question is different from the rest, on two counts: we have to add something to the code, and must find not one correct answer, but two. Once again, the quickest strategy is to eliminate the answers that are wrong. On this type of question, wrong answers most commonly fall into two categories: they are not part of the message, or they are already included in the code. All answers here are in the coded message—as 'disturb' means the same as 'alarm' in this context and 'noise' is the same as 'sound'. So eliminate those that are covered by the code: 'peril' means the same as 'danger', so eliminate answer **(A)**. A group of trees, or D6, would be a woodland, so eliminate **(B)**. And 'vulgar' also means 'common', which is the opposite of noble, or BF in the code. Eliminate **(D)**, which leaves the correct answers as **(C)** and **(E)**, as the code cannot cover the elements 'disturb' or 'noise'.

UKCAT Section 5 commentary

1. Appropriate, but not ideal
If you have concerns regarding the junior doctor's practice, it is appropriate to direct those concerns to the junior doctor in the first instance. This particular response is confrontational and more likely to antagonize the junior doctor than to successfully address the problem.

2. Inappropriate, but not awful
This attempt to plicate the junior doctor into completing his professional duties is inappropriate, and should not be necessary. You should not be expected to purchase coffee; the important point here is to address why the junior doctor is not responding to his pager.

3. Appropriate, but not ideal
It is reasonable to raise any concerns you have with your point of contact, but it would be more satisfactory to resolve your concerns more quickly, with the junior doctor or failing this with his clinical superiors.

4. A very inappropriate thing to do
You are not qualified to be able to respond to the doctor's paged requests, and volunteering to answer his pages in an effort to encourage his fulfilment of clinical duties is unnecessary.

5. Not important at all
While the additional knowledge of the junior doctor being under the influence of alcohol would not be unhelpful, this is not something you need to ascertain with certainty, and you should not hesitate to raise any genuine concerns.

6. Very important
It is essential to share any concerns that you may have regarding patient safety, with the responsible seniors.

7. Very important
There are various legitimate reasons why the junior doctor is not responding to his pager, and the option offered enables you to gauge this in an appropriate fashion before escalating the matter further. Perhaps the pager messages were mistakenly sent without a return number, or were group messages or test calls unintended for the junior doctor and not requiring a response. Ascertaining this before accusing the junior doctor of shirking his responsibilities is important for the professional standing and reputation of the junior doctor, and yourself.

8. Not important at all
This should have no implication to the way you handle this situation, as all practising doctors are considered competent and assumed clinically capable, and this would not be adequate justification for failing to perform one's clinical responsibilities.

BMAT section 1 questions

Time allowed 7 minutes

1 A conductor of an orchestra makes the following remarks about the composers that her musicians adore:

All musicians in the orchestra adore Handel. Some cellists adore Schumann and some adore Bach. All flautists adore Mozart and some adore Rimsky-Korsakov. No percussionist adores Bach and all percussionists adore Rimsky-Korsakov.

Based on the conductor's remarks, which of the following statements must be true?

A Some cellists adore Handel, but not Schumann or Bach.

B Some cellists adore both Schumann and Bach.

C Some flautists adore Bach.

D Some flautists adore three composers.

E Some percussionists adore three composers.

2 An electricals shop lowers the price of a digital camera each day of a bank holiday weekend. On Saturday, the price of the camera is lowered by 10 per cent from its price on Friday. On Sunday, the price is lowered 10 per cent from its price on Saturday. On Monday, the price is lowered by 10 per cent from its price on Sunday. The price of the camera on Monday is what percentage of its price on Friday?

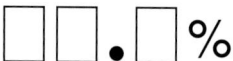

3 Media coverage of organ donation has increased as the Government considers making the donor registry 'opt-out', rather than 'opt-in'. Every week, newspapers and TV reports are filled with grim stories and statistics of waiting lists and deaths of those waiting for a transplant. Regardless of any changes to legislation, the media could do more to increase organ donation at present. For example, the frequent news reports on the need for more donated organs rarely mention how, exactly, members of the public can 'opt-in' to the donor registry. This practice stands in stark contrast to the presentation of such stories in other countries, such as the USA and Canada, where stories on the need for more organ donors almost always end with contact details for joining the donor registry. Providing viewers with a phone number or website for joining the registry is seen as a public service, part of the media's responsibility in calling attention to such a problem.

Which of the following best summarizes the main conclusion of the argument?

A It's easier to become an organ donor in the USA or Canada than in the UK.

B Sometimes the media can help to solve the problems it identifies.

C The Government wants to make organ donation compulsory.

D Many people die waiting for organs each year as there are too few donors opting-in to the registry.

E Everyone should be required to join the organ donor registry.

4 Shannon and Dave are hosting a dinner party for six friends. The surface of the dining table is circular, with chairs set out equal distances around its circumference. Each chair is directly opposite one other chair (see diagram).

Dave prefers to sit directly opposite Shannon. Rachael and James are a couple and prefer to sit next to each other. Ben fancies Lola, and he's a bit shy, so he prefers to sit directly opposite her. Dave and Shannon can't stand Patrick, whom Cindy is seeing, so neither of them will sit next to him.

If the seating plan meets everyone's preferences, what is the probability that Cindy will be seated directly opposite Rachael?

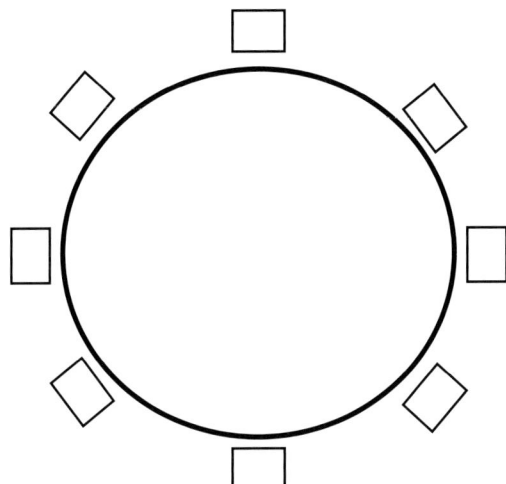

BMAT section 2 questions

Time allowed 4 minutes

1 Haemophilia B (Christmas disease) is an X-linked recessive disorder. Both Jane's father and maternal grandfather suffer from haemophilia B.

Which of Jane's relatives is neither a carrier of nor suffers from Christmas disease?

A Her sister

B Her father's monozygotic twin

C Her maternal uncle

D Her maternal aunt

E Her paternal grandmother

2 Concerning acids:

I   Citric acid ionizes partially in aqueous solution.

II A 1 M solution of ethanoic acid has the same concentration of $H+$(aq) as a 1 M solution of nitric acid.

III A 1 M solution of hydrochloric acid is a better conductor of electricity than a 1 M solution of lactic acid.

Which of the following choices lists the correct statements above?

A I only

B II only

C III only

D I and II only

E I and III only

F II and III only

G I, II, and III

3 Three points in the (x, y) coordinate plane lie at:(a, b)

(a + 3 $\sqrt{2}$, b)

(a + $\sqrt{2}$, b − 4$\sqrt{2}$)

What is the area of the triangle described by these coordinates?

A $\sqrt{2}$

B 6

C 5 $\sqrt{2}$

D 12

E 12 $\sqrt{2}$

4   A laser is shone through a small circular hole and the image is projected onto a screen.

Which of the following choices represents the pattern shown on the screen?

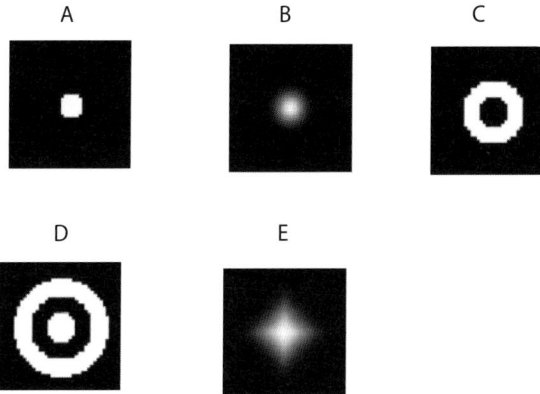

BMAT section 3 questions

Time allowed 30 minutes
Directions

- Answer ONE question.
- Handwrite your answer on a single page of A4.
- You are permitted to make any preparatory notes as needed, but time spent on such notes counts against the 30 minutes allowed for the essay.
- Essays are assigned a numerical score. To achieve a top mark, you must address all aspects of the question and write compellingly with few errors in logic or in use of English.

BMAT section 3: Questions

1 'A scientific man ought to have no wishes, no affections—a mere heart of stone.'

Charles Darwin

Write an essay in which you address the following points:

Why should those who practise science or medicine have 'no wishes, no affections'? What is the negative impact when scientists or doctors have 'hearts of stone'? How could a scientist or doctor best reconcile these competing concerns?

2 The self-inflicting diseases resulting from obesity should not be a burden for the National Health Service.

Explain the reasoning behind this statement and suggest arguments to the contrary. To what extent, if any, should the patient's responsibility of their disease shape clinical practice?

3 'The greatest enemy of knowledge is not ignorance; it is the illusion of knowledge.'

Stephen Hawking

Write an essay in which you address the following points:

In science, how is the illusion of knowledge an enemy of knowledge? Can you argue that ignorance is itself an enemy of knowledge? By what criteria could you assess the comparative impact of these two, to determine which is the greater enemy of scientific knowledge?

4 'I observe the physician with the same diligence as the disease.'

John Donne, English poet (1572–1631)

Write an essay in which you address the following points:

Why would a patient observe his physician with the same diligence as his disease? Under what circumstances might a patient be more concerned with his disease than with his physician? How would you advise a patient to best balance these two concerns?

BMAT answers and explanations

BMAT section 1 answers

1. (D) Some flautists adore three composers

This question is challenging as it hinges on the definition, in logic terms, of 'some', which simply means 'more than one'. The key, then, is in understanding what it means, and doesn't mean, to say that 'Some cellists adore Schumann and some adore Bach'. We know from the first sentence that all musicians adore Handel. Thus, we can divide cellists into at least two groups:

Those who adore Handel and Schumann	Those who adore Handel and Bach

But answers **(A)** and **(B)** suggest two additional groups:

Those who adore Handel, but neither Schumann nor Bach	Those who adore Handel, Schumann, and Bach

In fact, either of these groups *could* exist, without conflicting with the conductor's statements. She did not say that the 'some cellists' who adore Schumann and the 'some cellists' who adore Bach are mutually exclusive—nor did she say that they account for all the cellists in the orchestra. We can't infer beyond the logical meaning of her words, so the groups in **(A)** and **(B)** could exist, or they could not. But the key is that they don't *have to exist*, on the basis of the conductor's words—they aren't definitely true, so these two answers are wrong.

Similarly, answer **(C)** says that 'Some flautists adore Bach'—this might or might not be true, as the conductor has not mentioned Bach in reference to the flautists. Since we don't know for certain, the answer is out.

Answer **(D)** says that 'Some flautists adore three composers'. How does this stack up to our statements? We know that all musicians adore Handel and all flautists adore Mozart. So all flautists must adore at least two composers—that's something that must be true, based on the conductor's remarks. We can go a step further and see that some flautists must adore at least three composers, as some adore Rimsky-Korsakov in addition to Handel and Mozart. So statement **(D)** must be true.

We cannot conclude the statement made in answer **(E)**, as we don't know for sure that any percussionists adore more than three composers. They all adore Handel and Rimsky-Korsakov and none of them adores Bach, but we don't know about a third who any of them might adore. So this answer is out and our sole correct answer is **(D)**.

2. 72.9%

This question is tricky, for two reasons: 1) we're not told the starting price of the camera, and 2) there are no answer choices. There's potentially a third twist, in that we're asked to give our answer as a percentage to one decimal place and do so without a calculator!

Kaplan has a helpful technique for percentage questions without a starting value for the original: always pick 100 for the original value. This makes the maths a lot simpler. Here, we can start with £100 for the price of the camera on Friday. It's marked down by 10 per cent on Saturday, so the price on Saturday is £100—£10 = £90, as £10 is 10% of £100. Then, on Sunday, the £90 is marked down another 10%; 10% of £90 is £9, so the price on Sunday is £90—£9 = £81. Finally, on Monday, the price is marked down a further 10 per cent. Ten per cent of £81 is £8.10, so the final sale price on Monday is £81—£8.10 = £72.90.

We calculate the percentage by dividing the price on Monday, £72.90, by the price on Friday, £100, and $\frac{72.90}{100} \times 100 = 72.9\%$.

You could do the problem without picking a number, using a variable such as p for the initial price of the camera on Friday. The price on Saturday would be 90 per cent of the price on Friday, or .9p. The price on Sunday would be 90 per cent of the price on Saturday, or .9(.9p). Likewise, the price on Monday would be 90 per cent of the price on Sunday, so the final sale price would be .9(.9(.9p)). This would multiply out as .729p, which is equal to 72.9%. If you have trouble conceptualizing that, then it's definitely quicker to pick a number for the starting value.

3. (B)

The conclusion of the argument is the author's main point. The rest of the argument as stated is evidence, backing up this main point in some way. Sometimes the conclusion comes as the final sentence of the argument; on the BMAT, this is not always the case. Here, the author's main point comes in the middle of the argument: 'Regardless of any changes to legislation, the media could do more to increase organ donation at present'. The rest of the argument is an example of how the media's current practice is deficient, as they rarely mention how readers or viewers can 'opt-in' to the organ donor registry. This shortcoming is contrasted with standard media practice in the USA and Canada, where viewers are routinely given contact details for the donor registry following stories on the need for more donated organs. The conclusion is nicely summarized in answer **(B)**, which admittedly abstracts things a bit but matches the author's main point directly.

All the other answers here touch on relatively minor points of the author's argument, or are not really part of it at all. For instance, one might infer that it is effectively easier to become an organ donor in the USA or Canada than in the UK, as answer **(A)** states, but this is hardly the author's main point, as the argument is focused on media coverage of the need for organ donors. Answers **(C)** and **(D)** are certainly true, on the basis of our argument, but neither is the author's main point. Finally, answer **(E)** makes a conclusion that is outside the scope of our argument. Our author never goes so far as to suggest that membership on the organ donor registry should be compulsory.

4. (D)

This question is a good example of a BMAT question that seems a lot trickier than it actually is. That's not to say that it's easy, but it's definitely do-able and without requiring terribly complicated maths.

The question is slightly odd in that the table is circular and we're told which people are meant to be seated next to each other, or directly opposite each other. From these rules, we will get enough information to determine the probability of Cindy sitting directly opposite Rachael. (This will be expressed as a fraction, with the number of such seating arrangements divided by the total number of possible seating arrangements.)

The good news: this question has a built-in shortcut, of sorts. One option is to consider all possible arrangements for sitting the full group of eight. The other, simpler option is to consider the pairs who can sit directly opposite each other. Our rules may well let us determine the probability of Cindy sitting opposite Rachael on this basis.

We know from our rules that Dave will sit opposite Shannon and Ben opposite Lola. That leaves four people with seating to be determined: Rachael, James, Patrick, and Cindy. We know that Rachael and James will sit next to each other, which means one of them will sit opposite Cindy and the other will sit opposite Patrick. That means there are two possible people who could sit opposite Rachael: either Cindy or Patrick. Cindy is one of those two possibilities, so the probability of Cindy sitting opposite Rachael is ½, answer **(D)**.

BMAT Section 2 answers

1. (C) Her maternal uncle

As Christmas disease is an X-linked recessive disorder, every carrier or sufferer has inherited a faulty gene on the X-chromosome. As Jane's paternal grandfather suffers from the disease, all of his female offspring must also be carriers. Therefore Jane's mother and maternal aunt must carry the faulty gene on one X-chromosome. As Jane's father suffers from the disease, he must have inherited the faulty gene on the X-chromosome from Jane's paternal grandmother. Jane's father's monozygotic twin will have an identical genotype to Jane's father himself. We know Jane's mother and father both carry copies of the faulty gene on their X-chromosomes. Therefore Jane and her sister must be either carriers or suffer from the disease. Therefore Jane's maternal uncle is the only possible relative in these answer choices who can be free from disease. The correct answer is **(C)**.

2. (E) I and III only

Weak acids are only partially ionized in aqueous solution, while strong acids are almost completely ionized in aqueous solution. Citric acid is a weak acid so is only partially ionized in aqueous solution. Ethanoic acid is a weak acid, while nitric acid is a strong acid. So a 1 M solution of ethanoic acid will have a lower concentration of solvated protons than a 1 M solution of nitric acid. The electrical conductivity of a solution is greater when more ions are in solution. Hydrochloric acid is a strong acid and therefore will be almost completely ionized in aqueous solution, while lactic acid is a weak acid and will only be partially ionized in aqueous solution. So a 1M solution of hydrochloric acid will be a better conductor of electricity than a 1 M solution of lactic acid and the answer is **(E)**.

3. (D) 12

For a triangle, area = ½ × base × perpendicular height. The triangle in the question has one side parallel to the x-axis, as two of the points have an identical y-coordinate. This side is length $3\sqrt{2}$, the difference of the two x-coordinates. The perpendicular height of the third point is $4\sqrt{2}$. This is equivalent to its distance from b along the y-coordinate.

$$\text{Area} = \frac{3\sqrt{2} \times 4\sqrt{2}}{2} = \frac{3 \times 4 \times \sqrt{2} \times \sqrt{2}}{2} = \frac{3 \times 4 \times 2}{2} = 12,$$

or answer **(D)**.

4. (D)

The light passes through a circular hole, so the diffraction pattern will be circular. Light from the whole circumference of the circular hole will cause a pattern of overlapping waves, causing circular rings of constructive interference (bright) and destructive interference (dim). The point of strongest constructive interference will be in the centre of the pattern. Laser light is of a single wavelength so the size of the edges of the zones of interference will not be diffuse.

BMAT section 3 marking scheme

The essays will be marked by two examiners and if the marks are similar an average is taken; a third examiner is involved if there is a larger discrepancy. The content of the essay is scored out of a total of 5, while the quality of English used is graded A to E. The markers are instructed to assess content based on the following:

- Have they answered the questions? Markers are asked to consider three specific categories, which often correspond to the three questions asked:
  - Explore the implications of the phrase.
  - Suggest counter-arguments.
  - Suggest ways to evaluate the different opinions.
- Clearly organized cogent arguments.
- Appropriate use of general knowledge and opinions.
- Breadth of arguments leading to a carefully considered conclusion.

Remember to consider each argument from multiple viewpoints in order to produce a balanced argument. If you are proposing a counter-argument, consider what counter-claims could be made against each of your points and try to address them if appropriate.

Clear, concise, and fluent expression with the correct use of English spelling and grammar is scored from A (highest) to E (lowest). The composite mark of two scores, e.g. A and C, would be awarded a B. If there is a larger discrepancy than two adjacent scores the essay is marked for a third time by a senior assessor.

> ## Key points
>
> The full marking criteria for section 3 of the BMAT can be found at:
> www.admissionstestingservice.org/bmat

Useful resources

Chapter 18

Useful resources

Thinking about medicine

A deep insight into medicine comes from immersing yourself (as far as possible) in the culture of the profession you hope to join. Work experience (p. 49) will help but so will reading widely. Your understanding of how medicine works cannot help but pervade your personal statement and answers to interview questions.

Blogs

A number of doctors write blogs, i.e. online commentaries on their professional lives and issues affecting doctors. They are usually anonymous and so free to voice strong opinions on controversial topics. Take these for what they are and be cautious before reproducing the thoughts of these experienced (and often cynical) doctors at interview.

- KevinMD Insightful commentary on contemporary news and ideas, led by an American physician. www.kevinmd.com
- Bad Science Social commentary from self-styled 'evangelist for good science', Ben Goldacre. www.badscience.net
- The Jobbing Doctor A British GP muses about recent news and his own practice. http://thejobbingdoctor.blogspot.co.uk

Books

Lots of books have been written about the process of becoming a doctor. They are usually written for a popular audience and inject comedy as well as insight into the profession. These are worth reading but beware—they often reflect the experiences of doctors training years ago when the system was very different, although many important themes persist in the NHS today.

- Bedside Stories A collection of short, humorous (yet insightful) anecdotes describing life as a doctor in the NHS. *Bedside Stories: Confessions of a Junior Doctor*. Michael Foxton. Atlantic Books. ISBN 978-1843540328. £8.99.
- Trust Me, I'm A (Junior) Doctor Written in diary form describing the first couple of years as a new doctor. *Trust Me, I'm a (Junior) Doctor*. Max Pemberton. Hodder Paperbacks. ISBN 978-0340962053. £7.99.
- In Stitches Another book in diary format, this time describing life as a doctor in Accident and Emergency. *In Stitches: The Highs and Lows of Life as an A&E Doctor*. Nick Edwards. The Friday Project Ltd. ISBN 978-1905548705. £7.99.

There are also more serious accounts of working within healthcare. These all raise issues that could come up in medical school interviews:

- Complications A collection of thoughtful essays on various issues that are raised in medicine. A very easy read. *Complications: A Surgeon's Notes on an Imperfect Science*. Atul Gawande. Profile Books. ISBN 978-1846681325. £8.99.
- Bad Science This describes *how* we know treatments work. It is aimed at unravelling the debates around complementary medicine (e.g. homeopathy) but also explains the basis of clinical research. *Bad Science*. Ben Goldacre. HarperPerennial. ISBN 978-0007284870. £8.99.
- NHS Plc A thought-provoking analysis of the impact of recent government policies on the future of healthcare in the UK. *NHS Plc: The Privatisation of Our Healthcare*. Allyson Pollock. Verso Books. ISBN 978-1844675395. £9.99.

- Hippocratic Oaths A collection of essays covering various aspects of healthcare. It is a challenging read because many concepts are complicated and hard to grasp. But if you enjoy reading and want to think hard about medicine, this book is worth the effort. *Hippocratic Oaths: Medicine and its Discontents*. Raymond Tallis. Atlantic Books. ISBN 978-1843541271. £9.99.

Periodicals

It's worth subscribing to a good periodical. These lean towards either medicine (e.g. the *Student BMJ*) or science (e.g. *New Scientist*). Keeping abreast of what's happening in medicine (and science) is better preparation than cramming a week before interviews. Remember: if you subscribe, make a commitment to read every issue.

- Student BMJ A monthly magazine aimed at medical students. This is a good place to start thinking about the issues faced by medical students. It is available online or in print for subscribers. www.student.bmj.com
- BMJ This is a weekly medical journal read by most doctors in the UK. Much of the content will be difficult to follow but letters, commentaries, and opinion articles highlight what doctors are thinking about now. Reading something in the *BMJ* and talking intelligently about it at interview cannot fail to impress. www.bmj.com
- New Scientist A weekly international magazine covering recent advances in science. www.newscientist.com
- Scientific American Like *New Scientist*, a popular science magazine. Worth a subscription if you want to learn about science beyond the A-level curriculum. www.scientificamerican.com

TV shows

While most medical TV drama does not give an accurate representation of life in the NHS, one show does stand out:

- Getting On This BBC Four series, written by and starring Jo Brand, gives a cynical but extremely realistic portrayal of life on an NHS ward. Search the internet for 'Getting On Jo Brand' to find episodes.

Application resources

The internet provides a wealth of resources for improving your application.

Online forums

Forums are great for keeping in touch with what's going on in the world of medical school selection. They are also good for letting off steam to people who know what you're talking about. Medical school admissions tutors have been known to prowl forums as well. However, be warned that forums are a mine of gossip and hearsay. Just because a poster articulates their views clearly, this doesn't mean their perceptions are correct or that things haven't changed since their experience. If there is doubt, call medical school admissions offices for clarification.

- **New Media Medicine** Includes a separate forum for each medical school as well as specialist forums (e.g. work experience, personal statement). 60,000+ registered members. www.newmediamedicine.com/forum/forum.php
- **The Student Room** Probably the largest online resource for students with over a million members. Although not specific for medical applicants, it includes forums dedicated to every British university as well as medical applications. www.thestudentroom.co.uk

Learning about medical courses

- **Medschools Online** A frequently updated resource providing lots of information about different medical courses. www.medschoolsonline.co.uk
- **UCAS** Database of all medical schools in the UK with notes and entry requirements. www.ucas.com/students/coursesearch
- **Medical school websites** Web addresses for undergraduate and graduate courses begin on p. 107 and p. 217 respectively.

Improving your personal statement

- **Studential** An online student community with a database of personal statements. Over 80+ are for applications to medical school. Read these to gain an idea of how personal statements should look, but heed the plagiarism warning on p. 200. www.studential.com/personalstatements
- **The Student Room** Another database of 100+ medical personal statements. www.thestudentroom.co.uk/wiki/personal_statement_library

Admission tests

If you've exhausted the sample UKCAT (p. 306) and BMAT (p. 324) questions, see the following website for additional resources:

- **Kaplan Test Prep and Admissions** Provides online and classroom-based preparation for the admission tests; they supplied the test questions in this book. www.kaptest.co.uk

Useful news outlets

Keeping abreast of the news is almost as important as knowing what is going on in healthcare. You need to come across to course selectors as someone who is interesting, broad-minded, and informed.

- BBC The BBC website provides up-to-date and impartial news through its website. Set it (or an equivalent site) as your internet home page and read stories that interest you. www.bbc.co.uk or www.bbc.co.uk/health
- Newspapers Read a high quality newspaper. These include *The Times* (www.timesplus. co.uk), the *Daily Telegraph* (www.telegraph.co.uk), and the *Guardian* (www.guardian. co.uk). Most provide free content through their websites and publish a dedicated health section.
- The Economist This is an excellent way to keep up-to-date with current affairs; the articles are carefully researched and present thoughtful analyses of world events. www.economist.com

Money and careers

- Money 4 Medical Students A great resource to help plan your finances and budget at medical school. Information on student loans, the NHS Bursary, and other sources of income available to medical students. www.money4medstudents.org
- So you want to be a brain surgeon? The leading careers guide aimed at medical students. It is never too early to start thinking about your postgraduate career (p. 302) and this is a good place to begin. *So you want to be a brain surgeon?* 3rd edition. Simon Eccles and Stephan Sanders. Oxford University Press. ISBN 978-0199231966, £17.99.

Index

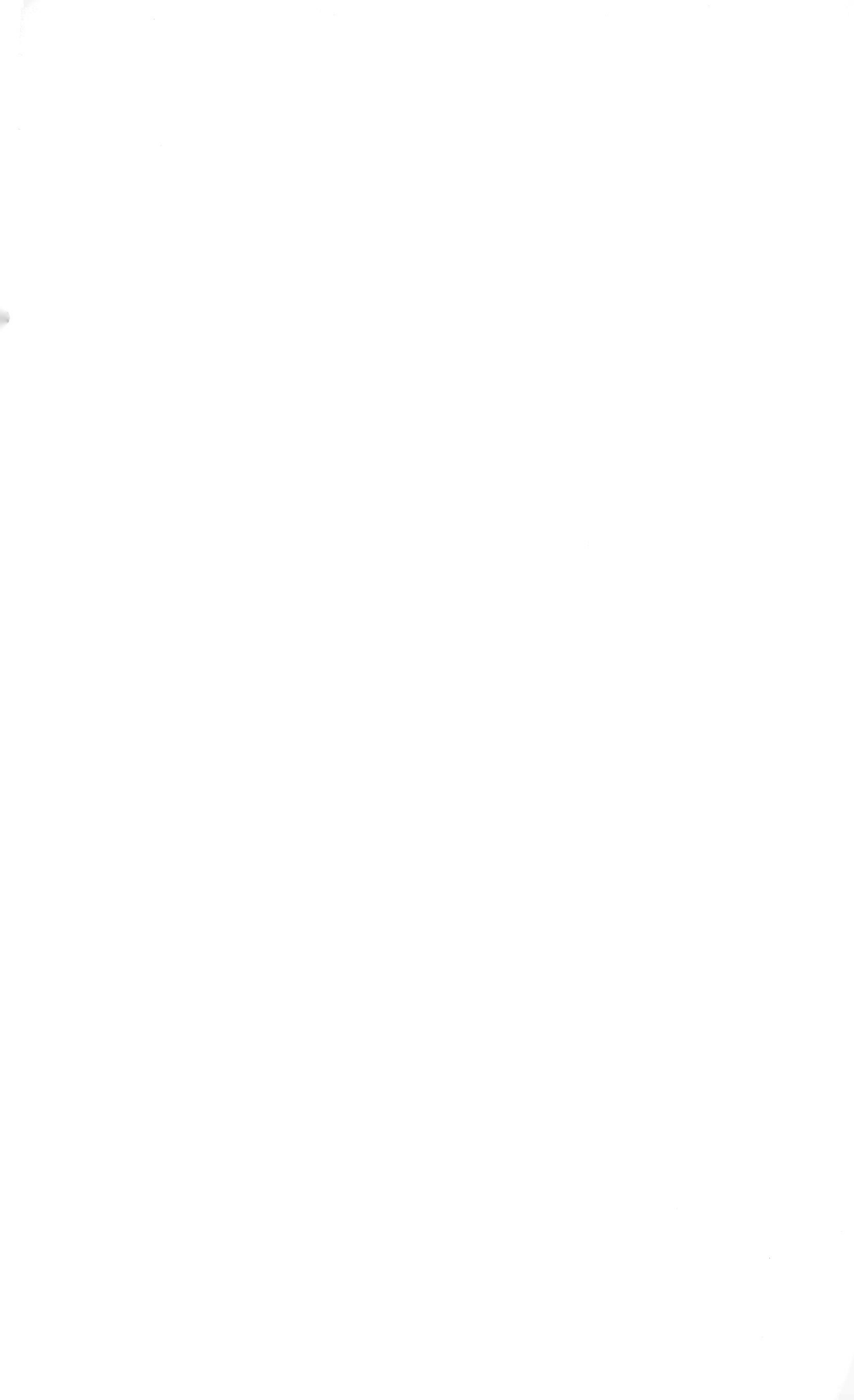